Lipid Metabolism and Health

Lipid Metabolism and Health

Edited by

Robert J. Moffatt
Bryant Stamford

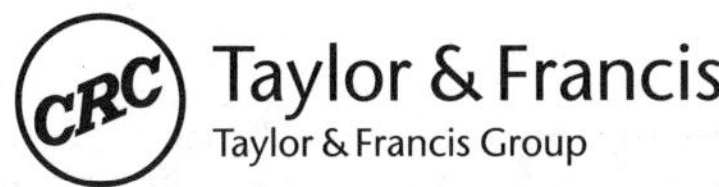

Taylor & Francis
Taylor & Francis Group

Boca Raton London New York

A CRC title, part of the Taylor & Francis imprint, a member of the Taylor & Francis Group, the academic division of T&F Informa plc.

Published in 2006 by
CRC Press
Taylor & Francis Group
6000 Broken Sound Parkway NW, Suite 300
Boca Raton, FL 33487-2742

CRC Press is an imprint of Taylor & Francis Group

Printed in the United States of America on acid-free paper
10 9 8 7 6 5 4 3 2 1

International Standard Book Number-10: 0-8493-2680-X (Hardcover)
International Standard Book Number-13: 978-0-8493-2680-6 (Hardcover)
Library of Congress Card Number 2005053181

Library of Congress Cataloging-in-Publication Data

Lipid metabolism and health / [edited by] Robert J. Moffatt and Bryant Stamford.
p. cm.
Includes bibliographical references and index.
ISBN 0-8493-2680-X (alk. paper)
1. Lipids--Metabolism. 2. Health. I. Moffatt, Robert J. II. Stamford, Bryant A.

QP751.L5475 2005
612.3'97--dc22 2005053181

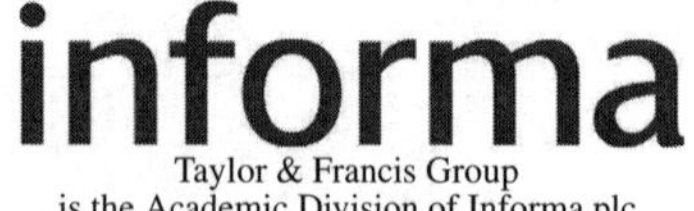

Taylor & Francis Group
is the Academic Division of Informa plc.

Visit the Taylor & Francis Web site at
http://www.taylorandfrancis.com

and the CRC Press Web site at
http://www.crcpress.com

Contributors

Sofiya Alhassan, Ph.D. Stanford University School of Medicine, Stanford, California

Theodore J. Angelopoulos, Ph.D., M.P.H. Exercise Physiology Laboratory, University of Central Florida, Orlando, Florida

Vic Ben-Ezra, Ph.D. Department of Kinesiology, Texas Women's University, Denton, Texas

Robert Carter III, Ph.D. Laboratory of Adaptation Physiology, Thermal and Mountain Medicine, United States Army Research Institute of Environmental Medicine, Natick, Massachusetts

Sarah Chelland, M.S. Department of Nutrition, Food and Exercise Sciences, Florida State University, Tallahassee, Florida

Yumei Coa, B.S. Department of Nutritional Sciences, Pennsylvania State University, University Park, Pennsylvania

Stephen F. Crouse, Ph.D. Texas A&M University, College Station, Texas

Paul G. Davis, Ph.D. Department of Exercise and Sport Science, University of North Carolina at Greensboro, Greensboro, North Carolina

Jacqueline L. Dupont, Ph.D., Hazel K. Stiebeling Professor, Department of Nutrition, Food and Exercise Sciences, Florida State University, Tallahassee, Florida

J. Larry Durstine, Ph.D. Department of Exercise Science, University of South Carolina, Columbia, South Carolina

Sarah Gebaur, B.S. Department of Nutritional Sciences, Pennsylvania State University, University Park, Pennsylvania

Peter W. Grandjean, Ph.D. Department of Health & Human Performance, Auburn University, Auburn, Alabama

Amy E. Griel, M.Ed. Department of Nutritional Sciences, Pennsylvania State University, University Park, Pennsylvania

Kirsten F. Hilpert, B.S. Department of Nutritional Sciences, Pennsylvania State University, University Park, Pennsylvania

Harlan P. Jones, Ph.D. Laboratory of Psychoneuro-Immunology, Department of Psychiatry and Behavioral Sciences, Emory University School of Medicine, Atlanta, Georgia

William B. Kannel, M.D., M.P.H., F.A.C.C. Boston University School of Medicine/Framingham Heart Study, Framingham, Massachusetts

Penny M. Kris-Etherton, Ph.D., R.D. Department of Nutritional Sciences, Pennsylvania State University, University Park, Pennsylvania

Michael R. Kushnick, Ph.D. School of Recreation and Sport Sciences, Ohio University, Athens, Ohio

Tom LaFontaine, Ph.D. PREVENT Consulting Services LLC, Columbia, Missouri

Robert J. Moffatt, Ph.D., MPH, Georgia A. Stamford Professor of Exercise Physiology, Department of Nutrition, Food and Exercise Sciences, Florida State University, Tallahassee, Florida

Sachin M. Navare, M.D. Division of Cardiology in the Henry Low Heart Center, University of Connecticut, School of Medicine, Hartford, Connecticut

Lynn B. Panton, Ph.D. Department of Food, Nutrition and Exercise Sciences, Florida State University, Tallahassee, Florida

Tricia Psota, B.S. Department of Nutritional Sciences, Pennsylvania State University, University Park, Pennsylvania

Jeffrey L. Roitman, Ed.D. Research Medical Center, Kansas City, Missouri

Bryant A. Stamford, Ph.D. Professor and Chair, Department of Exercise Science, Hanover College, Hanover, Indiana

Andrea C. Summer, B.S. Department of Exercise Science, University of South Carolina, Columbia, South Carolina

Paul D. Thompson, M.D. Division of Cardiology in the Henry Low Heart Center, University of Connecticut, School of Medicine, Hartford, Connecticut

Jason D. Wagganer, M.S. Department of Exercise and Sport Science, University of North Carolina at Greensboro, Greensboro, North Carolina

Table of Contents

1 **Lipids and Health: Past, Present, and Future** 1
Bryant A. Stamford and Robert J. Moffatt

2 **Cardiovascular Risk Assessment** 13
William B. Kannel

3 **Basic Lipidology** 31
Jacqueline L. Dupont

4 **Lipid and Lipoprotein Metabolism** 47
Paul G. Davis and Jason D. Wagganer

5 **The Vascular Biology of Atherosclerosis** 61
Robert Carter III and Harlan P. Jones

6 **Exercise Training and Endothelial Function in Patients at Risk for and with Documented Coronary Artery Disease** 85
Tom LaFontaine and Jeffrey L. Roitmann

7 **Essential Laboratory Methods for Blood Lipid and Lipoprotein Analysis** 117
Peter W. Grandjean and Sofiya Alhassan

8 **Metabolic Syndrome** 147
Vic Ben-Ezra

9 **Obesity, Lipoproteins, and Exercise** 173
Theodore J. Angelopoulos

10 **Pharmacological Treatments of Lipid Abnormalities** 183
Sachin M. Navare and Paul D. Thompson

11 **New Insights on the Role of Lipids and Lipoproteins in Cardiovascular Disease: The Modulating Effects of Nutrition** 211
Kirsten F. Hilpert, Amy E. Griel, Tricia Psota, Sarah Gebauer, Yumei Coa, and Penny M. Kris-Etherton

12 **Physical Activity, Exercise, Blood Lipids, and Lipoproteins** 265
J. Larry Durstine and Andrea C. Summer

13 **Acute Changes in Lipids and Lipoprotein-Lipids Induced by Exercise** 283
Stephen F. Crouse

14 **Smoking, Heart Disease, and Lipoprotein Metabolism** 299
Robert J. Moffatt, Sara Chelland, and Bryant A. Stamford

15 **Lipid and Lipoprotein Concentrations in Americans: Ethnicity and Age** 315
Michael R. Kushnick and Lynn B. Panton

Index 349

1

Lipids and Health: Past, Present, and Future

Bryant A. Stamford and Robert J. Moffatt

CONTENTS

Introduction 1
The Cholesterol Risk Factor 3
Lipoproteins 4
Atherosclerosis 6
Past, Present, and Future 7
Lipids and Health 8
References 9

Introduction

The German philosopher, Arthur Schopenhauer (1788–1860), once said that when new ideas are first introduced they are likely to be dismissed out of hand, then ridiculed, and finally, accepted as self evident. This natural progression is particularly applicable to the scrutinizing mind of the scientist who must dismiss new ideas as unacceptable, thus ensuring that acceptability will occur only when ample empirical evidence is provided. The acceptance of serum cholesterol as causally related to coronary artery disease (CAD) has traversed just such a gauntlet, and is now accepted as self-evident. Moreover, vigorous research efforts have revealed a relationship and interactions that are substantially more complex than imagined when this concept was introduced more than a half century ago.

In the 1930s, medical researchers were aware that extraordinarily high levels of serum cholesterol were associated with pathology. Xanthomatosis was known to be related to symptoms of heart disease (angina pectoris) and likely was a contributor to myocardial infarction.[1] Such cases were rare, however, and a relationship between cholesterol and CAD in those with high, but lesser, levels of cholesterol was dismissed. This, even though it was known that cholesterol was found in atherosclerotic lesions in persons not suffering from xanthomatosis. The cholesterol in lesions was considered to be incidental, as the lesions were, it was assumed, caused by degenerative alteration of the arterial wall.

At the time, the normal range for cholesterol was determined in the similar manner employed to judge other blood-borne components. The mean of the general population was assessed, standard deviations were calculated, and the normal range extended from minus two standard deviations of the mean, to plus two. This meant that only those individuals with blood cholesterol levels beyond two standard deviations above the mean were diagnosed as hypercholesterolemic.

The normal range extended to 300 mg/dl (7.76 mmol/L), and, thus, only approximately 2.5% of the population would be viewed as having a dangerously high level of cholesterol (greater than 300 mg/dl). And, given the tendency of practitioners to allow older patients a greater margin of error, it was not uncommon to extend the normal range by 10% in those at or above retirement age. Thus, persons 65 and older could be told that their cholesterol test results were "normal," notwithstanding an incredibly high level, reaching 330 mg/dl!

This interpretation logically excused serum cholesterol as a causal factor in CAD, because while only a tiny fraction of patients were labeled as hypercholesterolemic, legions were dying of CAD. Moreover, factors including cigarette smoking, high blood pressure, and diabetes had been identified and indicted as causal, pushing cholesterol further into the background. The well-respected 1948 text, *Quantitative Clinical Chemistry*, by Peters and VanSlyke[2] stated the case unequivocally: "There is no satisfactory evidence that the incidence of atherosclerosis bears any relationship to the concentration of cholesterol in the blood."

Once a seed is planted and takes root, it is difficult to stamp it out completely, even though the strength of evidence to the contrary is formidable. Indeed, today, although the role of cholesterol in the progression of CAD is taken for granted, not long ago offspring of the original seed continued to flourish, and many still questioned the extent of impact of cholesterol on atherosclerosis. And among those who accepted the basic premise, it was not clear that reducing cholesterol reduced mortality from CAD; and if it did, how much reduction was required? In addition, if there were a bona fide relationship, was the use of powerful medications warranted, or did available medications impose risks that were greater than those imposed by the high level of cholesterol itself?

The Cholesterol Risk Factor

The Framingham Heart Study was the key to elevating serum cholesterol to the status of CAD risk factor.[3–5] Thousands of men and women were studied prospectively and it was determined that, indeed, a relationship exists between cholesterol and CAD. As the concentration of blood cholesterol increases, the risk of CAD increases as well, the risk relationship defined as a continuous and curvilinear function (of the concentration of blood cholesterol). Many additional large-scale studies solidified the Framingham findings.

Despite the volume of data supporting blood cholesterol as problematic, skeptics required data supporting positive outcomes arising from intervention. Specifically, if cholesterol is a risk factor for CAD, reducing the concentration of cholesterol in the blood should reduce risk. The first step was determining safe and effective ways to reduce cholesterol. Dietary and drug intervention was studied and found to be effective.[6–9] Results from the Coronary Primary Prevention Trial[10] demonstrated that a drop in blood cholesterol of 9% reduced CAD risk by 19%. Results of this study combined with several others gave rise to national guidelines that replaced use of the "normal range" approach.

Impetus for change can be credited largely to efforts of the National Cholesterol Education Program (NCEP), launched by the National Heart, Lung and Blood Institute (NHLB) of the National Institutes of Health (NIH) in 1985. New guidelines set stricter goals as blood cholesterol levels below 200 mg/dl were deemed "healthy" and desirable, while those exceeding 240 mg/dl were viewed as clinically significant. Awareness of the risks associated with hypercholesterolemia increased greatly thanks to efforts of the NCEP and by 1995, 70–80 million more Americans sought to have their blood cholesterol concentrations determined, a 40% increase in ten years.

The above guidelines have been in place for nearly two decades. Many experts argue that such guidelines, while an improvement on the "normal range" approach, are far too liberal (given that the average total cholesterol level in the U.S. is 205 mg/dl). Moreover, such guidelines are viewed as deficient in many ways, particularly when considering the interplay between cholesterol and other risk factors. In addition, ample evidence has accumulated in recent years attesting to the clinical efficacy of so-called "statin" drugs to dramatically overhaul the cholesterol profile and, in turn, reduce the incidence of heart attacks and CAD deaths.

It would appear that continual redefining of guidelines would be the order of the day as new evidence accumulates. However, it must be taken into consideration that the creation, establishment, and acceptance of new guidelines add up to a ponderous and painstaking process. And when new guidelines are introduced, confusion often reigns because, in effect, at least for a while, two (or more) sets of guidelines are operating. The older guidelines continue to be followed faithfully by many practitioners on the front lines, while news of updated guidelines is disseminated directly to the public through various media outlets. Confronting such ominous circumstances ensures that the approach to new guidelines is calculated and cautious in the extreme.

This is a universal dilemma and is not peculiar to cholesterol. Serum triglycerides have traversed similar terrain. Traditionally, serum triglycerides have been viewed as lacking clinical significance until reaching 275–300 mg/dl, and even then there was some question as to the importance of such elevated levels. This is akin to the previous acceptance of the "normal range" criterion for cholesterol values. While it was known that triglycerides are adversely impacted by increased body fatness and uncontrolled diabetes, the facts that the role of triglycerides in CAD is controversial, and triglycerides are not recognized as an independent CAD risk factor, have inspired continued tolerance of such high levels.

Most recently, however, as metabolic syndrome has attracted increased attention, and owing to exploration of definitive diagnostic strategies, serum triglycerides seem to have elevated in status, leading to a tightening of guidelines. Diagnostic criteria for metabolic syndrome have been set forth that include a cluster of five characteristics. One of these is serum triglycerides (fasting) in excess of 150 mg/dl.

Regarding serum cholesterol and triglycerides as important health threats, each has gone through a stage of benign neglect in which very high levels were considered "normal." And now, each has captured the spotlight with emphasis focused on reducing levels to a fraction of what was previously deemed acceptable.

Efforts have been ongoing to further improve upon cholesterol guidelines for clinicians. New cholesterol guidelines have been proposed that address the need for placing blood cholesterol levels within the context of a global heart disease risk profile.[11] A risk score is computed referencing the probability of a heart attack within 10 years. The new guidelines recommend recurring assessment at five-year intervals beginning in young adulthood. Efforts in this direction not only broaden the scope of factors considered, they also have enhanced the sophistication of risk analysis by requiring a lipoprotein profile. Attention also has been focused on the interaction of serum triglycerides and lipoproteins.

Lipoproteins

Cholesterol is insoluble and, therefore, transportation of cholesterol in the blood is challenging. Over the years, considerable research has been conducted on cholesterol transport.[12–14] It was found that cholesterol is transported in combination with other substances as lipoproteins, with a hydrophobic lipid core, and a surrounding layer of apolipoproteins and phospholipids. The apolipoproteins were found to vary in size and density (labeled as high, low, and very low), and this, in turn, was found to be significant in determining the metabolic fate of the complex.[15–17]

The relative proportion of alpha (high-density HDL) to beta (low-density LDL) lipoproteins was found to be critical to the cholesterol/CAD relationship. The fraction of blood cholesterol transported as LDL contributes to atherosclerosis, whereas HDL is inversely related to risk. Vigorous research efforts have uncovered several more classes and subclasses of lipoproteins.[18] For utilitarian reasons in the clinical setting, the ratio of total cholesterol to HDL typically is employed, because direct assessment of LDL is difficult, and there exists a high correlation between LDL and total cholesterol.

But still, many questions remained unanswered as numerous exceptions to the rule surfaced. Intermediate-density lipoproteins (IDL) have been found to increase CAD risk, especially when IDL is the major lipoprotein.[19] Very-low-density lipoproteins (VLDL) also may be influential. However, the role of VLDL may be important because of the inverse relationship with HDL, and may reflect metabolic disorders (insulin resistance and diabetes, for example), rather than a direct impact.[19]

Despite progress, many inconsistencies associated with the prediction of CAD risk based upon serum cholesterol levels and the blood lipid profile remained. For example, if all risk factors are equal (or reasonably so), why is it that individuals with similar levels of LDL can have substantially different levels of risk for CAD? This would seem to be inconsistent with the notion that LDL entrance into the interior arterial wall (the endothelium) is gradient driven. The more LDL that is present the more interaction there will be between LDL and the arterial wall, resulting in greater LDL penetration of the endothelium, greater oxidation of LDL, and thus greater atherogenesis.

Unexplored until recently is the size and density of lipoprotein particles, and such explorations offer revealing insights.[20,21] At any given level of serum LDL, the size and density of LDL particles may be the determining factor that promotes CAD risk, because small, dense particles may enter the arterial wall more readily than larger, "fluffy" particles.[22,23] Those with small LDL particles have a substantially larger number of LDL particles and, thus, despite equal levels of serum LDL, gross differences in the particle size and density would appear to preserve the gradient driven aspects of atherogenesis. Unfortunately, when assessing LDL with a conventional blood lipid profile approach, the size and density of LDL particles escapes detection.

HDL is responsible for reverse cholesterol transport — the removal of cholesterol from developing lesions, which would reduce CAD risk.[24] Enzymes carried by HDL may also play a protective role, acting to retard oxidation of LDL (discussed below).[25] This would suggest that a high level of HDL is always helpful, and that a low level of HDL is always destructive. This is not the case, however, as inconsistencies have again been observed.

Particle sizing may be relevant to HDL as well as LDL and may help to explain some of these inconsistencies.[22,23] Larger HDL particles may be more effective in reverse cholesterol transport, and may interfere with interaction between LDL and the endothelium. Smaller HDL particles may be ineffective in this regard. Moreover, small HDL particles may actually contribute to atherosclerosis. Thus, a patient with a preponderance of larger HDL particles may be at lower risk than another patient with fewer large HDL particles, even though conventional blood lipid assessment reveals that the two are equal on the HDL scale.

Particle sizing may also have relevance with regard to VLDL.[22] Larger VLDL particles may increase CAD risk, because when insulin resistance is present, excess carbohydrate increases production of triglyceride. This results in VLDL that are loaded with triglyceride, which can lead to metabolism of large VLDL particles into small LDL and small HDL which, in turn, can promote atherosclerosis.

Atherosclerosis

The "injury" hypothesis of atherosclerosis was proposed by Ross in 1970.[26] The driving event in the process was thought to be damage to the endothelium, progressing to denuding of the delicate endothelial lining, and eventually progressing to the status of fibrous plaques. Major emphasis of the injury hypothesis was placed on smooth muscle proliferation.

Attention was focused on fatty streaks and the foam cells loaded with lipids. Because of the emphasis on smooth muscle proliferation, it was assumed that fatty streaks, the earliest of lesions, were associated with foam cells that were derived from smooth muscle cells exclusively. Later, it was determined that while some foam cells originate from smooth muscle, most arise from monocytes in the bloodstream. This finding challenged the injury hypothesis, because monocytes can penetrate an intact and functioning endothelium where they take up residence as macrophages and attract cholesterol.

Subsequent research efforts by Ross and Glomser[26] and others postulated the utility of both hypotheses — the endothelial injury, and monocyte (lipid infiltration) hypotheses in the progression of atherosclerosis.[27,28] Cholesterol may enter an uninjured endothelium that is fully functioning, and this could lead to the accumulation of foam cells. Damage to the endothelium may result, owing to secretion of local factors (such as cytokines and growth factor), and to an inflammatory response. This, in turn, would promote fibrous plaque development.

Progress in defining the steps of atherosclerosis was stymied, however, when it was discovered that isolation and incubation of monocytes in a medium loaded with cholesterol did not cause the monocytes to soak up cholesterol, and thus produce foam cells.[29] The same finding occurred with smooth muscle cells. This led to research that revealed the need for alteration of cholesterol prior to being taken up and accumulating. The cholesterol must experience oxidative damage.[30] In turn, animal research has indicated that antioxidants can retard progression of lesions substantially.[31] Research efforts into the impact of antioxidants (specifically vitamin E) in humans is ongoing, with mixed results.[32]

Integrity of the endothelium is a hot topic currently. Improved endothelial function has many advantages in that platelets and inflammatory cells are less likely to adhere, and the natural balance between locally derived vasodilating and vasoconstricting substances is preserved. Nitric oxide (NO) is a natural vasodilator, and it has been reported that in the presence of endothelial dysfunction, there is a paradoxical vasoconstriction response to vasodilator substances. This may be an important factor in initiating atherosclerosis.[33]

With all of the complexities associated with initiation and progression of atherosclerosis, it is clear that several factors conspire, conflict, and contribute. At first glance, it might appear that as the research movement in this area advances, the role of blood lipids has been demeaned. The role of a dysfunctional endothelium, the impact of NO, and the intricacies of the inflammatory response, have seized the focus. However, blood lipids retain their position in the spotlight as several studies have reported improved endothelial function when blood lipids are reduced.[34–36] And a profound and acute improvement in endothelial function was observed following LDL apheresis.[37]

Past, Present, and Future

Historically, in Japan decades ago, dietary fat intake was low, serum cholesterol levels were low (160 mg/dl),and the incidence of CAD was low.[38] This, despite a high incidence of hypertension and the immense popularity of cigarette smoking. Is it possible that a very low cholesterol level precluded atherosclerosis and development of CAD, even in the face of other significant CAD risk factors? Is there a protective threshold for cholesterol, and LDL in particular? Or, are other factors operating that have yet to be uncovered and elucidated.

Much still needs to be determined in the realm of lipoproteins and their role in promoting atherosclerosis, such as the role of lipoprotein (a), and specifics surrounding the increased risk associated with high serum triglyceride levels and low HDL. Further examination is needed of the notion that at any given level of serum LDL, the size and density of LDL particles may be the determining factor that promotes CAD risk. Particle sizing may be relevant to HDL as well as LDL, and may help to explain some of the current inconsistencies. A better understanding of homocysteine, HS-Crp, as a marker of the inflammatory response, the nature of receptor activity, the significance of nitric oxide, and elucidation of the roles of cytokines and growth factors, may lead to revision of current hypotheses and creation of new clinical strategies.

Lipids and Health

The purpose of this volume is to provide an overview and historical perspective of the evolution of serum lipids and lipoproteins from a mere curiosity, to acceptance as an established and major CAD risk factor, and, ultimately, to formulation of present clinical guidelines. Speculation regarding future developments and the further potential evolution of guidelines will be discussed.

Considerable attention has been focused on the fundamentals, such as basic lipidology. Lipids are the structural components of all living cells, and they play a number of critical roles. Lipid/lipoprotein metabolism is discussed with regard to the regulation, absorption, synthesis and excretion of cholesterol. The biology of atherosclerosis emphasizes arterial adaptations and the inflammatory response, as well as the impact of atherosclerosis on cerebral vascular and peripheral artery disease. A chapter on endothelial function as impacted by nitric oxide and exercise is included.

Clinical methodologies for measuring lipoproteins are a critical consideration given the many challenges associated with accurate determination of the number and size of circulating LDL (and HDL) particles and the CAD risk they confer. A critique of commonly employed assessment techniques and the implications of their potential inaccuracies is discussed. Clinical strategies, with emphasis on pharmacological treatments, are discussed with regard to managing unhealthy lipid levels.

Lipids and lipoproteins can be impacted by a number of factors, including obesity, diabetes and metabolic syndrome, diet/nutrition, exercise (acute and chronic effects), cigarette smoking and environmental tobacco smoke, alcohol consumption, heredity, age, gender, and race. These factors are discussed in detail.

In summary, the relationship between lipids and CAD risk is well established. The complexities associated with this relationship are continually being revealed and addressed, which has, among other things, instigated a shift toward more aggressive clinical management of unhealthy lipid levels. This is a highly positive step, and represents the first prong of a comprehensive approach. The second prong entails primary preventive intervention strategies that include emphasis on improving a variety of lifestyle factors (weight management, healthy dietary practices, daily exercise, etc.). Progress in these areas is greatly needed and is critical to reducing the incidence of the number one cause of death in the industrialized world today.

References

1. Muller C. Angina pectoris in hereditary xanthomatosis. *Arch Intern Med* 1939;64:675–700.
2. Peters JP, VanSlyke DD. *Quantitative Clinical Chemistry.* Baltimore, MD: Williams & Wilkins; 1948: pp 1931–1932.
3. Castelli WP. Epidemiology of coronary heart disease: the Framingham study. *Am J Med* 1984;76(suppl 2A):4–12.
4. Kannel WB, Castelli WP, Gordon T. Cholesterol in the prediction of atherosclerotic disease. New perspectives based on the Framingham study. *Ann Intern Med* 1979;90:85–91.
5. Stamler J. Lifestyles, major risk factors, proof and public policy. *Circulation* 1978;58:3–19.
6. Keys A, Ed. Coronary heart disease in seven countries: American Heart Association monograph 29. *Circulation* 1970;41(suppl 1):1–211.
7. Hegsted DM, McGrandy RB, Nyers ML, Stare FJ. Quantitative effects of dietary fat on serum cholesterol in man. *Am J Clin Nutr* 1965;17:281–295.
8. Keys A, Anderson JT, Grande F. Serum cholesterol response to changes in the diet. IV. Particularly saturated fatty acids in the diet. *Metabolism* 1965;14:776–787.
9. Mattson FH, Erickson BA, Kligman AM. Effect of dietary cholesterol on serum cholesterol in man. *Am J Clin Nutr* 1972;25:589–594.
10. Lipid Research Clinics Program. The Lipid Research Clinics Coronary Primary Prevention Trial results. *JAMA* 1984;251:351–374.
11. Pearlman BL. The new cholesterol guidelines. Applying them in clinical practice. *Postgrad Med* 2002;112:13–26.
12. Gofman JW, DeLalla O, Glazier, et al. The serum lipoprotein transport system in health, metabolic disorders, atherosclerosis and coronary artery disease. *Plasma* 1954;2:414–484.
13. Oncley JL, Harvie NR. Lipoproteins: a current perspective of methods and concepts. *Proc Natl Acad Sci USA* 1969;64:1107–1118.
14. Fredrickson DS, Levy RI, Lees RS. Fat transport in lipoproteins: an integrated approach to mechanisms and disorders. *N Engl J Med* 1967;276:34–44, 94–103.
15. Mahley RW, Innerarity TL, Rall SC Jr, Weisgraber KH. Lipoproteins of special significance in atherosclerosis: insights provided by studies of type III hyperlipoproteinemia. *Ann NY Acad Sci* 1985;454:209–221.
16. Brown MS, Goldstein JL. A receptor-mediated pathway for cholesterol homeostasis. *Science* 1986;232:34–47.
17. Langer T, Strober W, Levy RI. The metabolism of low-density lipoprotein in familial type II hyperlipoproteinemia. *J Clin Invest* 1972;51:1528–1536.
18. Yang CY, Chen SH, Gianturco SH, et al. Sequence, structure, receptor-binding domains and internal repeats of human apolipoprotein B-100. *Nature* 1986;323:738–742.
19. Steinberg D, Gotto AM. Preventing coronary artery disease by lowering cholesterol levels: fifty years from bench to bedside. *JAMA* 1999;282:2043–2050.
20. Stampfer MJ, Krauss RM, Ma J, et al. A prospective study of triglyceride level, low-density lipoprotein particle diameter, and risk of myocardial infarction. *JAMA* 1996;276:882–888.

21. Rosenson RS, Otvos JD, Freedman DS. Relations of lipoprotein subclass levels and low-density lipoprotein size to progression of coronary artery disease in the pravastatin limitation of atherosclerosis in the coronary arteries (PLAC-1) trial. *Am J Cardiol* 2002;90:89–94.
22. Sniderman AD. Putting low-density lipoproteins at center stage in atherogenesis. *Am J Cardiol* 1997;79:64–67.
23. Lamarch B. Prevalence of syslipidemic phenotypes in ischemic heart disease. *Am J Cardiol* 1993;75:1189–1195.
24. Pittman RC, Steinberg D. A novel mechanism by which high-density lipoprotein selectivity delivers cholesterol esters to the liver. In: Greten H, Windler E, Beisiegal J, Eds. *Receptor-Mediated Uptake in the Liver.* Berlin: Springer; 1986: pp 108–119.
25. Watson AD, Navab M, Hama SY, et al. Effect of platelet activating factor-acetylhydrolase on the formation and action of minimally oxidized low-density lipoprotein. *J Clin Invest* 1995;95:774–782.
26. Ross R, Glomser JA. Atherosclerosis and the arterial smooth muscle cell: proliferation of smooth muscle is a key event in the genesis of the lesions of atherosclerosis. *Science* 1973;180:1332–1339.
27. Steinberg D. Lipoproteins and atherosclerosis: a look back and a look ahead. *Arteriosclerosis* 1983;3:283–301.
28. Ross R. The pathogenesis of atherosclerosis: an update. *N Engl J Med* 1986;314:488–500.
29. Brown MS, Basu SK, Falck JR, Ho YK, Goldstein JL. The scavenger cell pathway for lipoprotein degradation: specificity of the binding site that mediates the uptake of negatively-charged LDL by macrophages. *J Supramol Struct* 1980;13:67–81.
30. Henriksen T, Mahoney EM, Steinberg D. Enhanced macrophage degradation of low-density lipoprotein previously incubated with cultured endothelial cells: recognition by receptors for acetylated low-density lipoproteins. *Proc Natl Acad Sci USA* 1981;78:6499–6503.
31. Steinberg D. Oxidative modification of LDL and atherogenesis. *Circulation* 1997;95:1062–1071.
32. The Alpha-Tocopherol, Beta Carotene Cancer Prevention Study Group. The effect of vitamin E and beta carotene on the incidence of lung cancer and other cancers in male smokers. *N Engl J Med* 1994;330:1029–1035.
33. Reddy KG, Nair RN, Sheehan HM, et al. Evidence that selective endothelial dysfunction may occur in the absence of angiographic or ultrasound atherosclerosis in patients with risk factors for atherosclerosis. *J Am Coll Cardiol* 1994;23:883–843.
34. Treasure CB, Klein JL, Weintraub WS, et al. Beneficial effects of cholesterol-lowering therapy on the coronary endothelium in patients with coronary artery disease. *N Engl J Med* 1995;332:481–487.
35. Anderson TJ, Meredith IT, Yeung AC, et al. The effect of cholesterol-lowering and anti-oxidant therapy in endothelial-dependent coronary vasomotion. *N Engl J Med* 1995;332:488–493.
36. O'Driscoll G, Green D, Taylor RR, et al. Simvastatin, an HMG-coenzyme A reductase inhibitor, improves endothelial function within 1 month. *Circulation* 1997;95:1126–1131.

37. Tamai O, Matsuoka H, Itabe H, et al. Single LDL apheresis improves endothelium-dependent vasodilation in hypercholesterolemic humans. *Circulation* 1997;95:76–82.
38. Mahley RW. The role of dietary fat and cholesterol in atherosclerosis and lipoprotein metabolism. *West J Med* 1981;134:34–42.

2

Cardiovascular Risk Assessment

William B. Kannel

CONTENTS

Introduction 13
Incidence of Atherosclerotic Cardiovascular Disease 14
Current Status of Risk Factors — Hypertension 15
Dyslipidemia 19
Diabetes and the Metabolic Syndrome 21
Obesity 22
Indicators of Pre-Symptomatic Arterial Ischemia 23
Indicators Suggesting Unstable Lesions 23
Novel Risk Factors 23
Multivariable Risk Assessment 24
Preventive Implications 25
References 27

Introduction

Five decades of epidemiologic research provides health workers with valuable insights into the factors predisposing to atherosclerotic cardiovascular disease (CVD), stimulating world-wide interest in preventive cardiology. This provoked public heath initiatives against smoking in the 1960s, hypertension in the 1970s and dyslipidemia in the 1980s.[1] It also stimulated clinical trials to demonstrate the efficacy of risk factor modification. The epidemiologic population approach provided an undistorted appraisal of the way CVD evolves in the population indicating that coronary heart disease (CHD) is extremely common, afflicting one in five persons before age 60 years.[2,3] It was demonstrated to be a highly lethal disease with unanticipated sudden death as a prominent feature of the mortality and a substantial fraction of myocardial infarctions that are silent or unrecognized.[2,4] Because of this clinical presentation, a more vigorous preventive approach is now advocated using multivariable risk assessment and trial data demonstrating the benefits of risk factor correction. Epidemiological research indicates that atherosclerotic vascular disease is multifactorial, giving rise to the risk factor concept. Certain living habits promote atherogenic traits in genetically susceptible persons that, after prolonged exposure, produce a compromised arterial circulation leading to clinical cardiovascular events. Atherosclerotic cardiovascular disease is now regarded as a multifactorial process involving a variety of factors each of which is best considered as an ingredient of a cardiovascular risk profile.

Incidence of Atherosclerotic Cardiovascular Disease

Data from the Framingham Study encompassing 44 years of surveillance of the original cohort and 20 years of the offspring indicate the hazard of this leading cause of death. Coronary disease is the most common manifestation, equaling in incidence all the others combined for persons aged 35–64 years. It is also dominant above age 65 (Table 2.1). Women lag behind men in incidence of CVD with a diminishing gap in incidence with advancing age. Because of the half-century duration of follow-up of the Framingham cohort it was possible to determine the actual lifetime risk of developing a coronary event. This indicates that a 40-year-old man has a 48.6% lifetime risk and for women the risk is 31.7%, which is three times the risk of breast cancer (Table 2.2). The lifetime risk diminishes the longer one survives without acquiring it, but even at age 70 the risk is 34.9% for men and 24.2% for women. Because the short-term mortality after onset of an initial myocardial infarction is so high (25% 1-year mortality for men and 38% for women),

TABLE 2.1

Incidence of Atherosclerotic Cardiovascular Events in the Framingham Study: 44-Year Follow-up of Original Cohort and 20-Year Follow-up of Offspring

	Average Annual Incidence per 1000			
	Age 35–64 Years		Age 65–94 Years	
	Men	Women	Men	Women
CVD (all types)	17	9	44	30
Coronary disease	12	5	27	16
Stroke	2	2	13	11
Heart failure	2	1	12	9
Peripheral artery	3	2	8	5

Average annual incidence rates are age adjusted.

TABLE 2.2

Lifetime Risk of Initial Coronary Events: Framingham Study Participants

	Lifetime Risk (95% Confidence Intervals)	
Age (Years)	**Men**	**Women**
40	48.6% (45.8–51.3)	31.7% (29.2–34.2)
50	46.9% (44.0–49.8)	31.1% (28.6–33.7)
60	42.7% (39.5–45.8)	29.0% (26.3–31.6)
70	34.9% (31.2–38.7)	24.2% (21.4–27.0)

Source: From Lloyd-Jones DM, et al. *Lancet* 1999; 34:381–385. With permission.

this disease must be diagnosed on its way to clinical expression and its predisposing risk factors corrected. One in six coronary events presents with sudden death as the first, last and only symptom.

Current Status of Risk Factors — Hypertension

Hypertension (> 140/90 mmHg) afflicts one in four Americans. About 4% of persons less than 30 years of age have the condition and it increases in prevalence to 71% beyond age 80 years.[5] Estimates of the prevalence of isolated systolic hypertension that rises with age, vary because of age, ethnicity, the definition used and whether clinical or population data are surveyed. Data from the SHEP trial, which used > 160/90 mmHg to define the condition, estimates the prevalence at 8% for age 60–69 years, 11% at 70–79 years and 22% at 80 years and over.[6] About 65% of hypertension in the elderly is of the isolated systolic variety, the prevalence in women exceeding that in men beyond age 55 years.[7]

Framingham Study estimates of the rate of progression to hypertension from non-hypertensive blood pressures indicate that over a 4-year period about 50% of the elderly with high–normal blood pressure can be expected to progress to hypertension (> 140/90 mmHg) a rate five times that of persons with optimal (120/80 mmHg) blood pressure.[8] The average blood pressure of the Framingham cohort declined progressively over five decades so that elevated blood pressure is currently only one-third as prevalent as formerly.[9] However, if treatment-normalized pressures are included hypertension prevalence appears to have *increased*. This is likely a result of earlier detection and institution of therapy at lower blood pressures. No decline in blood pressure over time was observed in participants not receiving treatment. Half a century of follow-up of Framingham Study participants indicates that the lifetime probability of receiving antihypertensive medication is 60% for men and 57% for women.[10]

TABLE 2.3

Percent of Hypertensive Persons Developing Overt CVD Prior to Indications of Target Organ Involvement: 20-year Follow-up to Framingham Study

	Age (Years)				
	35–44	45–54	55–64	65–74	All Ages
Men	75%	58%	48%	33%	50%
Women	33%	56%	38%	33%	39%

Target organ involvement: proteinuria, ECG abnormality, cardiomegaly.

The primary variety of hypertension was formerly believed to be *benign* and the rise in blood pressure with age *essential* in order to perfuse vital organs. Initiation of treatment was often delayed until there was evidence of target organ involvement. Framingham Study data indicated that this practice was imprudent because 40–50% of hypertensive persons developed overt CVD prior to evidence of proteinuria, cardiomegaly or ECG abnormalities (Table 2.3). Its cardiovascular consequences were believed to derive chiefly from the diastolic pressure and the isolated systolic hypertension of the elderly was regarded as an innocuous accompaniment of arterial stiffening. Treatment of this entity was considered fruitless, intolerable and dangerous. Blood pressures assigned as *normal* for the elderly (100 plus age mmHg) were substantially higher than for the middle-aged. Women were believed to tolerate hypertension better than men. It was believed that there were age-related critical thresholds for blood pressure regarding hypertensive cardiovascular hazards. Isolated systolic hypertension was considered an innocuous accompaniment of advanced age.[11,12]

Based on epidemiological data, the current concept of an *acceptable* blood pressure is now based on what is *optimal* for avoiding hypertension-related CVD rather than on what is *usual*. Epidemiological data from the Framingham Study and elsewhere clearly indicate that at all ages and in both sexes, CVD risk increases incrementally with the systolic blood pressure and at any given blood pressure the hazard is greater in the elderly (Table 2.4). Similar graded relationships of blood pressure to CHD and all-cause mortality have been reported in several other cohorts.[13–15] There is no threshold for blood pressure risk as claimed by some, and in the Framingham cohort, 45% of the CVD events in men occurred at a systolic blood pressure < 140 mmHg, the value recently claimed by some to be the threshold of risk.[17] Large datasets are needed to precisely estimate CVD incidence trends at low blood pressures. Both the MRFIT data on > 350,000 male screenees followed for CVD mortality, and the Prospective Studies Collaboration involving almost 1 million participants and 56,000 vascular deaths, found no indication of a threshold of risk down to 115/75 mmHg.[16,18] Persons aged 40–69 years had a doubling of stroke or CHD mortality with every 20 mmHg increment

TABLE 2.4

Average Annual Cardiovascular Disease Incidence by Systolic Blood Pressure: 30-Year Follow-up to Framingham Study

Systolic Blood Pressure (mmHg)	Men (Years Old)			Women (Years Old)		
	45–54	55–64	65–74	45–54	55–64	65–74
74–119	8	16	16	3	6	12
120–139	11	18	23	5	9	17
140–159	19	31	37	9	16	22
160–179	29	43	52	9	24	20
180–300	35	62	78	16	36	45

All systolic blood pressure CVD incidence trends statistically significant.

Source: From Cupples LA, D'Agostino RB. In: Kannel WB, Wolf PA, Eds. *The Framingham Study: an Epidemiological Investigation of Cardiovascular Disease*. Washington DC: NHLBI National Printing Office; 1971; section 34.

increase of systolic (or 10 mmHg diastolic) throughout the entire range of blood pressure. Recent examination of the relation of non-hypertensive blood pressure to the rate of development of CVD in the Framingham Study found a significant graded influence of blood pressure from optimal (< 120/80 mmHg) to normal (120–129/80–84 mmHg) to high–normal (130–139/85–89 mmHg) among untreated men and women.[19] Compared with optimal, high–normal blood pressure conferred a 1.6- to 2.5-fold age- and risk factor-adjusted risk of a CVD event.

The tenaciously held belief that the adverse consequences of hypertension derive chiefly from the diastolic blood pressure component has long been convincingly refuted by prospective epidemiological data demonstrating that the impact of systolic pressure is greater than the diastolic component.[12,16,20] Examination of the increment in CVD risk per standard deviation increment in systolic vs. diastolic blood pressure, to take into account the different range of values for each, at all ages in both sexes in the Framingham Study indicates a consistently greater impact for the systolic blood pressure (Table 2.5).

Although risk ratios are no larger than for other cardiovascular events, the most common hazard for hypertensive patients of all ages is coronary disease, equaling in incidence all the other hypertensive atherosclerotic consequences combined (Table 2.6). Although the CVD incidence rates appear to be higher for most adverse outcomes in men, the risk ratios comparing those with and without hypertension in each sex are no higher in men than women (Table 2.6). Hypertension predisposes to all clinical manifestations of CHD including myocardial infarction, angina pectoris and sudden death, imposing a 2- to 3-fold increased risk.

Because of progressive arterial stiffening with advancing age, isolated systolic hypertension comprises about two thirds of the hypertension of the elderly. Its chief determinants are a high–normal systolic blood pressure in middle-age and prior diastolic blood pressure elevation that disappears as the arteries lose compliance with advancing age.[11] Isolated systolic hypertension

TABLE 2.5

Risk of Cardiovascular Disease by Systolic vs. Diastolic Blood Pressure: Framingham Study 38-Year Follow-up

	Risk Factor-Adjusted Increment per Standard Deviation Increase			
	Systolic		Diastolic	
Age (Years)	Men	Women	Men	Women
35–64	40%	38%	37%	29%
65–94	41%	25%	25%	15%

Covariates: cholesterol, glucose, cigarettes, ECG-left ventricular hypertrophy.

All differences significant at $P < 0.001$.

Source: From Kannel WB. Hypertension. In: Aronow WS, et al., Eds. *Vascular Disease in the Elderly.* Futura; 1997. With permission.

TABLE 2.6

Risk of Atherosclerotic Cardiovascular Events in Hypertensive Persons: 36-Year Follow-up. Framingham Study

	Age 35–64 Years				Age 65–94 Years			
	Biennial Rate[a]		Risk Ratio[a]		Biennial Rate[a]		Risk Ratio[a]	
CVD Events	Men	Women	Men	Women	Men	Women	Men	Women
CHD	45	21	2.0*	2.2*	72	44	1.6*	1.9*
Stroke	12	6	3.8*	2.6*	36	38	1.9*	2.3*
PAD	10	7	2.0*	3.7*	17	10	1.6*	2.0*
H.F.	14	6	4.0*	3.0*	33	24	1.9*	1.9*

*$P < 0.0001$. Biennial rates per 1000.

CHD, coronary heart disease; PAD, peripheral artery disease; H.F., heart failure.

[a] Age-adjusted.

Source: Kannel WB. *Drugs Aging* 2003; 20(4):277–286. With permission.

is associated with excess development of CHD, stroke, heart failure, and peripheral artery disease, increasing cardiovascular events and mortality rates 2- to 3-fold.[11] The disproportionate rise in systolic blood pressure that results in isolated systolic hypertension produces a widening of the pulse pressure. This increase in pulse pressure is definitely not an innocuous accompaniment of advancing age as previously believed. Risk of cardiovascular events increases progressively by 20–23% per 10 mmHg increment in pulse pressure in men and 11–21% in women[21] (Table 2.7).

TABLE 2.7

Risk of Cardiovascular Events by Pulse Pressure (Age-Adjusted Rate per 1000): 30-Year Follow-up to Framingham Study

	Pulse Pressure (mmHg)				
	2–39	**40–49**	**50–59**	**60–69**	**70–182**
Men 35–64 years	9	13	16	22	33
Men 65–94 years	4	16	32	39	58
Women 35–64 years	4	6	7	10	16
Women 65–94 years	17	19	22	25	32

Increment per 10 mmHg: Men 35–64 years 20%; Men 65–94 years 23%; Women 35–64 years 21%; Women 65–94 years 11%.

Source: From Kannel WB. *Am J Cardiol* 2000; 85:251–255. With permission.

Dyslipidemia

Dyslipidemia is a fundamental aspect of accelerated atherogenesis.[22] Epidemiological, clinical, angiographic and postmortem investigations establish a causal relationship between dyslipidemia and vascular atherosclerosis and demonstrate that treating it reduces its occurrence.[23] Despite dietary advice, and the variety of lipid-modifying medications available, its prevalence in the general population remains unacceptably high. Each of the blood lipids influence the risk of CHD in a continuous graded fashion even within the range considered *normal.* Data from the MRFIT involving 356,000 screenees showed a continuous graded relationship of serum total cholesterol to coronary mortality.[24] The average lipid values at which CHD occurs in Framingham Study middle-aged men is only 227 mg/dl for total cholesterol, 43 mg/dl for high-density lipoprotein cholesterol (HDL-C), 151 mg/dl for low-density lipoprotein cholesterol (LDL-C) and 5.6 for the total/HDL cholesterol ratio.[25] The average lipid values at which CHD occurs are higher in women, decrease with age, and have been declining over the past five decades. Epidemiological population-based data and clinical trials suggest that each 1% increase in total cholesterol throughout its range confers a 2% increment in CHD and comparable reduction in LDL-C yields the same reduction in initial and recurrent CHD events.[26] The most efficient lipid profile for estimating CHD potential is the total/HDL cholesterol ratio that affords a practical reflection of the net effect of the cholesterol entering the arterial intima in the LDL and being removed in the HDL (Table 2.8). This ratio determines the CHD risk whether the total cholesterol is above or below 240 mg/dl. Optimal treatment of dyslipidemia should improve this ratio to a goal of 3.5 that corresponds to half the high average CHD risk. A high triglyceride

TABLE 2.8

Efficiency of Specified Blood Lipids in Predicting Coronary Disease in Framingham Study Subjects Aged 50–80 Years

	Age-Adjusted Q5/Q1 Risk Ratio	
	Men	Women
Total cholesterol	1.9	2.5
LDL cholesterol	1.9	2.5
HDL cholesterol	0.4	0.5
Total/HDL cholesterol	2.5	3.1
LDL/HDL cholesterol	2.5	2.6

Q, quintiles of the distribution of the lipids.

Source: From Kannel WB, Wilson PWF. *Am Heart J* 1992; 124:768–774. With permission.

(> 150 mg/dl) in association with a reduced HDL-C signifies presence of insulin resistance and more atherogenic small-dense LDL.

The dyslipidemic CHD risk imposed is strongly influenced by the burden of associated risk factors.[27] Measurement of other risk factors such as blood pressure blood glucose, and weight is important because these cluster with dyslipidemia about 80% of the time and profoundly influence the risk imposed by dyslipidemia (Table 2.9). Dyslipidemia also tends to cluster with thrombogenic risk factors such as PAI-1, and when associated with inflammatory markers such as CRP, is especially dangerous.[28,29] The lack of a clear demarcation of high-risk coronary candidates based solely on lipid values indicates the need to evaluate dyslipidemia in the context of multivariable risk assessment. Global risk assessment is recommended by the ATP III guidelines for evaluation of dyslipidemic risk and treatment.[30] Multivariable CHD risk assessment using Framingham Study multivariable risk formulations is recommended to estimate the 10-year probability of CHD events for

TABLE 2.9

20-Year Risk of Coronary Disease Associated with Lipid Abnormalities by Extent of Risk Factor Clustering in Framingham Study Offspring: Age-Adjusted Incidence per 1000

	High Cholesterol		High Triglyceride		Low HDL-C	
No. of Risk Factors	Men	Women	Men	Women	Men	Women
None	103	110	88	37	172	21
One	232	141	190	52	228	74
≥ Two	313	177	309	186	306	179

Associated risk factors: other lipids, elevated blood pressure, body mass index, glucose.

dyslipidemic persons depending on the burden of other risk factors. Dyslipidemic persons at high global risk (> 20% 10 year risk) are assigned more stringent goals for LDL cholesterol.[30]

Diabetes and the Metabolic Syndrome

Atherosclerotic cardiovascular disease is a major hazard of Type 2 diabetes. Its prevalence in the general population has been rising.[31] Persons with the metabolic syndrome, a condition characterized by disturbed glucose and insulin metabolism, visceral adiposity, dyslipidemia and hypertension, appear to have a prediabetic state.[32]

Diagnostic criteria for this metabolic syndrome were promulgated by the 3rd Adult Treatment Panel,[33] requiring three or more of the aforementioned variables as specified in Table 2.10. Recent estimates indicate that the condition is highly prevalent in the U.S. population, affecting 24% of adults.[34] About 50% of diabetic men and 62% of women in the Framingham Study had the metabolic syndrome whereas among persons with the metabolic syndrome, only 15% of men and 17% of women had overt diabetes. The hazard for CVD in persons with the metabolic syndrome is estimated to be substantial: 3-fold increased risk of CHD and stroke, and 5-fold increased risk of CVD mortality.[35]

TABLE 2.10

NCEP ATP III Criteria for Designation of the Metabolic Syndrome

Risk Factor	Defining Level
3 or More of the Following:	
Abdominal obesity	Waist circumference
Men	> 40 inches (102 cm)
Women	> 35 inches (88 cm)
Triglycerides	150 mg/dl
HDL-cholesterol	
Men	< 40 mg/dl
Women	< 50 mg/dl
Blood pressure	≥ 130/85 mmHg
Fasting glucose	≥ 110 mg/dl

Source: From NCEP ATP III. *Circulation* 2002; 106:3134–3421. With permission.

Obesity

Overweight (body mass index [BMI] 25–29) and obesity (BMI > 29) are now epidemic, posing a major threat to the public health. Adiposity is the most prevalent metabolic disorder in the United States. At any given time 40% of women and 25% of men are attempting to lose weight.[36] The high average weight of Americans carries a substantial health penalty of hypertension, dyslipidemia, diabetes, cardiovascular disease, gallstone disease, and prostate and colon cancer. Following considerable prior skepticism about obesity it is no longer regarded as an innocent accompaniment of CVD risk factors.

After longer periods of observation, consideration of patterns of adiposity and the clear and consistent demonstration that changes in weight are mirrored by changes in multiple atherogenic risk factors,[37] the true role of obesity as a cardiovascular hazard has become accepted. The burden of cardiovascular risk factors is substantially greater in the obese than in lean persons and the greater the adiposity the higher the blood pressure, level of dyslipidemia, blood glucose insulin resistance and left ventricular hypertrophy. The average number of risk factors that cluster with any particular risk factor increases, the greater the associated BMI (Table 2.11). Weight gain leading to abdominal obesity promotes many of the atherogenic traits that in aggregate have been characterized as the *metabolic syndrome*. The hazard of obesity varies widely depending on the accompanying burden of CVD risk factors. Weight loss improves insulin sensitivity and reduces the amount of atherogenic risk factor clustering. If optimal weight is defined as that weight which optimizes the cardiovascular risk profile it would correspond to a BMI of 22.6 for men and 21.1 for women.[38] Estimates from the Framingham Study indicate that if everyone could be maintained at optimal weight there would be 25% less CHD and 35% fewer strokes and heart failure.[39] Unfortunately, sustained weight reductions in the obese have been difficult to achieve.

TABLE 2.11

Risk Factor Clustering with Elevated Cholesterol According to BMI: Framingham Offspring Cohort Subjects Aged 30–70 years

Men		Women	
BMI	Av. No. of Risk Factors	BMI	Av. No. of Risk Factors
<23.6	1.5	<20.6	1.7
23.7–25.4	1.7	20.6–22.2	1.6
25.5–27.1	2.0	22.3–23.8	1.9
27.2–29.3	2.1	23.9–26.5	1.9
>29.3	2.5	>26.5	2.6

BMI, body mass index. Elevated cholesterol: men 232 mg/dl; women 224 mg/dl (upper quintile values).

Indicators of Pre-Symptomatic Arterial Ischemia

There are a number of indicators of arterial ischemia that greatly affect the risk of established risk factors. A compromised coronary arterial circulation may be manifested prior to symptoms by ECG abnormalities such as nonspecific repolarization abnormalities, left ventricular hypertrophy, blocked intraventricular conduction and myocardial infarction. Myocardial infarctions in hypertensive persons are surprisingly often silent or unrecognized. In the Framingham Study, 49% of myocardial infarctions are unrecognized.[40] In order not to overlook these myocardial infarctions, that are hazardous despite lack of symptoms, biennial ECG examinations should be done.

Carotid and femoral vascular bruits usually signify diffuse atherosclerosis and are associated with not only stroke and intermittent claudication, but CHD as well.[41] Framingham Study data indicated that it is imprudent to await indications of target organ involvement because 40–50% of hypertensive persons developed overt CVD prior to evidence of proteinuria, cardiomegaly or ECG abnormalities.

Indicators Suggesting Unstable Lesions

Elevated fibrinogen and leukocyte count within the purported "normal" range and level of C-reactive protein (CRP) tend to coexist and predict atherosclerotic CVD events. They appear to reflect the presence of unstable lesions that are undergoing inflammatory lipid infiltration and fissuring portending thrombotic arterial occlusion.[42–44] Levels of these risk factors are likely to be elevated in persons who smoke, are hypertensive, diabetic or dyslipidemic.

Novel Risk Factors

It has been claimed that only half the coronary disease incidence is explained by the standard major risk factors, but a recent report based on 120,000 patients enrolled in clinical CHD trials indicated that at least one major risk factor is present in 85% of men and 81% of women.[45] Another report derived from 400,000 persons enrolled in three cohort studies showed that among those suffering fatal CHD events, 87–100% had exposure to at least one major risk factor.[46] Nevertheless, epidemiological research continues to find and evaluate additional risk factors that contribute to the occurrence of CVD, and warrant further evaluation.

Subgroups of HDL and LDL are shown to be associated with CHD but the utility of these refinements over the standard lipoprotein determinations is not established.[47,48] Similarly, lipoprotein (a) is associated with CHD and stroke in some, but not all studies.[49] Elevated triglyceride is consistently associated with increased CHD risk, but its predictive power is often lost or attenuated when HDL cholesterol and triglycerides or diabetes are taken into account. However, a recent meta-analysis of 17 studies strongly suggests an independent incremental triglyceride CHD risk, particularly when the LDL or total/HDL cholesterol ratio is high.[50]

C-reactive protein is a confirmed risk factor for CHD along with other circulating markers of inflammation.[51] A recent meta-analysis of CRP investigations indicates that the independent relative risk of an elevated CRP is less than suggested in earlier reports. It appears that the predictive value of CRP adds relatively little to multivariable risk estimation based on the standard risk factors.[52]

Homocysteine, an amino acid regulated by vitamins B-12 and folate, found in higher concentration in 29% of the elderly Framingham Study participants and 5% of subjects in the Physicians' Health Study has been found to be associated with increased risk of cardiovascular disease.[53,54] However, no clinical trials have thus far tested whether reducing homocysteine by vitamin supplementation decreases risk of developing atherosclerotic cardiovascular disease.

Multivariable Risk Assessment

Epidemiological investigation has long contended that atherosclerotic CVD is of multifactorial etiology. There are faulty lifestyles that promote atherogenic traits in susceptible persons, indicators of unstable lesions, and signs of a compromised arterial circulation that strongly indicate impending clinical events. The cardiovascular risk factors seldom occur in isolation of each other because they are metabolically linked, tending to cluster, and the extent of this clustering profoundly influences the CVD hazard of any particular risk factor. Weight gain leading to visceral adiposity promotes most of the components of the cluster of risk factors characterized as the insulin-resistant metabolic syndrome. The hazard of obesity varies widely depending on the burden of atherogenic risk factors that accompany it. Multivariable analysis of the influence of established and potential risk factors is undertaken to explore clues to the pathogenesis of CVD, and for estimation of the independent effect of risk factors and the global risk of candidates for CVD events. The set of risk factors employed for the former is constrained by the hypothesis to be tested, and for the latter by the availability of reliable noninvasive tests for the risk factors, cost, and whether the risk factors used can be safely modified with the expectation of benefit.

Major established risk factors have been synthesized into composite scoring algorithms based on Framingham Study data for the cardiovascular disease outcomes of coronary disease, stroke, peripheral artery disease and heart failure.[55–58] The risk factors chosen had to be independent contributors to risks that are not highly intercorrelated, and obtainable by ordinary office procedures and readily available reliable laboratory tests.

When confronted with a patient with any particular CVD risk factor it is essential to test for the others that are likely to coexist with it. Such coexistence can be expected 80% of the time. Now that guidelines for dyslipidemia, hypertension and diabetes recommend treating modest elevations of risk factors, candidates for treatment are best targeted by global risk assessment to reduce the number needed to treat to prevent one event.

Preventive Implications

Awaiting overt signs and symptoms of cardiovascular disease before initiating treatment of hypertension, dyslipidemia or glucose intolerance is no longer justified. The occurrence of symptoms is more properly regarded as a medical failure than the first indication for therapy. As stated by Chobanian, "Intensified efforts to alter modifiable cardiovascular risk factors such as blood pressure, lipoprotein levels, smoking, blood glucose levels, weight and physical activity levels must become a national priority."[59]

Overwhelming evidence indicates a continuous incremental influence of systolic blood pressure on CVD mortality at all ages in both men and women. Optimal blood pressure for avoiding CVD is less than 140/90 mmHg with no discernible critical blood pressure that delineates normal from abnormal. For cost-effective treatment of blood pressure in the high–normal prehypertensive range multivariable risk assessment is required and the goal of therapy should be to improve global CVD risk.[60] Because the hazard of any degree of blood pressure elevation is increased when there is concomitant dyslipidemia, diabetes, proteinuria, or the metabolic syndrome, more rigorous blood pressure control is recommended. In this circumstance and when there is already existing overt renal disease, coronary disease or peripheral artery disease, the importance of what appear to be trivial increases in blood pressure, even within the high–normal rage, should not be underestimated. The effort needed to lower the blood pressure to the goals recommended for avoiding CVD is worthwhile.

Notwithstanding the abundant evidence of the benefits of treatment of systolic hypertension, this is the type of hypertension least likely to be treated, and when treated is seldom treated to the recommended goal.[61,62] Despite the variety of antihypertensive agents for controlling elevated blood pressure by different mechanisms, many patients are failing to reach the JNC 7 recommended goals of therapy.[63] This is due to failure to achieve goals for

TABLE 2.12

Control of Systolic and Diastolic Blood Pressure in Framingham Study Participants 1990–1995

Control of	All Hypertensives	On Treatment
Systolic (<140 mmHg)	33%	49%
Diastolic (<90 mmHg)	83%	90%
Both (<140/90 mmHg)	30%	48%
	(n = 1995)	(n = 1189)

Source: Lloyd-Jones DM, Evans JC, Larson MG, et al. Differential control of systolic and diastolic blood pressure: factors associated with lack of blood pressure control in the community. *Hypertension* 2000; 36:594–599.

systolic blood pressure. The Framingham Study reports that, whereas 90% of hypertensive persons on treatment have their diastolic blood pressure reduced to below 90 mmHg, only 48% have their systolic pressure controlled to below 140 mmHg (Table 2.12). This failure applies to all subgroups of hypertensive persons including African Americans, the elderly, and patients with diabetes. Failure to control systolic pressure adequately in the elderly and diabetics is particularly unfortunate because the benefits are greatest in these patients.

Poor control of blood pressure is attributable to the need for long-term adherence to treatment of an asymptomatic condition, adverse symptomatic side effects when there were none to begin with, and the high cost of medications. About half of patients prescribed blood pressure medications stop taking them by the end of the first year.[64] Physicians' knowledge and attitudes concerning vigorous control of blood pressure also appear to be problematic.

Lipid correction has been consistently shown by numerous trials to bestow benefit for atherosclerotic CVD. Lipid-modifying agents, particularly the statins, reduce coronary and stroke events, modify endothelial dysfunction, decrease platelet aggregation, stabilize plaques and promote coronary vasodilation.[22,23] The benefit of correcting dyslipidemia for decreasing the hazard of coronary morbidity and mortality has been demonstrated with and without established coronary disease, and whether lipids are distinctly abnormal or only average. Recently reported results of the Heart Protection Study indicate that high-risk patients, including those with LDL-cholesterol values under 100 mg/dl, benefit from aggressive lipid-modifying therapy.[65] The VA-HIT trial showed that even a modest fibrate-induced increase in HDL cholesterol results in a reduction in CHD events.[66]

As clinicians cope with the task of implementing preventive measures for avoiding or delaying development of atherosclerotic CVD by modifying correctable risk factors, they must remember that the goal is to target high-risk persons and reduce their global (multivariable) risk as well as the particular risk factor under scrutiny. This requires getting familiar with multivariable risk factor algorithms to assess risk before, during and after treatment.

References

1. Report of the Intersociety Commission of Heart Disease Resources. Resources for primary prevention of atherosclerotic disease. *Circulation* 1984; 70 (suppl): 155A–205A.
2. Gordon T, Kannel WB. Premature mortality from coronary heart disease. The Framingham Study. *JAMA* 1971; 215:1617–1625.
3. Lloyd-Jones DM, Larson MG, Beiser A, Levy D. Lifetime risk of developing coronary heart disease. *Lancet* 1999; 353:89–92.
4. Kannel WB, Abbott RD. Incidence and prognosis of unrecognized myocardial infarction. An update on the Framingham Study. *N Engl J Med* 1984; 311:1144–1147.
5. *Morbidity and Mortality: Chartbook on Cardiovascular, Lung and Blood Diseases.* NIH, NHLBI; 2000.
6. SHEP Cooperative Research Group. Prevention of stroke by antihypertensive drug treatment in older persons with isolated systolic hypertension: final results of the Systolic Hypertension in the Elderly Program (SHEP). *JAMA* 1991; 265:3255–3264.
7. Kannel WB. Prospects for prevention of cardiovascular disease in the elderly. *Prev Cardiol* 1998; 1:32–39.
8. Vasan RS, Larson MG, Leip EP, Kannel WB, Levy D. Assessment of frequency of progression to hypertension in non-hypertensive participants in the Framingham Study; a cohort study. *Lancet* 2001; 358:1682–1686.
9. Kannel WB. Blood pressure as a cardiovascular risk factor: prevention and treatment. *JAMA* 1996; 275:1571–1576.
10. Vasan R, Beiser A, Seshadri S, et al. Residual lifetime risk of developing hypertension in middle-aged women and men; the Framingham Heart Study. *JAMA* 2002; 287:1003–1010.
11. Wilking SVP, Belanger AJ, Kannel WB, et al. Determinants of isolated systolic hypertension. *JAMA* 1988; 260:3451–3455.
12. Kannel WB, Gordon T, Schwartz MJ. Systolic versus diastolic blood pressure and risk of coronary heart disease: the Framingham Study. *Am J Cardiol* 1971; 27:335–345.
13. The Pooling Project Research Group. Relationship of blood pressure, cholesterol, smoking habit, relative weight and ECG abnormalities to incidence of major coronary events: final report of the Pooling Project. *J Chron Dis* 1978; 201–206.
14. Lew EA. High blood pressure, other risk factors and longevity. The insurance viewpoint. *Am J Med* 1973; 55:281–294.
15. Cupples LA, D'Agostino RB. Some risk factors related to the annual incidence of cardiovascular disease and death using pooled biennial measurements: 30-year follow-up. In: Kannel WB, Wolf PA, Eds. *The Framingham Study: an Epidemiological Investigation of Cardiovascular Disease.* Washington DC: NHLBI National Printing Office; 1971; section 34.
16. Neaton JD, Kuller L, Stamler J, Wentworth DN. Impact of systolic and diastolic blood pressure on cardiovascular mortality. In: Laragh JH, Brenner BM, Eds. *Hypertension: Pathophysiology, Diagnosis and Management*, 2nd ed. New York: Raven Press; 1995; 127–144.

17. Port S, Demer L, Jennrich R, Walter D, Garfinkle A. Systolic blood pressure and mortality. *Lancet* 2000; 355:175–180.
18. Prospective Studies Collaboration. Age-specific relevance of usual blood pressure to vascular mortality; a meta-analysis of individual data for one million adults in 61 prospective studies. *Lancet* 2002; 360:1903–1913.
19. Vasan RS, Larson MG, Leip EP, et al. Impact of high-normal blood pressure on the risk of cardiovascular disease. *N Engl J Med* 2001; 345:1291–1297.
20. Kannel WB, Dawber TR, McGee DL. Perspectives on systolic hypertension. The Framingham Study. *Circulation* 1980; 61:1179–1182.
21. Kannel WB. Elevated blood pressure as a cardiovascular risk factor. *Am J Cardiol* 2000; 85:251–255.
22. Knopp RH. Drug therapy: drug treatment of lipid disorders. *N Engl J Med* 1999; 341–511.
23. Levine GN, Keaney JF Jr, Vita JA. Cholesterol reduction in cardiovascular disease. *N Engl J Med* 1995; 332:512–521.
24. Stamler J, Wentworth D, Neaton JD. Is the relationship between serum cholesterol and risk of premature death from coronary heart disease continuous or graded? Results in 356,222 primary screenees of the Multiple Risk Factor Intervention Trial (MRFIT). *JAMA* 1986; 256:2823–2828.
25. Kannel WB. Range of serum cholesterol values in the population developing coronary artery disease. *Am J Cardiol* 1995; 76:69C–77C.
26. Grundy SM. Approach to lipoprotein management in 2001 national cholesterol guidelines. *Am J Cardiol* 2002; 90(suppl): 11i–21i.
27. Kannel WB, Wilson PWF. Efficacy of lipid profiles in predicting coronary disease. *Am Heart J* 1992; 124:768–774.
28. Ridker PM. Evaluating novel cardiovascular risk factors. Can we better predict heart attacks? *Ann Intern Med* 1999; 130:933–937.
29. Libby P, Ridker PM. Novel inflammatory markers of coronary risk: theory versus practice. *Circulation* 1999; 100:1148–1150.
30. Executive summary of the Third Report of the National Cholesterol Education Program (NCEP) Expert Panel on Detection, Evaluation, and Treatment of High Blood Cholesterol in Adults (Adult Treatment Panel III). *JAMA* 2001; 285:2486–2497.
31. Mokdad AH, Ford ES, Bowman BA, Dietz WH, et al. Prevalence of obesity, diabetes, and obesity-related health risk factors. *JAMA* 2110; 289:76–79.
32. Reaven GM. Banting Lecture. 1988; role of insulin resistance in human disease. *Diabetes* 1988; 37:1595–1607.
33. Third Report of the National Cholesterol Education Program (NCEP) Expert Panel on Detection, Evaluation and Treatment of High Blood Cholesterol in Adults (Adult Treatment Panel III). Final report. *Circulation* 2002; 106:3143–3421.
34. Ford ES, Giles WH, Dietz WH. Prevalence of the metabolic syndrome among U.S. adults: findings from the third National Health and Nutrition Examination Survey. *JAMA* 2002; 287:356–359.
35. Isomaa B, Almgren B, Tuomi T, et al. Cardiovascular morbidity and mortality associated with the metabolic syndrome. *Diabetes Care* 2001; 24:683–689.
36. Clinical Guidelines on the Identification, Evaluation and Treatment of Overweight and Obesity in Adults. The Evidence Report. Bethesda, MD: National Institutes of Health; 1998. Publication 98-4083.

37. Ashley F, Kannel WB. Relation of weight change to changes in atherogenic traits. The Framingham Study. *J Chron Dis* 1974; 27:103–114.
38. Garrison RJ, Kannel WB. A new approach for estimating healthy body weights. *Int J Obes* 1993; 17:417–423.
39. Gordon T, Kannel WB. The effects of overweight on cardiovascular disease. *Geriatrics* 1973; 28:80–88.
40. Kannel WB, Dannenberg AL, Abbott RD. Unrecognized myocardial infarction and hypertension; the Framingham Study. *Am Heart J* 1995; 109:581–585.
41. Kannel WB, McGee DL. Update on some epidemiologic features of intermittent claudication: the Framingham Study. *J Am Geriatr Soc* 1985; 33:13–18.
42. Ernst E, Hammerschmidt DE, Bagge U, et al. Leukocytes and risk of ischemic diseases. *JAMA* 1987; 257:2318–2324.
43. Fuster V, Badimon L, Badimon JJ, et al. The pathogenesis of coronary artery disease and the acute coronary syndromes (Part 1). *N Engl J Med* 1992; 326:310–318.
44. Ernst E, Resch KL. Fibrinogen as a cardiovascular risk factor: a meta-analysis and review of the literature. *Ann Intern Med* 1993; 118:956–963.
45. Khot UN, Khot MB, Bajer CT, et al. Prevalence of conventional risk factors in patients with coronary heart disease. *JAMA* 2003; 290:898–904.
46. Greenland P, Knoll MD, Stamler J, et al. Major risk factors as antecedents of fatal and non-fatal coronary heart disease events. *JAMA* 2003; 290:891–897.
47. Wilson PWF. Relation of high-density lipoprotein subfractions and apolipoprotein isoforms to coronary disease. *Clin Chem* 1995; 41:165–169.
48. Austin MA, Hokanson JE, Brunzell JD. Characterization of low-density lipoprotein subclasses: methodological approaches and clinical relevance. *Curr Opin Lipidol* 1994; 5:395–403.
49. Ridker PM, Hennekens CH. Lipoprotein (a) and the risks of cardiovascular disease. *Ann Epidemiol* 1994; 4:360–362.
50. Hokanson JE, Austin MA, Edwards KL. Hypertriglyceridemia as a cardiovascular risk factor independent of high-density lipoprotein: a meta-analysis of population-based prospective studies. *J Cardiovasc Risk* 1996; 3:213–219.
51. Danesh J, Wheeler JG, Hirschfield GM, et al. C-reactive protein and other circulating makers of inflammation in the prediction of coronary heart disease. *N Engl J Med* 2004; 350:1387–1397.
52. Tall AR. C-reactive protein reassessed (Editorial). *N Engl J Med* 2004; 350:1450–1452.
53. Stampfer MJ, Malinow MR, Willett WC, et al. A prospective study of plasma homocysteine and risk of myocardial infarction in U.S. physicians. *JAMA* 1992; 268: 877–881.
54. Genest JJ Jr, McNamara JR, Salem DN, et al. Plasma homocysteine levels in men with premature coronary artery disease. *J Am Coll Cardiol* 1990; 16:1114–1119.
55. Wilson PWF, D'Agostino RB, Levy D, et al. Prediction of coronary heart disease using risk factor categories. *Circulation* 1998; 97:1837–1847.
56. Wolf PA, D'Agostino RB, Belanger AJ, et al. Probability of stroke: a risk profile from the Framingham Study. *Stroke* 1991; 3:312–318.
57. Murabito JM, D'Agostino RB, Levy D, et al. Intermittent claudication: a risk profile from the Framingham Heart Study. *Circulation* 1997; 6:44–49.
58. Kannel WB, D'Agostino RB, Silbershatz H, Belanger A, Wilson PWF, Levy D. Profile for estimating risk of heart failure. *Arch Intern Med* 1999; 159:1197–1204.

59. Chobanian AV. Control of hypertension — an important national priority. *N Engl J Med* 2001; 345:534–535.
60. Kannel WB. Risk stratification of hypertension. *Am J Hypertens* 2000; 13:3S–10S.
61. Coppola WG, Whincup PH, Walker M, et al. Identification and management of stroke risk in older people; a national survey of current practice in primary care. *J Hum Hypertens* 1997; 11:185–197.
62. Berlowitz DR, Ash AS, Hickey EC, et al. Inadequate management of high blood pressure in a hypertensive population. *N Engl J Med* 1998; 339:1957–1963.
63. Chobanian AV, Bakris GL, Black HR, et al. Seventh report of the Joint National Committee on prevention, detection, evaluation and treatment of high blood pressure: the JNC 7 report. *JAMA* 2002; 289:2560–2527.
64. Bloom BS. Continuation of initial antihypertensive medication after 1 year of therapy. *Clin Ther* 1998; 20:671–681.
65. Heart Protection Collaborative Group MRC/BHF Heart protection study of cholesterol lowering with simvastatin in 20,536 high-risk individuals: a randomized placebo controlled trial. *Lancet* 2002; 360:7–22.
66. Rubens HB, Robins SJ, Collins D, et al. For the Veterans Affairs High-density cholesterol lipoprotein Intervention Trial study group. Gemfibrozil for the secondary prevention of coronary heart disease in men with low levels of high-density lipoprotein cholesterol. *N Engl J Med* 1999; 341:410–418.

3

Basic Lipidology

Jacqueline L. Dupont

CONTENTS

Introduction 31
Lipid Classes 32
Acylglycerides 32
Fatty acids 32
Phospholipids and Sphingolipids 34
Sterols and Steroids 36
Lipid Digestion 37
Regulation of Cholesterol Synthesis 38
Essential Fatty Acids and Eicosanoids 41
Lipid Peroxidation 43
References 45

Introduction

Lipids are structural components of all living cells. They are integral to membranes, providing a water barrier that gives form to cellular components. Major classes and functions of lipids are: (a) acylglycerides, energy source and storage, (b) phospholipids, metabolically active cellular lipids, (c) fatty acids, essential metabolites and precursors of autocoids, and (d) sterols and their metabolites including hormones and bile acids. The metabolism of lipids includes ingestion of lipids from foods, digestion and transport, and functions of cholesterol and essential fatty acids. Lipid transport is not included in this chapter as it is considered extensively elsewhere.

Lipid Classes

Acylglycerides

The most abundant form of lipids in plants and animals is triacylglycerides made up of fatty acids esterified to glycerol (Figure 3.1). Di- and monoacylglycerides exist in small quantities and are important in metabolic transformations of the glycerides. The fatty acids may be attached to any of the three glycerol carbons and their positions are designated by the stereospecific numbering of the glycerol molecule. In the esterified form the molecules have no polar constituents and are thus quite hydrophobic. The characteristics of the fatty acyl chains determine the nature of the acylglycerides.

Fatty acids

Fatty acids are hydrocarbon chains of from 2 to 20 and more carbons with a carboxyl at one end. The nomenclature has evolved over time from known chemistry and from sources from which they are isolated (Table 3.1). Those of two or three carbons are volatile, 4–6 carbons are called short chain, 8–12 carbons are medium chain and 14–18 carbons are long chain. A group of 20 carbon and longer chain fatty acids is important in metabolism and is referred to as a very long chain or by their individual names. The short-chain fatty acids are water soluble, and as the chains lengthen, the water solubility declines. The melting point is the opposite, with melting points rising as chain length increases. Fatty acids may be saturated, i.e., having all carbons in single linkage to other carbons or hydrogens, or monounsaturated, or polyunsaturated (Figure 3.2). The natural double bonds formed

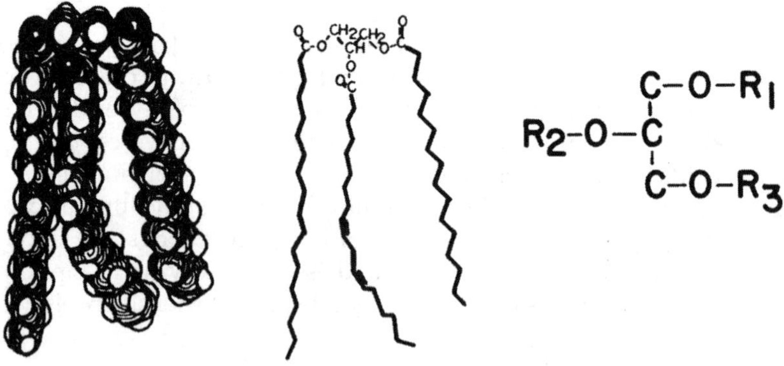

FIGURE 3.1
Space-filling and conventional models of triacylglycerols: (A) space filling; (B) conformational; (C) stereospecific numbering (sn) of glycerides. If the R_3 substituent is PO_4, the compound is phosphatidic acid.

TABLE 3.1

Fatty Acids Important in Nutrition

Symbol[a]	Systematic Name[b]	Common Name	Melting Point (°C)	Sources
Saturated Fatty Acids (SFA)				
2:0	*n*-Ethanoic	Acetic	16.7	Many plants
3:0	*n*-Propanoic	Propanoic	–22.0	Rumen
4:0	*n*-Butanoic	Butyric	–7.9	Rumen and milk fat
6:0	*n*-Hexanoic	Caproic	–8.0	Milk fat
8:0	*n*-Octanoic	Caprylic	12.7	Milk fat, coconut
10:0	*n*-Decanoic	Capric	29.6	Milk fat, coconut
12:0	*n*-Dodecanoic	Lauric	42.2	Coconut, palm kernel
14:0	*n*-Tetradecanoic	Myristic	52.1	Milk fat, coconut
16:0	*n*-Hexadecanoic	Palmitic	60.7	Most common SFA in plants and animals
18:0	*n*-Octadecanoic	Stearic	69.6	Animal fat, cocoa butter
20:0	*n*-Eicosanoic	Arachidic	75.4	Widespread minor
22:0	*n*-Docosanoic	Behenic	80.0	Minor in seeds
24:0	*n*-Tetracosanoic	Lignoceric	84.2	Minor in seeds
Monounsaturated (Monoenoic) Fatty Acids				
10:1 n-1	*cis*-9-Decanoic	Caproleic		Milk fat
12:1 n-3	*cis*-9-Dodecanoic	Lauroleic		Milk fat
14:1 n-5	*cis*-9-Tetradecanoic	Myristoleic		Milk fat
16:1 n-7*t*	*trans*-Hexadecanoic	Palmitelaidic		HVO[c]
16:1 n-7	*cis*-9-Hexadecanoic	Palmitoleic	1	Most fats and oils
18:1 n-9	*cis*-9-Octadecanoic	Oleic	16	Most fats and oils
18:1 n-9*t*	*trans*-9-Octadecanoic	Elaidic	44	Ruminant fat, HVO
18:1 n-7*t*	*trans*-11-Octadecanoic	*trans* Vaccenic	44	Ruminant fat
20:1 n-11	*cis*-9-Eicosanoic	Gadoleic		Fish oils
20:1 n-9	*cis*-11-Eicosanoic	Gondoic	24	Rapeseed, fish oils
22:1 n-9	*cis*-13-Docosanoic	Erucic	24	Rapeseed, mustard oil
Polyunsaturated (Polyenoic) Fatty Acids				
Dienoic				
18:2 n-9	*cis,cis*-6,9-Octadecadienoic		–11	Minor in animals
18:2 n-6	*cis,cis*-9,12-Octadecadienoic	Linoleic	–5	Most plant oils
Trienoic				
18:3 n-6	All-*cis*-6,9,12-Octadecatrienoic	γ-Linolenic		Evening primrose, borage oils
18:3 n-3	All-*cis*-9,12,15-Octadecatrienoic	α-Linolenic	–11	Soybean and Canola oils
20:3 n-6	All-*cis*-8,11,14-Eicosatrienoic	Dihomo-gammalinolenic		

(continued)

TABLE 3.1 (CONTINUED)

Fatty Acids Important in Nutrition

Symbol[a]	Systematic Name[b]	Common Name	Melting Point (°C)	Sources
Tetra-, Penta-, Hexanoic				
20:4 n-6	All-*cis*-8,11,14-Eicosatetranoic	Arachidonic	–49.5	Meat
20:5 n-3	All-*cis*-5,8,11,14,17-Eicosapentanoic	EPA, Timnodonic		Fish oils
22:4 n-6	All-*cis*-7,10,13,16-Docosatetranoic	Adrenic		Brain
22:5 n-6	All-*cis*-7,10,13,16,19-Docosapentanoic	DPA, Clupanodonic		Brain
22:6 n-3	All-*cis*-4,7,10,13,16,19-Docosahexanoic	DHA		Fish

[a] Number of carbons: number of double bonds, location of first double bond from the methyl carbon; *t* = *trans*.

[b] Geometric isomer-Δ positions of double bonds.

[c] Hydrogenated vegetable oil.

by removal of hydrogens are primarily in the *cis* configuration and in methyl interrupted positions (three carbons apart) rather than in conjugated positions. Enzymes exist in mammalian systems to insert double bonds between the C-9 position and the carboxyl carbon. Plant enzymes synthesize 18 carbon fatty acids with double bonds at the n 3 (methyl carbon minus 3) or ω-3 (omega carbon minus 3) and the n-6 positions. Because those fatty acids are required in metabolism, they are essential components of human diets. Some *trans* fatty acids are naturally occurring but most in the human diet are formed by chemical hydrogenation of vegetable oils. The *cis* or *trans* configuration (Figure 3.3) is very important in metabolism, conveying major aspects of physical conformation and therefore reactivity to the molecule (Figure 3.2). The melting points of *cis* unsaturated fatty acids are lower than saturated or *trans* unsaturated fatty acids (Table 3.1).

Phospholipids and Sphingolipids

The glycerol molecule is the backbone of the major group of phospholipids or glycerophosphatides (Figure 3.4). Phosphatidic acid is the building block to which fatty acids are esterified at the C1 and C2 positions, with the C1 position having a saturated and the C2 position an unsaturated fatty acid. Individual phospholipids have different patterns of fatty acids and are further characterized by their derivatives with the compounds choline, ethanolamine, serine, inositol and others. Phosphatidylcholine is better known by its common name of lecithin. The presence of polar constituents makes phospholipids both neutral and polar and they are therefore amphipathic, reacting at hydrophobic and hydrophilic interfaces.

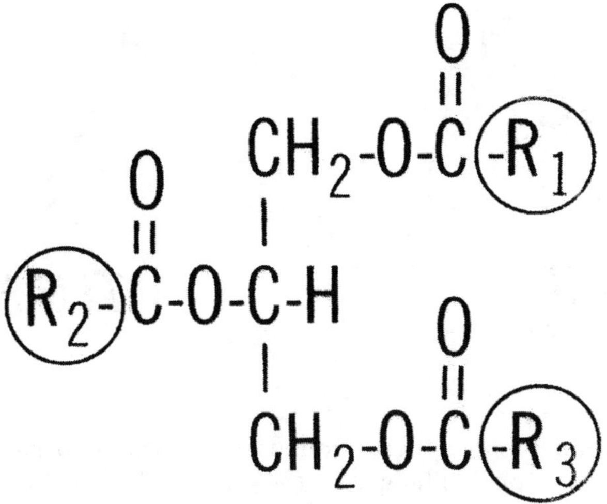

TRIACYLGLYCEROL

FIGURE 3.2
Space-filling and conventional models of fatty acids: (A) stearic acid (18:0), space-filling; (B) stearic acid, conformational; (C) elaidic acid (18:1n-9*t*) *trans*, conformational; (D) α-linolenic acid, all-*cis*, conformational.

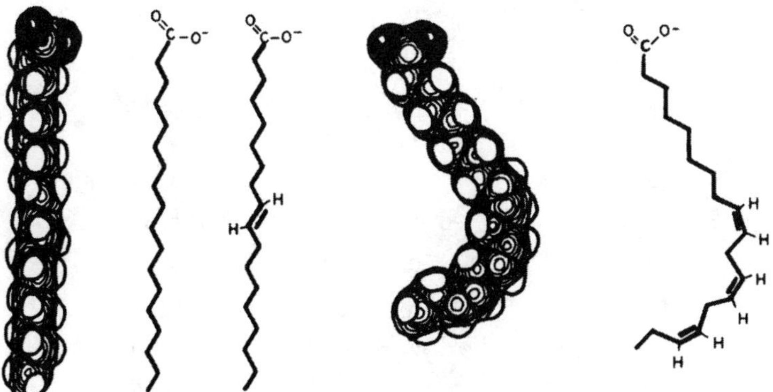

FIGURE 3.3
Hydrogenation of *cis* and *trans* double bonds.

CIS TRANS

FIGURE 3.4
Structure of common phospholipids.

Another group of phosphorus-containing lipids is formed from the 18-carbon amino alcohol sphingosine (Figure 3.5). Linked to a long-chain fatty acid, it forms ceramide and with the inclusion of sugar molecules it forms cerebrosides and gangliosides. Some of the glycosphingolipids have sialic (*N*-acetyl neurominic) acid linked to one or more of the sugar residues of a ceramide oligosaccharide. These compounds are functional in membranes, particularly in nervous tissue.

Sterols and Steroids

Steroids are hydrocarbons with a rigid ring structure and, having few sites with reactive groups, are quite hydrophobic (Figure 3.6). Plant sterols are called phytosterols and the major animal sterol is cholesterol. The structure

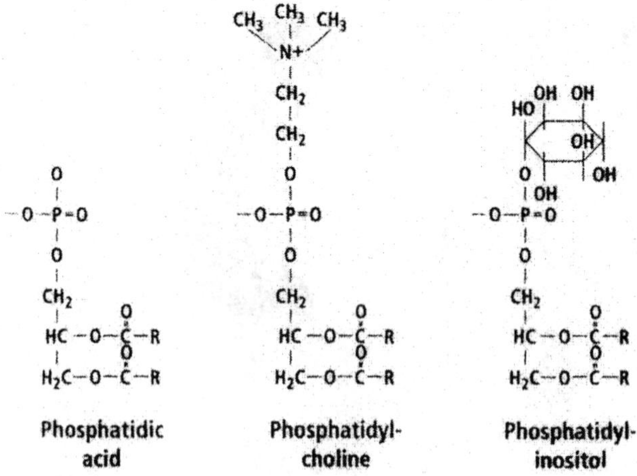

FIGURE 3.5
General structure of sphingolipids.

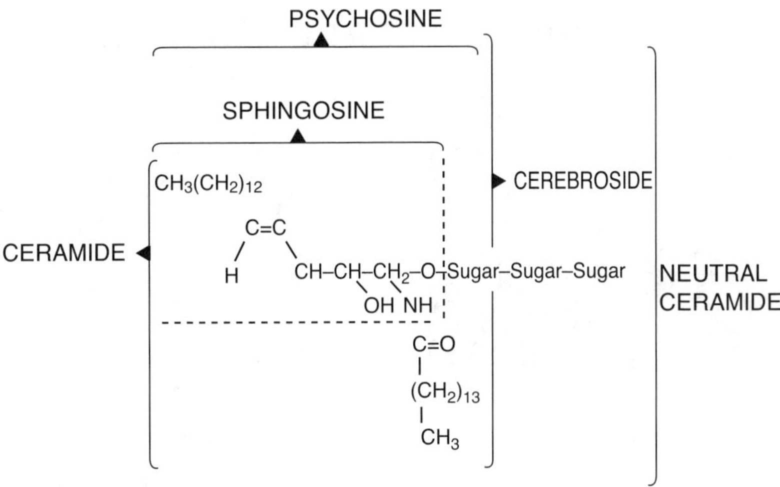

FIGURE 3.6
Space-filling and conventional models of cholesterol. (A) conventional; (B) space-filling.

accounts for its dielectric characteristic and its functions in nerve tissues and membranes. Steryl esters do not cross membranes, whereas free cholesterol crosses by passive diffusion. Cholesterol is converted to bile salts by hydroxylation and conjugation. It is the precursor to steroid-based hormone systems, sex hormones and adrenocorticoid hormones. As 7-dehydrocholesterol, cholesterol is the precursor to vitamin D, the only biological conversion of cholesterol that breaks the ring structure. Because it cannot be degraded, cholesterol must be excreted as free cholesterol or bile acids.

Lipid Digestion

The average American diet contains about 150 g of fat daily, mainly as triacylglycerols with cholesterol making up 300–600 mg. Digestive enzymes, being proteins, are water soluble and the dietary fat is hydrophobic. The beginning of digestion is the secretion of lingual lipase, which acts on mainly short-chain acylglycerols in the mouth and stomach. Partial emulsification occurs by muscular action and the presence of phospholipids, polysaccharides and peptides. The major digestive activity occurs in the duodenum and the ilium. There the presence of bile acids and pancreatic phospholipids effects further emulsification and formation of micelles (Figure 3.7). Bile salts adhere to the surface of lipid droplets and prevent access by lipase (Figure 3.8). Lipolysis occurs because procolipase is secreted with lipase and is activated to colipase by pancreatic trypsin; the colipase complexes with lipase and also binds to the lipid droplets, permitting lipase to come in

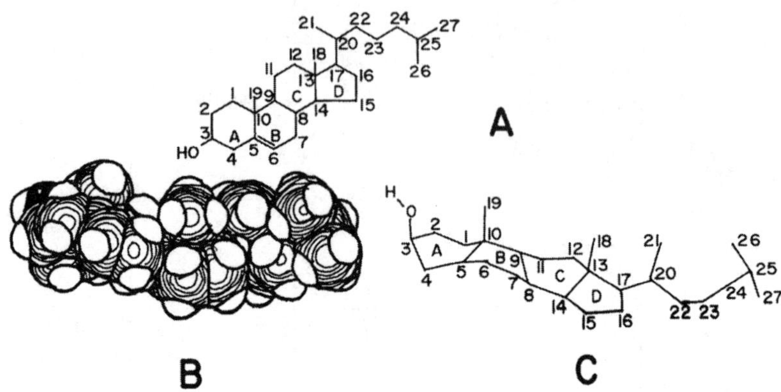

FIGURE 3.7
Orientation of fatty acids in micellar configuration.

contact with the triacylglycerols. Hydrolysis of fatty acids occurs, yielding free fatty acids and sn2-monoaclyglycerols. Bile micelles are formed when bile acids and phospholipids reach a critical micellar concentration. Water-soluble micellar aggregates engulf free fatty acids and monoacylglycerols and the micelles diffuse through the unstirred water layer. Passage through the unstirred water layer is the rate-limiting step in lipid absorption. The free fatty acids and monoacylglycerols diffuse freely through the mucosal membrane and are re-esterified into triacylglycerols that do not passively diffuse in the reverse direction.

Phospholipids are hydrolyzed by pancreatic phospholipase A2, cleaving the fatty acid at the sn2 position. The resulting lysophospholipid, along with the free fatty acids, diffuse into the mucosal cell where the remaining fatty acid is cleaved from the lysophospholipid. Inside the mucosal cell the phospholipid is reformed by acylation. Cholesterol from the diet is hydrolyzed and free cholesterol in micelles from biliary secretion is subjected to the same micellar transport through the unstirred water layer and into mucosal cells as fatty acids. Free cholesterol is re-esterified and the cholesteryl ester does not diffuse in the reverse direction.

Regulation of Cholesterol Synthesis

The metabolism of cholesterol contains a system of controls that are, of course, maintained by genetic coding. The metabolic systems are described

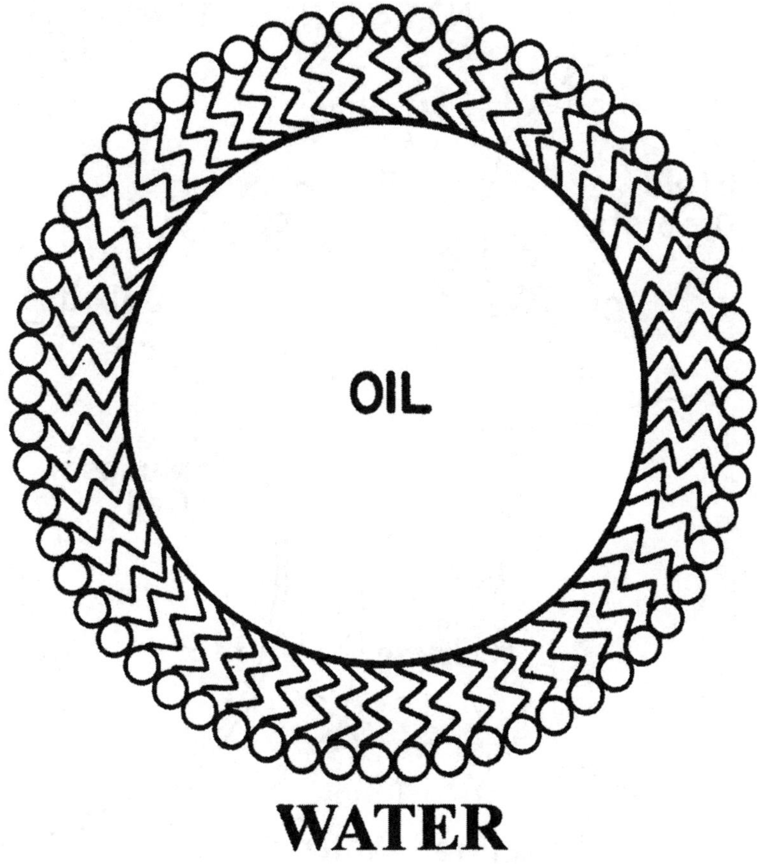

FIGURE 3.8
Processes of digestion and absorption of dietary fat. Hydrolyzed fatty acids and monoacylglycerides are made water soluble by incorporation into micelles and thereby cross the unstirred water layer, then diffuse into mucosal cells where they are re-esterified.

here and much research is underway to determine the genetic regulatory elements. Cholesterol synthesis occurs in the liver, although all mammalian cells examined have the capacity to synthesize cholesterol and extrahepatic tissues account for most synthesis in humans. The necessary precursor is acetyl coenzyme A (CoA). It is generated within the mitochondria and converted into citrate, which diffuses into the cytosol and is hydrolyzed by citrate lyase to yield acetyl-CoA and acetoacetate (Figure 3.9). Three molecules of acetyl CoA are converted to β-hydroxy-β-methyl glutaryl (HMG) CoA. The action of HMG CoA reductase produces mevalonic acid, and that enzymic step is the major site of regulation of cholesterol synthesis. Statin drugs are inhibitors of HMG CoA reductase. Mevalonate is phosphorylated

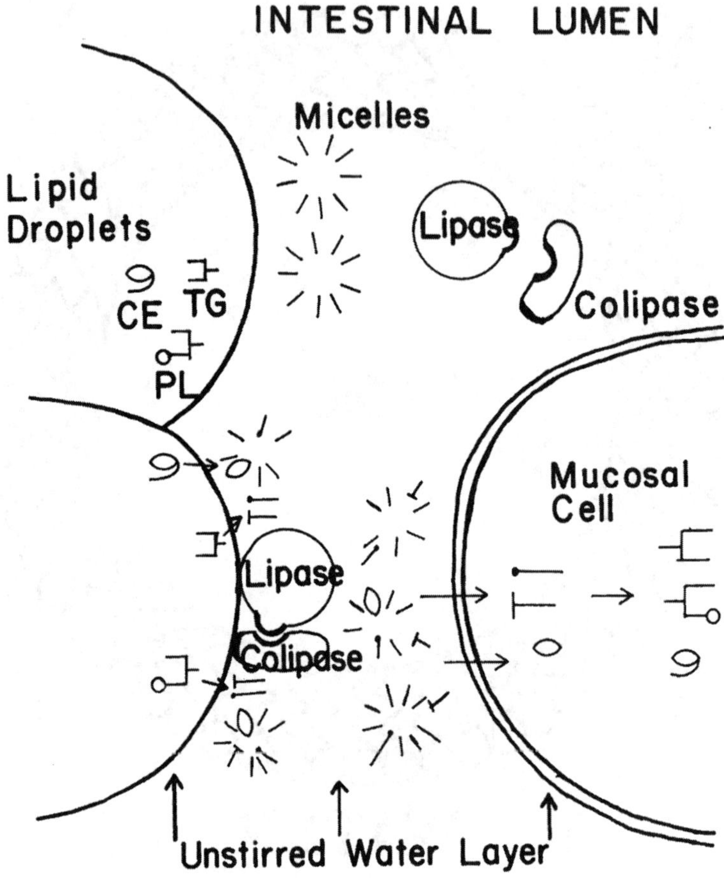

FIGURE 3.9
Synthesis of cholesterol. Three molecules of acetyl CoA form HMG CoA which is reduced to mevalonate by an irreversible step; three mevalonate molecules condense to form farnesyl pyrophosphate, and two of those condense to form squalene. Squalene is cyclized to form lanosterol. Many reactions remove three methyl groups and transfer the double bond from the 8–9 to the 5–6 position.

and three molecules are combined to produce farnesyl pyrophosphate and two molecules of it unite to produce the 30-carbon squalene. Squalene is oxidized and cyclized to form the steroid ring lanosterol in a reaction that is not reversible in mammalian systems. Loss of three methyl groups completes the formation of cholesterol, a total process involving more than 20 steps.

The other significant step in the regulation of cholesterol synthesis is the formation of bile acids (Figure 3.10). The irreversible synthetic enzyme of bile salts is 7α-hydroxylase. Bile acids are secreted via the gallbladder and

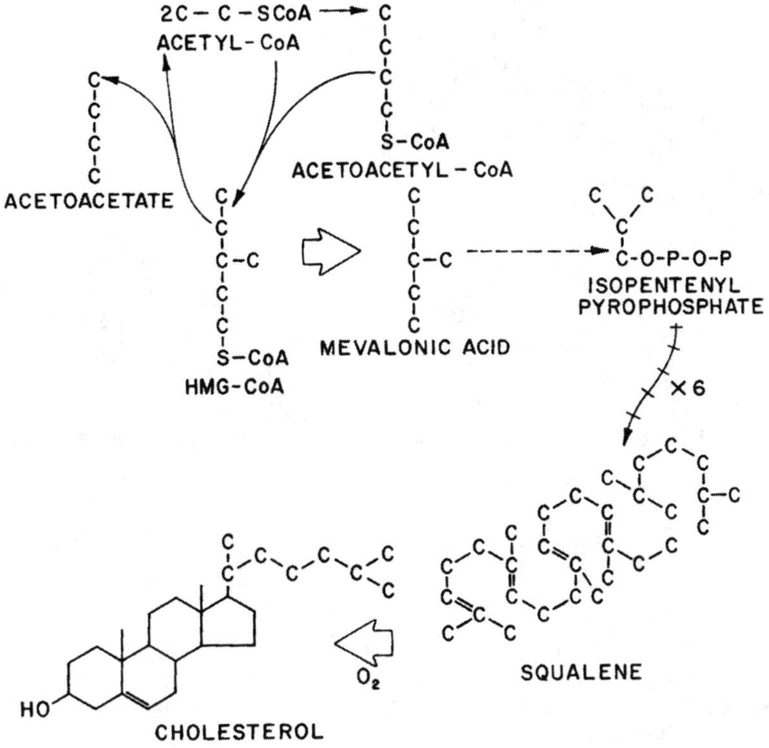

FIGURE 3.10
Structural formulas of cholesterol, cholanoic acids, and two commonly occurring primary bile acids.

bile duct into the intestine and a large portion is reabsorbed. This enterohepatic circulation is a factor in regulation of cholesterol synthesis by controlling the demand for bile acid formation for digestion. Cholesterol itself is also reabsorbed and the system of synthesis and absorption constitutes a continuous self-regulating cycle of cholesterol metabolism. Factors that impinge on one factor have cascading effects on the complete cycle to maintain a constant whole body cholesterol balance.

Essential Fatty Acids and Eicosanoids

Linoleic and α-linolenic (18:2 n-6 and 18:3 n-3) are called essential fatty acids. They cannot be synthesized by mammalian organisms because of the absence of enzymes that can introduce double bonds beyond the Δ^9 (9th carbon from

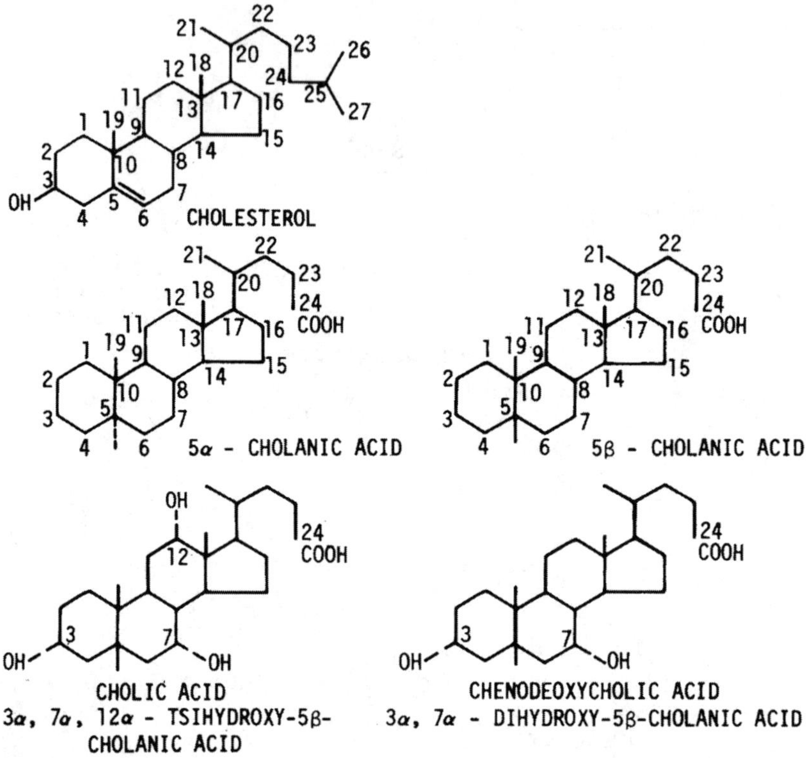

CHOLESTEROL

5α - CHOLANIC ACID

5β - CHOLANIC ACID

CHOLIC ACID
3α, 7α, 12α - TSIHYDROXY-5β-CHOLANIC ACID

CHENODEOXYCHOLIC ACID
3α, 7α - DIHYDROXY-5β-CHOLANIC ACID

FIGURE 3.11
Families of fatty acids formed from C18 precursors by desaturation (D) and elongation (E). The n-9 pathway is exhibited only in mammals deficient in dietary n-6 fatty acids.

the carboxyl) position. The n-minus 3 or 6 nomenclature is used instead of delta because it makes reference to the fatty acid families clearer (Figure 3.11). Linoleate is essential in skin integrity and other membrane functions. The elongation and desaturation of 18:2 n-6 to the 20 carbon fatty acid arachidonic acid (20:4 n-6) is the precursor for the family of autocoids known as eicosanoids (Figure 3.12). Oxygenation of the arachidonate by cyclooxygenase results in cyclization to form prostaglandins and thromboxanes. Action of lipoxygenase in linear reactions produces leukotrienes. These compounds are formed in extremely small amounts and have potent metabolic functions.

They participate in physiological reactions regulating blood pressure, diuresis, blood platelet aggregation, the immune system, gastric secretions, reproduction, smooth muscle contractions and others. Excess production is associated with adverse reactions such as inflammation. Their study is a major activity in lipid metabolism research.

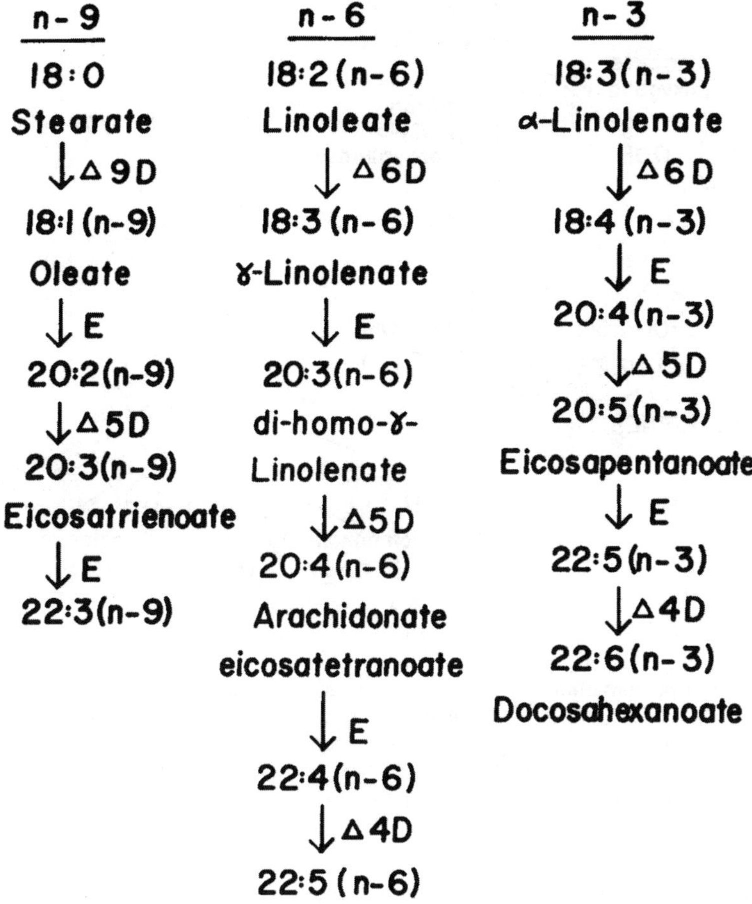

FIGURE 3.12
Eicosanoid synthesis from arachidonate (C20:4n-6). HETE (hydroxyeicosatetranoic acid), PETE (peroxyeicosatetranoic acid), PG (prostaglandin), GSH (glutathione), and MDA (malondialdehyde).

Lipid Peroxidation

The presence of methyl-interrupted double bonds creates a methyl group in the polyunsaturated fatty acid chain that is vulnerable to oxidation. Removal of a hydrogen results in formation of a free radical that is very reactive and starts a chain reaction that propagates in a cascade (Figure

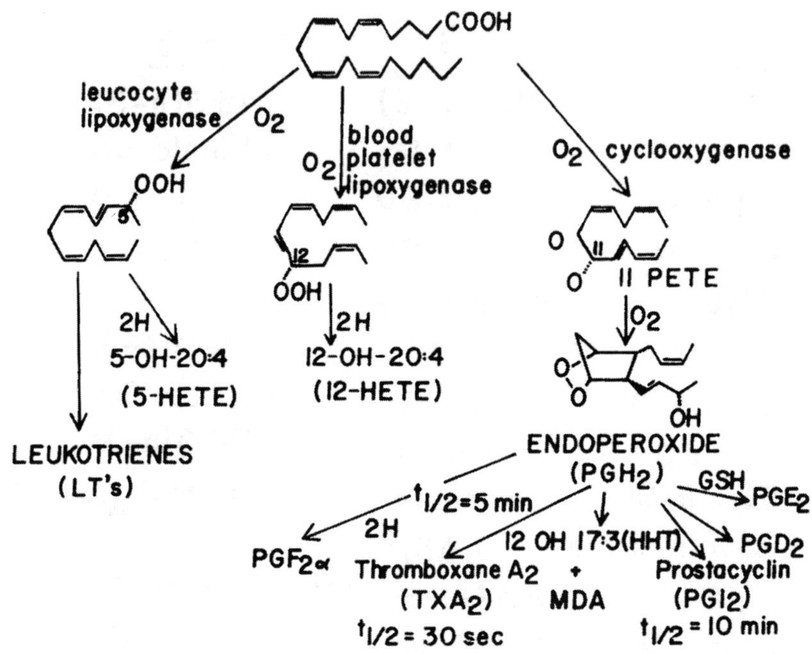

FIGURE 3.13
Peroxidation of polyunsaturated fatty acids. Autoxidation results when a hydrogen atom is removed by an oxidizing agent from a methylene group between two double bonds leaving a resonating free radical that can be reduced by an antioxidant such as tocopherol. The free radical can propagate additional free radicals or be oxidized by molecular oxygen to a peroxide that can degrade to many smaller compounds or polymerize.

3.13 and Figure 3.14). This process is called peroxidation and it is controlled *in vivo* by antioxidants. The products of the oxidation can react with proteins and DNA, causing deleterious changes. Oxidation is obviously necessary for such reactions as formation of eicosanoids, but if there is not sufficient antioxidant capacity at the cellular level metabolic damage is done. Tocopherols are major cellular antioxidants. and many newly described plant components are being investigated as contributors to control of peroxidation.

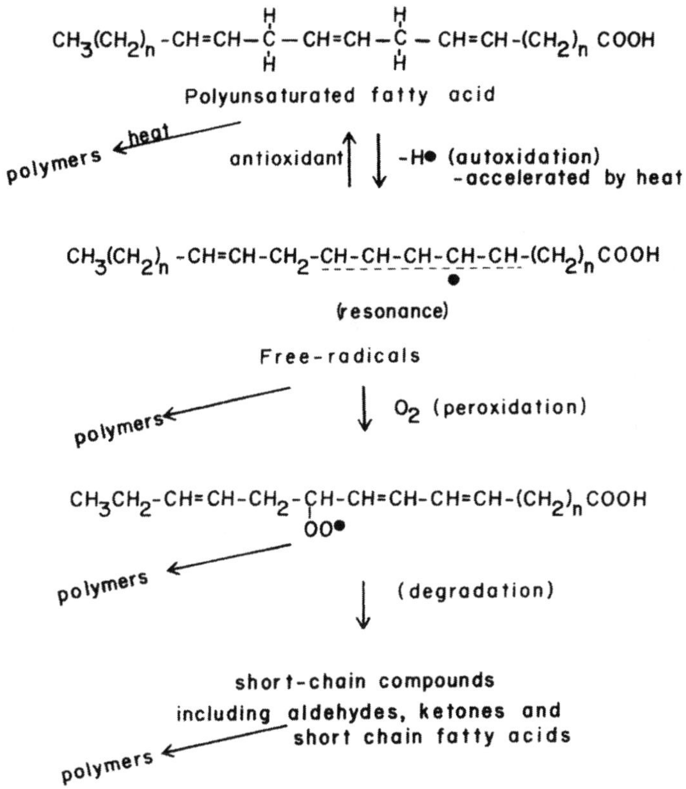

$CH_3(CH_2)_n$-CH=CH-CH_2-CH=CH-CH_2-CH=CH-$(CH_2)_n$COOH

Polyunsaturated fatty acid

polymers ← heat

antioxidant ↑ ↓ -H• (autoxidation) -accelerated by heat

$CH_3(CH_2)_n$-CH=CH-CH_2-CH-CH-CH-CH-CH-$(CH_2)_n$COOH

(resonance)

Free-radicals

polymers ←

↓ O_2 (peroxidation)

CH_3CH_2-CH=CH-CH_2-CH(OO•)-CH=CH-CH=CH-$(CH_2)_n$COOH

polymers ←

↓ (degradation)

short-chain compounds including aldehydes, ketones and short chain fatty acids

polymers ←

FIGURE 3.14
Peroxidation of polyunsaturated fatty acids.

References

1. Dupont, J. Lipids, in *Present Knowledge in Nutrition,* Brown, M.L., Ed. International Life Sciences, Washington, DC, 1990, chap.7.
2. Dupont, J. Saturated and hydrogenated fats in food in relation to health, *J. Am. Coll. Nutr.,* 10:577–592, 1991.
3. Jones, P.J.H. and Papamandjaris, A. Lipids: Cellular metabolism, in *Present Knowledge in Nutrition*, Bowman, B.A. and Russell, R.M., Eds. International Life Sciences, Washington, DC, 2001, chap. 10.
4. Lichtenstein, A.H. and Jones, P.J.H. Lipids: Absorption and transport, in *Present Knowledge in Nutrition*, Bowman, B.A. and Russell, R.M., Eds. International Life Sciences, Washington, DC, 2001, chap. 9.
5. Gropper, S.S., Smith, J.L. and Groff, J.L. *Advanced Nutrition and Human Metabolism,* 4th ed. Thomson Wadsworth, Belmont, CA, 2005, chap. 6.
6. Gurr, M.I., Harwood, J.L. and Frayn, K.N. *Lipid Biochemistry, An Introduction,* 5th ed. Blackwell Science, Iowa State Press, Ames, IA, 2002.

4

Lipid and Lipoprotein Metabolism

Paul G. Davis and Jason D. Wagganer

CONTENTS

Introduction 47
Lipoprotein Classification 50
Lipid Transport 51
    Lipid Transport: Exogenous Pathway 51
    Lipid Transport: Endogenous Pathway 53
Reverse Cholesterol Transport 54
    Formation of HDL 54
    Reverse Cholesterol Transport: Direct Pathway 56
    Reverse Cholesterol Transport: Indirect Pathway 57
    Other Anti-Atherogenic Roles of HDL 58
References 58

Introduction

Due to their hydrophobic nature (insoluble in water), cholesterol and triglyceride (or triacylglycerol), the major lipids in the blood, must be transported within lipoproteins. Lipoproteins constitute a packaging of electrically neutral lipid (triglyceride and esterified cholesterol) within a monolayer shell consisting of mostly phospholipids and also of proteins (apolipoproteins) and a small amount of unesterified or "free" cholesterol. The components of this outer shell are amphipathic (charged on one end and neutral on the other). With their neutral ends facing the hydrophobic core and the charged ends facing outward, the outer shell components make the lipoprotein particles water soluble, allowing them to be transported through the circulatory system.

Lipoproteins are classified by *density* (high-density, low-density, etc.). The density is dictated by both the lipid content (i.e., the amount of cholesterol and triglyceride) and the ratio of the amounts of lipid and protein in the lipoprotein. For example, high-density lipoprotein (HDL) contains approximately equal amounts of lipid and protein, while lipoproteins of lower density contain much larger amounts of lipid than protein, making them larger and more buoyant. Lipoproteins are most commonly classified based on their density gradients following ultracentrifugation. Characteristics of the lipoproteins and their major subfractions isolated through this method are listed in Table 4.1. Other common methods of lipoprotein classification include (1) *non-denaturing polyacrylamide gradient gel electrophoresis*, in which lipoproteins of different sizes migrate different distances across the gel; (2) *agarose gel electrophoresis*, in which lipoproteins migrate different distances based upon their different surface charges; and (3) *nuclear magnetic resonance (NMR) spectroscopy*, in which "signals" emitted from the terminal methyl groups of the lipids within the lipoproteins are read and lipoproteins are classified based upon this lipid content.

Although lipoproteins are generally classified by density, it is primarily the *apolipoprotein* content of a lipoprotein that determines both its function, as well as types and quantities of its lipid content. In addition to serving as important structural components of the different lipoproteins, different apolipoproteins also serve as ligands for specific receptors and as cofactors for specific enzymes. Conversely, change in the lipid content (and size) of a given lipoprotein particle can alter the tertiary structure of an apolipoprotein, resulting in either an increased or decreased affinity for a particular receptor or enzyme. Therefore, both the lipid and the apolipoprotein contents are key factors in determining a lipoprotein's "behavior." The major plasma apolipoproteins are described in Table 4.2 and will be discussed below. All, with the exception of the B class, are "exchangeable," meaning that they may leave one lipoprotein particle and be incorporated into particle of another.[1]

The remainder of this chapter begins with a brief description of the composition of the different lipoproteins and will then discuss the coordinated role of these lipoproteins in transport of lipid to tissues throughout the body (including atherosclerotic plaque) and the process of *reverse cholesterol transport*, in which lipid is harvested from atheroma and catabolized. This chapter discusses atherosclerosis only to the extent that lipid transport is involved. More detailed mechanisms of atherosclerosis, as well as the effects of various interventions on lipoprotein metabolism, are detailed in other chapters of this text.

TABLE 4.1

Characteristics of Major Lipoproteins

Lipoprotein Class	Density (g/ml)	Electrophoretic Mobility	Diameter (nm)	Approximate NMR Classification	% Composition				
					TG	CE	FC	PL	apo
Chylomicron	<0.94	Origin	75–1200	–	86	3	2	7	2
VLDL	0.94–1.006	Pre-beta	30–80	V6-V1	55	12	7	18	8
IDL	1.006–1.019	Slow pre-beta	25–35	IDL	23	29	9	19	19
LDL	1.019–1.063	Beta	18–25	L3-L1	6	42	8	22	22
HDL_2	1.063–1.125	Alpha	9–12	H5-H3	5	17	5	33	40
HDL_3	1.125–1.21	Alpha	5–9	H2-H1	3	13	4	35	55

VLDL, very low-density lipoprotein; IDL, intermediate-density lipoprotein; LDL, low-density lipoprotein; HDL, high-density lipoprotein; TG, triglyceride; CE, cholesteryl ester; FC, free cholesterol; PL, phospholipids; apo, apolipoprotein.

Source: Adapted from Burnett, J.R., Barrett, P.H.R., *Crit. Rev. Clin. Lab. Sci.*, 39, 89, 2002. With permission.

TABLE 4.2

Major Apolipoproteins

Apolipoprotein	Major Sites of Synthesis	Associated Lipoproteins	Major Functions
A-I	Liver, intestine	Chylomicron, HDL	Accepts cholesterol from peripheral cells through ABCA1; cofactor for LCAT; facilitates lipid uptake through SR-BI
A-II	Liver	HDL	Facilitates lipid uptake through SR-BI; displaces apo A-I from HDL
B-48	Intestine	Chylomicron	Structural component
B-100	Liver	VLDL, IDL, LDL	Facilitates lipid uptake through LDL receptor
C-I	Liver, lung, skin, testes, spleen	Chylomicron, VLDL, HDL	Inhibits HL activity; activates LPL activity; inhibits apo E-mediated lipid uptake by LDL receptor and LRP
C-II	Liver, intestine	Chylomicron, VLDL, HDL	Cofactor for LPL
C-III	Liver, intestine	Chylomicron, VLDL, HDL	Inhibits LPL and HL activity; may stimulate CETP activity
E	Liver, brain, skin, testes, spleen	Chylomicron, VLDL, HDL	Facilitates lipid uptake through LDL receptor and LRP
(a)	Liver	Lp(a)	Most likely inhibits fibrinolysis through competing with plasminogen for binding with fibrin

HDL, high-density lipoprotein; VLDL, very low-density lipoprotein; IDL, intermediate-density lipoprotein; LDL, low-density lipoprotein; ABCA1, adenosine triphosphate-binding cassette-A1; LCAT, lecithin:cholesteryl acyltransferase; SR-BI, scavenger receptor BI; HL, hepatic lipase; LPL, lipoprotein lipase; LRP, LDL receptor-related protein; CETP, cholesteryl ester transfer protein.

Lipoprotein Classification

The major lipoproteins are chylomicrons, very low-density lipoprotein (VLDL), intermediate-density lipoprotein (IDL), low-density lipoprotein (LDL), and high-density lipoprotein (HDL) (Table 4.1). In short, chylomicrons and VLDL are the major carriers of triglyceride and are synthesized and released by the intestine (chylomicrons) and liver (VLDL). Chylomicrons and VLDL contain approximately 85% and 55% triglyceride, respectively, with smaller amounts of cholesterol, protein, and phospholipids. As explained below, the primary apolipoproteins are apolipoprotein (apo) B-48 for chylomicrons and apo B-100 for VLDL. Apo C-II and apo C-III also have important regulatory roles. NMR spectroscopy divides VLDL into six subclasses (V1–V6), with V6 being the largest and most triglyceride-laden. With the exception of those with exceptionally high triglyceride concentrations, chylomicrons are present in only trace amounts in fasted plasma or serum samples.

After a brief transition through IDL, which has a relatively small concentration in plasma/serum, VLDL may be converted to LDL. LDL is the most cholesterol-rich of the lipoproteins, containing approximately 50% cholesterol and 4% triglyceride, although these proportions vary with different-sized LDL particles. All VLDL, IDL, and LDL particles, regardless of size, contain exactly one apo B-100. Apo E also resides on both VLDL, IDL, and LDL, as well as HDL. NMR spectroscopy divides LDL into three subclasses (L1–L3), with L1 being the smallest, densest, and containing the most triglyceride and least esterified cholesterol. LDL subfractions (as many as six) can also be derived by polyacrylamide gradient gel electrophoresis.

HDL contains the largest amount of protein (~50%) and smallest amount of lipid of all the lipoproteins. The vast majority of lipid contained in HDL is cholesterol ester. Ultracentrifugation preparations typically divide HDL into two main subfractions, HDL_2 and HDL_3, with HDL_3 being the more dense of the two (a less dense "HDL_1" has been described, but is not commonly found in discernable amounts). All HDL particles contain at least one apo A-I, and most HDL_3 particles also contain apo A-II. It is important to note that, since lipoprotein fractions and subfractions are classified by density, they exist on a continuum, meaning that a certain amount of heterogeneity exists (e.g., apolipoprotein content) within each classification. NMR spectroscopy divides HDL into five subclasses (H1–H5), with H1 and H2 corresponding roughly to HDL_3 and H3–H5 approximating the HDL_2 subfraction.[2]

Lipid Transport

Lipid transport to tissues via the lipoproteins is summarized in Figure 4.1. Separate pathways exist for the transport of exogenous (dietary) and endogenous (hepatic) lipids. The two pathways are similar, in that large lipid-laden lipoproteins secreted from the intestine or liver are "trimmed" into smaller lipoproteins or remnants, which provide lipid to the liver or other tissues through receptor-mediated mechanisms.

Lipid Transport: Exogenous Pathway

In the exogenous pathway, apo B-48 is synthesized by intestinal cells and, incorporated with mostly triglyceride, enters the lymphatic system and eventually the circulatory system in the form of chylomicrons. Although they play a more minor role in the structure and metabolism of chylomicrons,

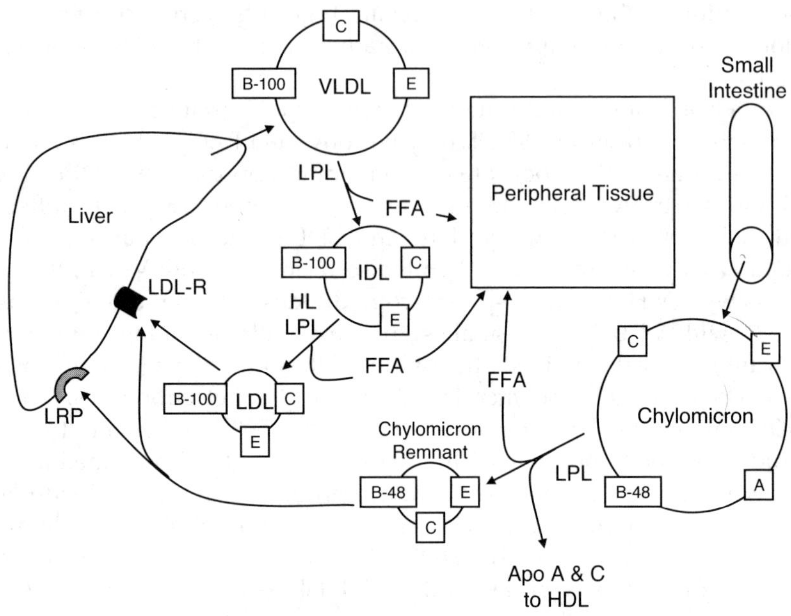

FIGURE 4.1
Lipid transport. Dietary lipid is secreted from the small intestine in chylomicrons. The triglycerides of chylomicrons are hydrolyzed by lipoprotein lipase (LPL). Free fatty acids (FFA) are then taken up by numerous body tissues while chylomicron remnants are catabolized primarily by the liver through both the low-density lipoprotein (LDL) receptor (LDL-R) and the LDL receptor-related protein (LRP) through recognition of apolipoprotein (apo) E. *De novo* synthesized lipid is released from the liver primarily through very low-density lipoprotein (VLDL). LPL hydrolyzes the triglyceride of VLDL, reducing the lipoprotein to an intermediate-density lipoprotein (IDL), which is subsequently hydrolyzed by LPL and hepatic lipase (HL) into LDL. Hepatic catabolism of LDL occurs mainly through apo B-100 recognition by the LDL receptor.

apo A-I and A-IV are also included in these lipoproteins when released from the intestine, while apo C-I, C-II, C-III, and E are incorporated into the lipoprotein within the circulation as a result of transfer from HDL.[3] The incorporation of apo C-II into the chylomicron particle is essential for the catabolism of triglyceride, as this apolipoprotein is a cofactor for the enzyme *lipoprotein lipase* (LPL). LPL, which is attached to the luminal surface of capillary endothelial cells via heparin sulfate-proteoglycans, hydrolyzes the fatty acids of triglyceride at the first and third positions, allowing them to be taken up by adjacent tissue (usually muscle or adipose tissue) or to be bound and transported within circulation to other tissues, including the liver, by albumin.[4] *Hepatic lipase* (HL; also termed *hepatic triglyceride lipase*) also performs this function, although its activity does not depend upon an apolipoprotein co-activator, as does LPL's.[5] Left over are "remnants" consisting of cholesterol, phospholipids, apolipoproteins, and much less triglyceride. Most of the apo A and a portion of the apo C are transferred to HDL and the remaining remnants are available for catabolism by the liver. This can occur through an *LDL receptor* or through an *LDL receptor-related protein* (LRP), both of which endocytose the remnants into lysosomes, where hydrolysis of the remaining lipoprotein components takes place.[3] Apo E serves as the ligand for both of these receptors. Three major alleles for apo E exist, with ε3 being the most common. Protein expressed by the ε2 allele does not bind the LDL receptor and results in increased plasma VLDL-cholesterol concentration. Conversely, ε4 produces a protein with abnormally strong binding to the LDL receptor. The prolonged binding inhibits other apo E-containing from binding the receptor, resulting in increased LDL-cholesterol concentration.[6] In addition, apo C-I inhibits apo E-mediated lipid uptake by both the LDL receptor and LRP.[7] Apo B-48 is not recognized by the hepatic receptors. However, an apo B-48-specific receptor has been found to be expressed by macrophages, indicating a possible mechanism for hypertriglyceridemia-induced atherosclerosis.[8] Nearly all chylomicrons are absent from circulation within 12 h following a fatty meal.[9]

Lipid Transport: Endogenous Pathway

Transport of cholesterol and triglyceride synthesized by the liver (endogenous pathway) takes place through release of VLDL, which contain apo B-100 (a "longer" version of apo B-48) and apo C-I, C-II, C-III, and E. As with chylomicrons, apo C-II serves as a cofactor for LPL, which hydrolyzes much of the triglyceride within VLDL. This hydrolysis results in a less buoyant IDL particle. Further hydrolysis by both LPL and *hepatic lipase* (HL) results in the loss of most of the triglyceride, as well as apo E, leaving an even less buoyant LDL particle, which contains esterified cholesterol as its major lipid component and apo B-100 as its primary apolipoprotein. Apo B-100 is recognized by the LDL receptor on the liver and other tissues, which internalizes the lipoprotein, making the cholesterol available for cell membrane structure and steroid hormone synthesis. Regarding both chylomicron and VLDL metabolism, just as apo C-II is a cofactor for LPL, apo C-III *inhibits* LPL and HL activity.[7] Therefore, the ratio of apo C-II to apo C-III is important in regulating plasma concentrations of triglyceride, as well as VLDL and LDL.

When an insufficient number of LDL receptors are synthesized or the receptors do not possess proper affinity for apo B (genetic abnormalities resulting in *familial hypercholesterolemia*), or when dietary fat intake is high (which causes down-regulation of LDL receptor synthesis), plasma cholesterol concentration is abnormally high. This excess cholesterol contained in apo B-containing lipoproteins, particularly LDL, can be internalized in macrophages and foam cells in the vascular intima through scavenger receptors (CD36, SR-A), which do not require specific apolipoprotein ligands. These scavenger receptors have a much higher affinity for LDL in the oxidized form. Oxidized LDL also contributes to vascular inflammation and inhibits nitric oxide, a potent vasodilator.[10]

In addition to the above, *lipoprotein (a)* [Lp(a)] transports cholesterol, is often present in atherosclerotic plaque, and may be particularly atherogenic. Lp(a) is a variant of LDL and is characterized by the covalent attachment of the glycoprotein *apo(a)* to apo B-100. Due to one or more proposed mechanisms, apo(a) is most likely responsible for Lp(a)'s atherogenic effect. Apo(a) consists of repeated coils of protein called "kringles" with amino acid sequencing very similar to that of plasminogen. Because of this homology, Lp(a) may inhibit fibrinolysis through interference at the binding site of fibrin.[11] Second, Lp(a) may accelerate wound healing by transporting lipid to the vascular intima to combine with extracellular matrix components.[12] As such, Lp(a) may act as a "repairer" of endothelial injury. Third, the LDL receptor does not appear to play a major role in clearance of Lp(a) from plasma.[13] This may result in the cholesterol of Lp(a) being more available for uptake by scavenger receptors. In addition, the LDL component of Lp(a) is the smaller, denser phenotype associated with higher cardiovascular disease risk (see *Reverse Cholesterol Transport* section). Finally, apo(a) may contribute to atherogenesis by increasing monocyte chemotactic activity in the vasculature,[14] possibly through up-regulation of intracellular adhesion molecule-1 (ICAM-1).[15] Lp(a)'s relationship with cardiovascular disease varies across races. For example, blacks commonly have higher plasma Lp(a) concentrations than whites, yet Lp(a) concentrations are not typically related to cardiovascular disease risk in blacks.[16] The number of kringle repeats present in Lp(a) is highly variable and may explain differences in the relation of Lp(a) to cardiovascular disease among races.[17]

Reverse Cholesterol Transport

While excess cholesterol carried by LDL and VLDL is associated with atherosclerosis due to its uptake by scavenger receptors in vascular lesions, HDL may *protect* against atherosclerosis through a process termed *reverse cholesterol transport*, whereby HDL harvests cholesterol from arterial plaque (and other body tissues, as well) and transports it to the liver where it may be catabolized and secreted as bile. As simple as this concept appears, successful reverse cholesterol transport relies upon the availability and activity of a collection of apolipoproteins, enzymes, transfer proteins, and receptors. The process of reverse cholesterol transport is summarized in Figure 4.2.

Formation of HDL

The formation of HDL is dependent upon release of apo A-I from the liver and intestines and upon formation of remnants containing apo A-I following

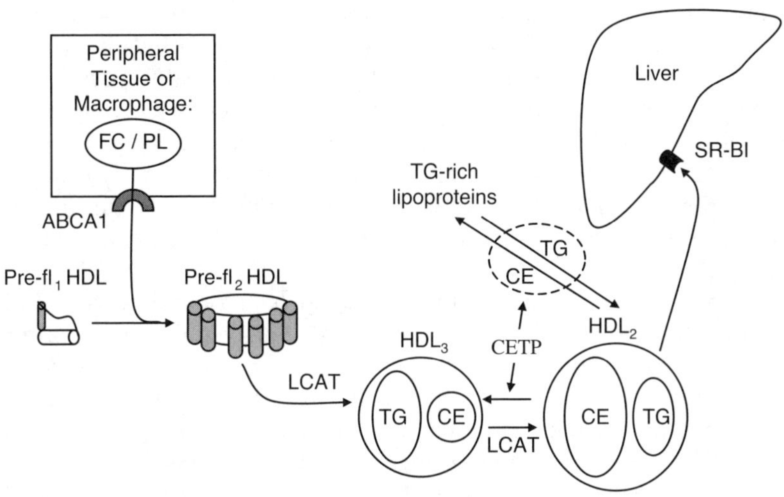

FIGURE 4.2
Reverse cholesterol transport. Lipid-poor pre-beta$_1$ high-density lipoprotein (pre-β_1 HDL), composed primarily of apolipoprotein (apo) A-I, sequesters free cholesterol (FC) and phospholipid (PL) from peripheral tissues and arterial macrophages via the adenosine triphosphate-binding cassette-A1 (ABCA1) transporter. Incorporation of the FC and PL allows HDL to assume a more discoidal shape (pre-β_2 HDL). HDL associated apo A-I and apo C-I permit lecithin:cholesteryl ester transferase (LCAT) and facilitate esterification and internalization of cholesterol, allowing HDL to become more spherical (HDL$_3$). Further esterification of cholesterol by LCAT transforms HDL$_3$ into the less dense HDL$_2$. Cholesteryl ester transfer protein (CETP) facilitates transfer of CE from HDL to triglyceride (TG)-rich lipoproteins in exchange for TG. Adding and removing CE to/from HDL, LCAT and CETP, respectively, cause HDL particles to be in constant flux between HDL$_2$ and HDL$_3$. Hepatic catabolism of HDL occurs mainly through apo A-I and apo A-II recognition by the scavenger receptor B-I (SR-BI).

chylomicron, VLDL, and HDL catabolism. While most analytical techniques quantify HDL primarily in its spherical forms (e.g., HDL$_2$, HDL$_3$), formation of HDL begins with an immature, non-spherical particle that migrates to form a small pre-beta band via agarose gel electrophoresis (as opposed to the alpha band formed by the larger HDL species). The *pre-beta$_1$ HDL* particle, which is often formed in lymph and delivered to circulation, is a loosely formed apo A-I bound to small amounts of phospholipid and cholesterol. The apo A-I may be newly synthesized or may be derived from previous catabolism of chylomicrons, VLDL, or HDL. The lipid-poor pre-beta$_1$ HDL crosses the vascular endothelium and enters both interstitial spaces and the vascular intima where it can interact with various peripheral cells and arterial plaque components, respectively. With the help of the *adenosine triphosphate-binding cassette-A1* (ABCA1) transporter present in various cells, including arterial macrophages, pre-beta$_1$ HDL then begins to accumulate phospholipid and cholesterol from these cells. Through mechanisms not fully understood, ABCA1 transports phospholipid and cholesterol from intercellular depots to extracellular apolipoproteins, allowing phospholipid and cholesterol to become incorporated into the HDL particle. The major

HDL apolipoproteins (A-I, A-II, A-IV, C, and E), all of which contain amphipathic alpha helices, can participate in cholesterol and phospholipid efflux through ABCA1.[18] However, apo A-I of the immature HDL particle, which can freely traverse the endothelium, is the major acceptor of cholesterol and phospholipid from peripheral tissues and arterial macrophages. Tangier Disease patients, who do not synthesize ABCA1, have abnormally low plasma concentrations of HDL-cholesterol and are at high risk for cardiovascular disease. ABCA1's role in cellular cholesterol removal has been reviewed in detail by Oram.[19]

As the pre-beta$_1$ HDL incorporates more cholesterol and phospholipid, it transforms into *pre-beta$_2$ HDL*, which has a more discoidal shape. In pre-beta$_2$ HDL, apo A-I takes on a more "formal" shape and, along with the phospholipids, "wraps around" the outer edge of the lipoprotein while the cholesterol is incorporated into the inner "core." This alteration of apo A-I's tertiary structure allows it to become a stronger cofactor for the enzyme *lecithin:cholesterol acyltransferase* (LCAT). Apo C-I, to a lesser extent, also stimulates LCAT activity.[7] LCAT facilitates transfer of a fatty acid from a phospholipid to free cholesterol, resulting in esterified cholesterol (cholesteryl ester). Since cholesteryl ester is particularly hydrophobic, the LCAT reaction results in further "packaging" of cholesterol within HDL and the previously discoidal pre-beta$_2$ HDL particle takes on a more spherical shape. This *HDL$_3$* particle (along with *HDL$_2$*) is one of the two main HDL species typically analyzed in human plasma.

The end result of reverse cholesterol transport is the delivery of cholesteryl ester and other lipoprotein components to the liver. As described below, this is accomplished both through direct and indirect pathways.

Reverse Cholesterol Transport: Direct Pathway

In the *direct* pathway, LCAT continues to facilitate loading of cholesteryl ester into the HDL$_3$ particle, converting it to the less dense HDL$_2$. Phospholipase transfer protein (PLTP) also participates in conversion of HDL$_3$ to HDL$_2$ by displacing apo A-I and phospholipid from HDL$_3$ to form pre-beta particles. Although PLTP's role in HDL$_3$ to HDL$_2$ conversion has not been fully elucidated, loss of some of the apo A-I may result in "unstable" particles. It has been hypothesized that these unstable particles may combine to form the less dense HDL$_2$.[20] Alternatively, these unstable particles may combine with pre-beta *apo A-II*-containing particles.[21]

HDL delivers cholesterol into cells mainly through the *scavenger receptor class B type I* (SR-BI). SR-BI participates in *selective uptake* of cholesterol, meaning that it binds HDL and takes in the cholesterol without degrading the lipoprotein.[22] This receptor can bind most of the various lipoproteins, but has particularly high affinity for both apo A-I and A-II, although conflicting reports exist as to which of these two apolipoproteins has the highest binding affinity and which facilitates the most cholesterol uptake.[23,24] Since

SR-BI operates on a concentration gradient, the larger, less dense HDL particles are able to deliver more cholesterol to the cells. In addition to hepatic cells, SR-BI is also expressed in steroid-producing cells and in sub-endothelial macrophages. Since SR-BI can facilitate cholesteryl ester transport both into and out of cells, depending upon the concentration gradient, cholesterol efflux out of macrophages and foam cells may be an additional mechanism that SR-BI can contribute to reverse cholesterol transport and protect against atherosclerosis.[25]

Reverse Cholesterol Transport: Indirect Pathway

The *indirect* pathway of reverse cholesterol transport involves the transfer of cholesteryl ester to the apo B-containing lipoproteins, which then deliver the cholesterol to the liver as described in the previous section. *Cholesteryl ester transfer protein* (CETP), which has a particularly high affinity for HDL, transfers cholesteryl ester from one lipoprotein to another in exchange for triglyceride. Since the lipids are transported by CETP on a concentration gradient, the most common action of this protein is to transfer cholesteryl ester from HDL to VLDL and LDL in exchange for triglyceride. By exchanging cholesteryl ester for triglyceride, a given HDL particle will become more dense. A portion of the triglyceride added to HDL through CETP is hydrolyzed by hepatic lipase. Through the opposite actions of LCAT and CETP (i.e., adding and removing cholesteryl ester to or from HDL), it is possible for HDL to shift back and forth between density ranges (e.g., from HDL_3 to HDL_2 and vice versa).

Barter et al. have reviewed the metabolism of CETP and its potential roles in atherosclerosis in detail.[26] Briefly, in plasma with normal lipid concentrations, much of the cholesteryl ester from HDL is transferred to LDL. However, in hypertriglyceridemic conditions, which result in greater VLDL concentrations, more lipid exchange takes place between HDL and VLDL, leaving smaller HDL particles which do not transport as much cholesterol to the liver for catabolism.[27] In addition, more exchange takes place between VLDL and LDL (cholesteryl ester to VLDL; triglyceride to LDL), leaving less cholesterol to be taken up through apo B-100 recognition.

The above scenario results in a smaller, denser LDL particle that may be more atherogenic. A plasma profile consisting of more small dense LDL (*pattern B*) than large buoyant LDL (*pattern A*) is a byproduct of the atherogenic combination of high triglyceride and low HDL-cholesterol concentrations. In fact, although persons having a pattern B profile are more prone to cardiovascular disease, this relationship has been shown to disappear when controlling statistically for triglyceride concentration.[28] However, other longitudinal research has shown the pattern B profile to be independently related to cardiovascular disease incidence.[29] Potential mechanisms by which small dense LDL may contribute to cardiovascular disease include (1) increased ability to cross the vascular endothelium and enter the intima,

(2) increased ability to be oxidized, and (3) lower affinity for the LDL receptor due to altered conformation of apo B-100.[30]

Other Anti-Atherogenic Roles of HDL

Although reverse cholesterol transport is HDL's most recognized and possibly most dominant role, this lipoprotein likely participates in the prevention of atherosclerosis through other mechanisms as well. Protective mechanisms of HDL independent of reverse cholesterol transport have been reviewed by Barter et al.[31] HDL-associated paraoxonase (a detoxifying enzyme) can inhibit oxidation of LDL[32] and various cell membranes, including those of erythrocytes.[33] HDL can also inhibit expression of vascular and intercellular adhesion molecules for monocytes.[34] In addition, HDL increases prostacyclin synthesis[35,36] and apo A-I stabilizes its existence in plasma.[37,38] Prostacyclin may protect against CAD through vasodilation, inhibition of platelet aggregation, and inhibition of endothelin-1 synthesis.[39] (Endothelin-1 is a potent vasoconstrictor and smooth muscle mitogen.) Furthermore, in patients with early development of atherosclerosis, Zeiher et al. demonstrated less acetylcholine-induced vasoconstriction in patients with the highest HDL-cholesterol concentrations.[40]

In conclusion, lipoproteins represent a complicated, multi dimensional pathway of lipid transport to and away from various body tissues. The metabolism of lipoproteins and their effect in contributing to or protecting against atherosclerosis are highly dependent upon genetic and behavioral factors that alter the availability and activity of lipids, various apolipoproteins, enzymes, and transfer proteins.

References

1. Bolanos-Garcia, V.M., Miguel, R.N., On the structure and function of apolipoproteins: more than a family of lipid-binding proteins, *Prog. Biophys. Mol. Biol.*, 83, 47, 2003.
2. Kwiterovich, P.O., Jr., The metabolic pathways of high-density lipoprotein, low-density lipoprotein, and triglycerides: a current review, *Am. J. Cardiol.*, 86, 5L, 2000.
3. Burnett, J.R., Barrett, P.H.R., Apolipoprotein B metabolism: tracer kinetics, models, and metabolic studies, *Crit. Rev. Clin. Lab. Sci.*, 39, 89, 2002.
4. Mead, J.R., Irvine, S.A., Ramji, D.P., Lipoprotein lipase: structure, function, regulation, and role in disease, *J. Mol. Med.*, 80, 753, 2002.
5. Connelly, P.W., The role of hepatic lipase in lipoprotein metabolism, *Clin. Chim. Acta*, 286, 243, 1999.
6. Brown, M.L., Ramprasad, M.P., Umeda, P.K., et al., A macrophage receptor for apolipoprotein B48: cloning, expression, and atherosclerosis, *Proc. Nat. Acad. Sci. USA*, 97, 7488, 2000.

7. Ginsberg, H.N., Lipoprotein physiology, *Endocrinol. Metab. Clin. North Am.*, 27, 503, 1998.
8. Jong, M.C., Hofker, M.H., Havekes, L.M., Role of apoCs in lipoprotein metabolism: functional differences between apoC1, apoC2, and apoC3, *Arterioscler. Thromb. Vasc. Biol.*, 19, 472, 1999.
9. Mahmood Hussain, M., Kancha, R.K., Zhou, Z., et al., Chylomicron assembly and catabolism: role of apolipoproteins and receptors, *Biochim. Biophys. Acta*, 1300, 151, 1996.
10. Lusis, A.J., Atherosclerosis, *Nature*, 407, 233, 2000.
11. Harpel, P.C., Gordon, B.R., Parker, T.S., Plasmin catalyzes binding of lipoprotein (a) to immobilized fibrinogen and fibrin, *Proc. Natl. Acad. Sci. USA*, 86, 3847, 1989.
12. Rath, M., Pauling, L., Hypothesis: lipoprotein(a) is a surrogate for ascorbate, *Proc. Natl. Acad. Sci. USA*, 87, 6204, 1990.
13. Dieplinger, H., Kroenberg, F., Genetics and metabolism of lipoprotein(a) and their clinical implications (part 1), *Wein. Klin. Wochenschr.*, 111, 5, 1999.
14. Poon, M., Zhang, X., Dunsky, K.G., et al., Apolipoprotein(a) induces monocyte chemotactic activity in human vascular endothelial cells, *Circulation*, 96, 2514, 1997.
15. Takami, S., Yamashita, S., Kihara, S., et al., Lipoprotein(a) enhances the expression of intercellular adhesion molecule-1 in cultured human umbilical endothelial cells, *Circulation*, 97, 721, 1998.
16. Howard, B.V., Le, N.A., Belcher, J.D., et al., Concentrations of Lp(a) in black and white young adults: relations to risk factors for cardiovascular disease. *Ann. Epidemiol.*, 4, 341, 1994.
17. Marcovina, S.M., Albers, J.J., Wijsman, E., et al., Differences in Lp(a) concentrations and apo(a) polymorphs between black and white Americans, *J. Lipid Res.*, 37, 2569, 1996.
18. Remaley, A.T., Stonik, J.A., Demosky, S.J., et al., Apolipoprotein specificity for lipid efflux by the human ABCA1 transporter, *Biochem. Biophys. Res. Commun.*, 280, 818, 2001.
19. Oram, J.F., HDL apolipoproteins and ABCA1: partners in removal of excess cellular cholesterol, *Arterioscler. Thromb. Vasc. Biol.*, 23, 720, 2003.
20. Lusa, S., Jauhiainen, M., Metso, J., The mechanism of human plasma phospholipid protein-induced enlargement of high-density lipoprotein particles: evidence for particle fusion, *Biochem. J.*, 313, 275, 1996.
21. Clay, M.A., Pyle, D.H., Rye, K.A., Barter, P.J., Formation of spherical, reconstituted high density lipoproteins containing both apolipoproteins A-I and A-II is mediated by lecithin: cholesterol acyltransferase, *J. Biol. Chem.*, 275, 9019, 2000.
22. Acton, S., Rigotti, A., Landschulz, K.T., et al., Identification of scavenger receptor SR-BI as a high density lipoprotein receptor, *Science*, 271, 518, 1996.
23. De Beer, M.C., Durbin, D.M., Cai, L., et al., Apolipoprotein A-II modulates the binding and selective lipid uptake of reconstituted high density lipoprotein by scavenger receptor BI, *J. Biol. Chem.*, 276, 15832, 2001.
24. Pilon, A., Briand, O., Lestavel, S., et al., Apolipoprotein AII enrichment of HDL enhances their affinity for class B type I scavenger receptor but inhibits specific cholesteryl ester uptake, *Arterioscler. Thromb. Vasc. Biol.*, 20, 1074, 2000.
25. Ji, Y., Jian, B., Wang, N., et al., Scavenger receptor BI promotes high density lipoprotein-mediated cellular cholesterol efflux, *J. Biol. Chem.*, 272, 20982, 1997.

26. Barter, P.J., Brewer, B., Jr., Chapman, J., et al., Cholesteryl ester transfer protein: a novel target for raising HDL and inhibiting atherosclerosis, *Arterioscler. Thromb. Vasc. Biol.*, 23, 160, 2003.
27. Guerin, M., Le Goff, W., Lassel, T.S., et al., Atherogenic role of elevated CE transfer from HDL to VLDL (1) and dense LDL in type 2 diabetes: impact of the degree of hypertriglyceridemia, *Arterioscler. Thromb. Vasc. Biol.*, 21, 282, 2001.
28. Stampfer, M.J., Krauss, R.M., Blanche, P.J., et al., A prospective study of triglyceride level, low-density lipoprotein particle diameter, and risk of myocardial infarction, *J.A.M.A.*, 276, 882, 1996.
29. Lamarche, B., St. Pierre, A.C., Ruel, I.L., et al., A prospective, population-based study of low density lipoprotein particle size as a risk factor for ischemic heart disease in men, *Can. J. Cardiol.*, 17, 859, 2001.
30. Krauss, R.M., Heterogeneity of plasma low-density lipoproteins and atherosclerosis risk, *Curr. Opin. Lipidol.*, 5, 339, 1994.
31. Barter, P., Kastelein, J., Nunn, A., et al., High density lipoproteins (HDLs) and atherosclerosis; the unanswered questions, *Atherosclerosis*, 168, 195, 2003.
32. Mackness, M.I., Arrol, S., Abbott, C., Durrington, P.N., Protection of low-density lipoprotein against oxidative modification by high-density lipoprotein associated paraoxanase, *Atherosclerosis*, 104, 129, 1993.
33. Ferretti, G., Bacchetti, T., Busni, D., et al., Protective effect of paraoxanase activity in high-density lipoproteins against erythrocyte membranes peroxidation: a comparison between healthy subjects and type I diabetic patients, *J. Clin. Endocrinol. Metab.*, 89, 2957, 2004.
34. Cockerill, G.W., Rye, K.A., Gamble, J.R., et al., High density lipoproteins inhibit cytokine-induced expression of endothelial cell adhesion molecules, *Arterioscler. Thromb. Vasc. Biol.*, 15, 1987, 1995.
35. Fleisher, L.N., Tall, A.R., Witte, L.U., et al., Stimulation of arterial endothelial cell prostacyclin synthesis by high density lipoproteins, *J. Biol. Chem.*, 257, 6653, 1982.
36. Tamagaki, T., Sawada, S., Imamura, H., et al., Effects of high-density lipoproteins on intracellular pH and proliferation of human vascular endothelial cells, *Atherosclerosis*, 123, 73, 1996.
37. Aoyama, T., Yui, Y., Morishita, H., Kawai, C., Prostacyclin I_2 half-life regulated by high density lipoprotein is decreased in acute myocardial infarction and unstable angina pectoris, *Circulation*, 81, 1784, 1990.
38. Yui, Y., Aoyama, T., Morishita, M., et al., Serum prostacyclin stabilizing factor is identical to apolipoprotein A-I (apo A-I): a novel function of apo A-I, *J. Clin. Invest.*, 82, 803, 1988.
39. Prins, B.A., Hu, R.-M., Nazario, B., et al., Prostaglandin E_2 and prostacyclin inhibit the production and secretion of endothelin from cultured endothelial cells, *J. Biol. Chem.*, 269, 11938, 1994.
40. Zeiher, A.M., Schächinger, V., Hohnloser, S.H., et al., Coronary atherosclerotic wall thickening and vascular reactivity in humans: elevated high-density lipoprotein levels ameliorate vasoconstriction in early atherosclerosis, *Circulation*, 89, 2525, 1994.

5

The Vascular Biology of Atherosclerosis

Robert Carter III and Harlan P. Jones

CONTENTS

Introduction 61
Anatomical Structure of the Normal Human Artery 63
Endothelial Dysfunction 64
A Tale of Two Hypotheses: Lipids vs. Endothelium 66
Chronic Endothelial Injury Hypothesis 66
Lipid Hypothesis 67
Stages of Atherosclerosis 68
Initiation of LDL-Mediated Atherogenesis (Lipid Accumulation) 68
LDL Oxidative Modification and Fatty Streak Formation 68
Foam Cell Formation (Intracellular Lipid Accumulation by Macrophages) 72
Immigration of Smooth Muscle Cells 73
Immune Responsiveness during Atherosclerotic Development 74
Plaque Formation 75
Summary 77
Acknowledgments 77
References 77

Introduction

Cardiovascular disease is the leading cause of mortality in the United States, Europe, the vast majority of Asia, and is likely to be the greatest threat to overall health worldwide.[1,2] As a major cause of cardiovascular disease, the development of atherosclerosis starts early in childhood.[3] Despite this fact, most individuals are asymptomatic until many decades later. Autopsy studies of coronary arteries from healthy, young American soldiers killed during

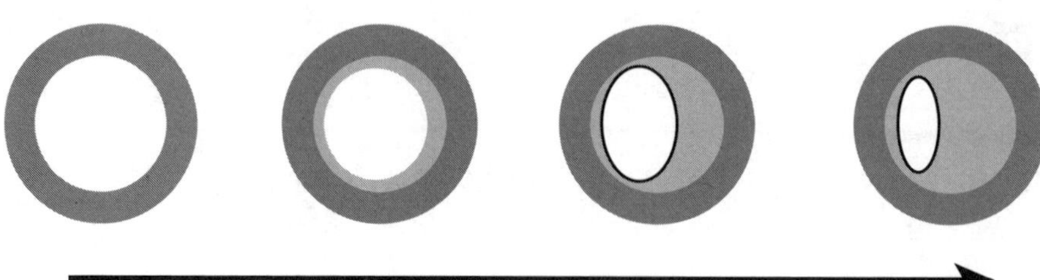

FIGURE 5.1
The progression of atherosclerosis. As the atheroma matures the lumen diameter is reduced which leads to decreased blood flow, thrombosis complications, and unstable plaques. The clinical presentations may be peripheral artery disease, cerebrovascular disease, or ischemic heart disease.

the Korean conflict revealed surprisingly advanced atherosclerotic lesions.[4] Intimal lesions were discovered in more than 50% of the right coronary arteries of the youngest group (15–19 years of age). More recently, fatty streaks, an early marker of atherosclerosis, have been found in the intima of infants.[5] More advanced atherosclerotic lesions are first identified in the intima of three primary target vessels: the carotid and coronary arteries and the aorta.[6,7] Figure 5.1 illustrates the progressive narrowing of the artery during atherosclerosis. Although there is significant disparity in the evolution of lesion formation, ischemic coronary disease, stroke, peripheral artery disease, and transient ischemic attacks are among the clinical presentations of matured lesions and ruptured plaques.[8, 9]

Emerging epidemiologic studies[1,10] have shown that elevated low-density lipoprotein (LDL), male gender, increased homocysteine, and ethnicity are among the many risk factors and markers involved in the pathogenesis of atherosclerosis (Table 5.1). In a recent study of 557 first-generation immigrants, it was concluded that acculturation into western societies may also be an independent risk factor for coronary artery disease and atherosclerotic lesion development.[11] Nevertheless, among the consequences of acculturation are stress, dietary patterns, and physical inactivity which also have been identified as major risk factors for atherosclerosis and cardiovascular disease.

This chapter reviews the recent literature regarding the biology of atherosclerosis and considers in detail: (1) anatomical structure of the normal and diseased artery, (2) chronic endothelial injury and lipid hypotheses, and (3) the events that contribute to formation of the atherosclerotic lesion. The authors hope that this chapter will serve as a basic tutorial for the understanding of the biology of atherosclerosis, and provide an appreciation for the complexity of this disease by introducing new and exciting research contributions to this area.

TABLE 5.1

Risk Factors for Atherosclerotic Lesion Formation

Physical inactivity
Smoking
Infectious agents
Family history
Elevated LDL and VLDL
Low levels of HDL
Elevated lipoprotein (a)
Hypertension
Diabetes mellitus
Male gender
Homocysteine
Ethnicity
Obesity
Age

LDL, low-density lipoprotein; VLDL, very low-density lipoprotein; HDL, high-density lipoprotein.

Anatomical Structure of the Normal Human Artery

The structure of the normal artery consists of three layers: the intima, the media, and the adventitia (Figure 5.2). The intima, the innermost layer, is composed of an endothelial monolayer lying on the basement membrane with elastic fibers comprised of type IV collagen, laminin, and heparin sulfate proteoglycans.[12] This layer also contains smooth muscle cells (SMCs) embedded in sulfated polysaccharide, hyaluronic acid intimal thickenings.[13]

The endothelium of a normal, healthy artery functions as a non-thrombogenic surface and serves as a selectively permeable barrier, which regulates the transport of solutes across the arterial wall. Importantly, the vascular endothelium is also essential in the regulation of vascular tone, coagulation, and inflammatory responses.[14–16] Changes in shear stress and blood flow lead to phosphorylation of endothelial nitric oxide synthase (eNOS), which generates nitric oxide (NO), which then produces vasodilation.[17] The intima is separated from the media by an internal elastic lamina comprised primarily of the protein polymer elastin.[12]

The tunica media, the middle layer, is primarily comprised of SMCs surrounded by its own basement membrane. The media's basement membrane is anchored within an interstitial matrix composed of type I collagen, fibronectin, dermatan, and chondroitin sulfate proteoglycans.[12,18] This interstitial matrix is intertwined with perforated sheets of elastic fibers.

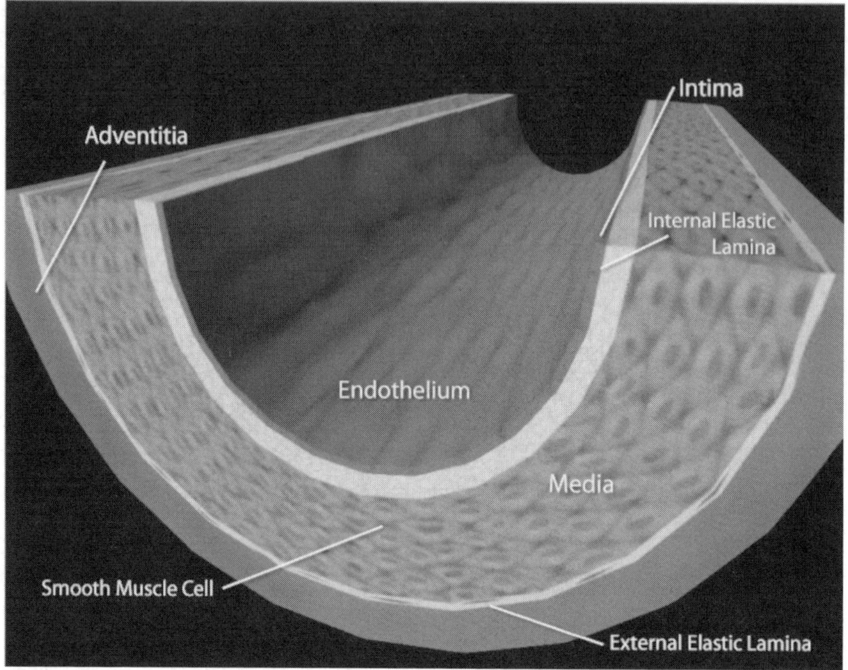

FIGURE 5.2
Anatomical structure of the normal artery. This illustration displays the three distinct layers of the vessel wall: intima, media, and adventitia as well as the endothelium and the external and internal elastic lamina.

The adventitia attaching the vessel to the surrounding tissue is made up of capillaries, fibroblasts, fat cells, proteoglycans, connective tissue, and elastic and collagen bundles. The adventitia is separated from the tunica media by the external elastic lamina.[12] The connective tissue in the adventitia is very compressed where it borders the tunica media, but it changes to loose connective tissue near the periphery of the vessel.[19]

Endothelial Dysfunction

In humans, the normal endothelium has many unique anti-atherosclerotic properties, including vasoregulation of conductive and resistance vessels, monocyte disadhesion, and vessel growth.[14,20] The pathophysiological consequences of disruption of these factors serve as hallmarks of endothelial dysfunction. Endothelial dysfunction as a result of injury leads to compensatory responses that modify the normal physiological characteristics of the endothelium and become the foundation for the disease process.[13]

Endothelial dysfunction is characterized as a systemic, reversible disorder and is associated with an impairment in endothelium-dependent vasodilation and recruitment of inflammatory cells to the vessel wall.[14,21] Potential causes of endothelial dysfunction include hypercholesterolemia, diabetes,[22] smoking,[23] hypertension,[24] and infectious microorganisms[25] such as *Chlamydia pneumoniae*,[26] cytomegaloviral infection, *Helicobacter pylori* infection, and herpes virus infection,[27] many of which are associated with a reduction in availability of vasodilators such as NO, decreased flow-induced vasodilation, and increased endothelium-derived contracting factors.[23] Lipid and cell permeability, lipoprotein oxidation, inflammation, platelet activation, and thrombus formation are all promoted by endothelial dysfunction.[28,29] The paradigm of endothelial dysfunction propagates a proatherogenic milieu that favors atheroma formation.[30]

Ludmer and colleagues, using a selective agonist acetylcholine test, provided the first evidence in humans of impaired endothelium-dependent vasodilation in the presence of atherosclerosis,[31] which is now attributed to a reduced bioavailability of NO.[15,32,33] In large arteries of humans,[23] rabbits,[34] pigs,[35] and monkeys,[36] reduced endothelium-dependent vasodilation due to atherosclerosis and hypercholesterolemia has been reported. However, the sensitivity of injured endothelial cells is not homogeneous for all vasoactive agonists.[37] For example, the responsiveness of the endothelial cells to acetylcholine, substance P, serotonin, and alpha-adrenergic agonists is severely decreased, while the responsiveness to bradykinin and adenosine diphosphate is only mildly attenuated. In contrast, endothelium-independent vasodilation to nitro-containing vasodilators is not altered.[37]

Endothelium dysfunction is also involved in the activation of endothelial-leukocyte adhesion molecules.[38,39] Specifically, P-selectin, E-selectin, intracellular adhesion molecule-1 (ICAM-1), and vascular cell adhesion molecule (VCAM-1) are adhesion molecules known to be involved with the recruitment of leukocytes.[40] VCAM-1 plays a role in the binding of both monocytes and leukocytes to endothelial cells. In lesion-prone areas (e.g., endothelial cells exposed to long duration, high shear stress), VCAM-1 is up-regulated and occurs in response to inflammatory cytokines.[38] Increased expression of ICAM-1 on endothelial cells has been detected in both lesion-prone areas as well as on endothelial cells exposed to normal shear stress.[41] In humans, E-selectin is only upregulated on injured endothelial cells and is important in the regulation of adhesive interactions between certain blood cells and the endothelium,[40,42] whereas P-selectin is involved in adhesion of certain leukocytes and platelets to the endothelium.[43–45] The importance of P-selectin during atherosclerosis has also been demonstrated in animal models.[46] For example, P-selectin is expressed on endothelial cells overlying active atherosclerotic plaques, and inactive atherosclerotic plaques lacking in P-selectin expression.[43] Furthermore, animals lacking P-selectin have a decreased tendency to form atherosclerotic plaques.[40]

Several potential mechanisms by which statin therapy, angiotensin receptor blockers, and aspirin might improve endothelial dysfunction have been suggested, including up-regulation of nitric oxide production, reduction of oxidative stress, and increased adhesion molecule expression.[12,33,47] More recently, the finding that the insulin-sensitizing thiazolidinediones (TZDs), peroxisome proliferator-activated receptor-gamma (transcription factor) agonists have antiproliferative and anti-inflammatory effects has led to the investigation of their possible role in the treatment of endothelial dysfunction and atherosclerotic lesion formation.[12,48]

A Tale of Two Hypotheses: Lipids vs. Endothelium

The chronic endothelial injury and the lipid hypotheses are the two main proliferative mechanisms postulated to explain the underlying pathogenesis of atherosclerosis. These two hypotheses are not mutually exclusive and are closely linked by the culmination of molecular and cellular events. The roles of cell types of the vessel wall in healthy and diseased (atherosclerosis) states are summarized in Table 5.2. Although others[49–53] have postulated alternative hypotheses about the development of atherosclerosis, the chronic endothelium injury hypothesis is the one most widely accepted.

Chronic Endothelial Injury Hypothesis

Based on pathophysiological evidence in animals and humans, Ross and Glomset introduced the endothelial injury hypothesis of atherosclerosis, which initially postulated that endothelial cell uncovering was the initial step in the development of atherosclerosis.[54] However, endothelial dysfunction is presently considered to be the precursor that initiates the atherosclerotic process and is associated with increased lipoprotein accumulation at

TABLE 5.2

Role of Cell Type of the Vessel Wall in Healthy and Diseased (Atherosclerosis) States

Cellular Components	Healthy	Diseased
Endothelial cell	NO production Vasoreactivity Anti-adhesive	Loss of NO production Paradoxical vasoconstriction Leukocyte adhesion
T-cell	Inflammatory signals	Macrophage stimulation Cytokine production
Macrophage	Lipid uptake	Cytokine release MMP production
Smooth muscle cell	Structural Vasoreactivity	Intimal migration Proliferation

NO, nitric oxide; MMP, matrix metalloproteinases.

the site of injury.[13,29] The response to the chronic endothelial injury hypothesis or "response to injury hypothesis" of atherosclerosis states that the protective, inflammatory response followed by the formation of fibroproliferative response begins as a protective mechanism that with time and continuing insult may become excessive.[55,56] Due to release of chemoattractants and growth regulatory molecules by the altered endothelium,[57] leukocytes,[58] monocytes, and T lymphocytes[59] attach to the endothelial cell surface. The leukocytes migrate to the subendothelial space, between the tiny junctions of the endothelial cells, and aggregate within the intima.[56] The presence of elevated levels of oxidized low-density lipoproteins (oxLDL) is the basis of conversion of monocytes to macrophages, and is a fundamental factor responsible for injury to the vascular wall.[60] Through scavenger cell receptors, macrophages accumulate modified lipid particles and become foam cells. As the process persists, foam cell and lymphocyte accumulation forms the basis for the fatty streak.[61,62] It is believed that fatty streaks frequently form at sites with significant intimal smooth muscle accumulation.[63] More advanced lesions develop as a result of continued cell migration and proliferation[56] which eventually turn into a fibrous plaque.[64] This hypothesis is based on the notion that repeated insult to the endothelium leads to dysfunction, which is followed by a cascade of pathophysiological consequences.

Lipid Hypothesis

In 1913, Nikolai N. Anitschkow demonstrated that cholesterol feeding of rabbits could induce vascular lesions consistent with the characteristics of human atherosclerotic lesions.[65,66] Unknowingly, his research and others established the principles of what is now commonly referred to as the "lipid hypothesis." Through decades of research and much controversy, the "lipid hypothesis" is still believed to be one of the prominent mechanisms contributing to atherosclerosis.[66] Based upon its principles, many discoveries have been made in understanding the pathogenesis of atherosclerosis and the fight against cardiovascular disease.

Although elevated LDL cholesterol is associated with increased risk for cardiovascular disease and the pathogenesis of atherosclerosis, LDL has an essential biological role to transport cholesterol to peripheral tissues.[67] Serum cholesterol is transported by lipoprotein particles that perform important tasks of carrying both dietary and endogenously produced lipids.[68] While the transport of endogenous lipids is mediated by LDL, very low-density lipoproteins (VLDL), and high-density lipoprotein (HDL), the dietary lipids are carried primarily by chylomicrons. For the most part, LDL particles transport the vast majority of serum cholesterol.

The lipid hypothesis postulates that an elevation in LDL levels results in penetration of LDL into the arterial wall, leading to lipid accumulation in SMCs and in macrophages (foam cells).[69] LDL also augments smooth muscle cell hyperplasia and migration into the subintimal and intimal region in response to growth factors. LDL is modified or oxidized in this environment and is rendered more atherogenic. Small dense LDL cholesterol particles are also more susceptible to modification and oxidation. The modified or oxidized LDL is chemotactic to monocytes, promoting their migration into the intima, their early appearance in the fatty streak,[28] and their transformation and retention in the subintimal compartment as macrophages. Scavenger receptors on the surface of macrophages facilitate the entry of oxidized LDL into these cells, transferring them into lipid-laden macrophages and foam cells. As cell migration and proliferation continues, advanced lesions are formed which leads to plaque formation.

Stages of Atherosclerosis

Initiation of LDL-Mediated Atherogenesis (Lipid Accumulation)

As postulated by the "lipid hypothesis," atherosclerotic lesion development begins with the accumulation of LDL cholesterol levels within the circulation. The studies of Brown and colleagues[70] elucidated that the molecular mechanisms controlling LDL-cholesterol uptake were instrumental in this determination. Under pathologic conditions where LDL levels are elevated, lipid accumulation is noticeable along the lining of the arterial wall termed the tunica lamina (Figure 5.3). The aggregates of lipid particles form intimate associations with epithelia moieties such as proteoglycans and become embedded in the tunica lamina structure (Figure 5.4). In defense, the arterial epithelium fortifies itself with self-protective structural and biochemical mechanisms that maintain a homeostatic environment in the presence of lipid accumulation. The expression of molecules such as heparin sulfate constituents, which provide arterial integrity and blood fluidity and the expression of many antithrombin molecules,[70] are instrumental in protection against atherogenesis.[70] However, under hypercholesterolemic conditions, the protective integrity of the epithelium falls prey to initiation of lesion development.

LDL Oxidative Modification and Fatty Streak Formation

Atherosclerotic lesions present initially in the form of fatty streaks forming along the endothelium of arteries (Figure 5.4). The major contributing event believed to be responsible in fatty streak development is oxidative modifications of the lipid and apolipoprotein B (apo B) components of LDL.[71]

The precise molecular mechanisms responsible for LDL oxidation are largely unknown. Studies have identified several plausible mechanisms supportive of LDL modification. The enzymatic activity of nitric oxide synthase,

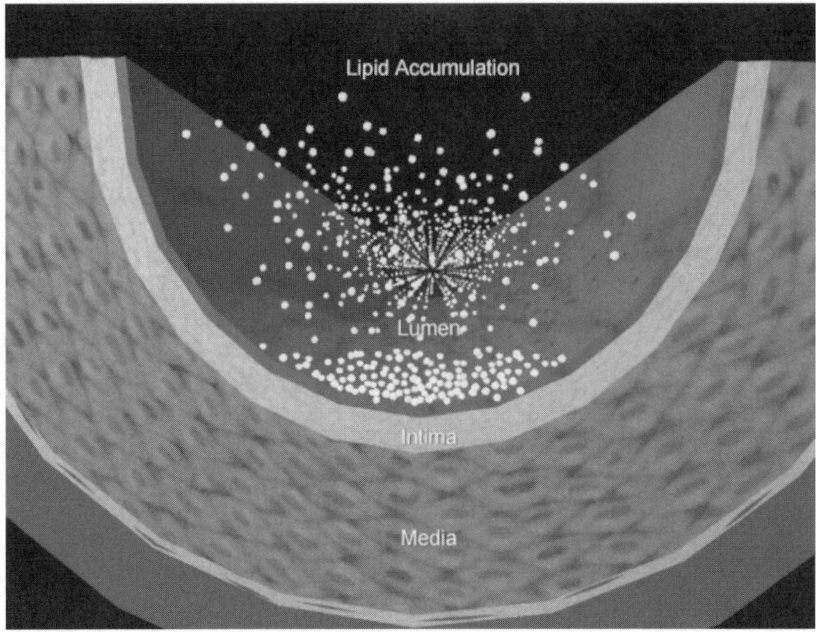

FIGURE 5.3
Initiation of LDL-mediated atherogenesis (lipid accumulation). Atherosclerotic lesion development begins with the accumulation of LDL. Lipid accumulation is noticeable along the lining of the arterial wall.

15-lipoxengenase activity,[72] as well as nitric oxide production by epithelial cells and macrophages[73] have been shown to be capable of LDL modification. Recent findings supporting their proatherogenic role have been documented using gene knockout models.[74–76] Despite formidable evidence that LDL oxidation confers lesion formation, data regarding antioxidant therapy to date have not shown promise.[77] In broad terms, atherosclerosis can be characterized as a chronic inflammatory disease. As such, cellular responses such as cellular adhesion and recruitment during lesion development are central components as in other chronic inflammatory diseases.

The recruitment of monocytes occurs at the sites of lipid accumulation and function in uptake of various lipids and apolipoprotein components produced from oxidative stress and other biochemical breakdown products of LDL (Figure 5.4). Such recruitment is known to be regulated by chemotactic factors[10] as well as being attracted by oxidative-LDL species.[10] Chemokines are small proteins subdivided into three major groups based upon the structural positions of the first two cysteines at the amino terminus of the molecule.[78–80] Chemokines stimulate the migration and activation of cells, especially phagocytic cells and lymphocytes. Most notable is the release of macrophage chemotactic protein 1 (MCP-1) found to be produced locally by endothelial cells[71] and the coordinate expression of chemokine receptor 2 (CCR2), the receptor for MCP-1 by monocytes. In fact, it has been shown

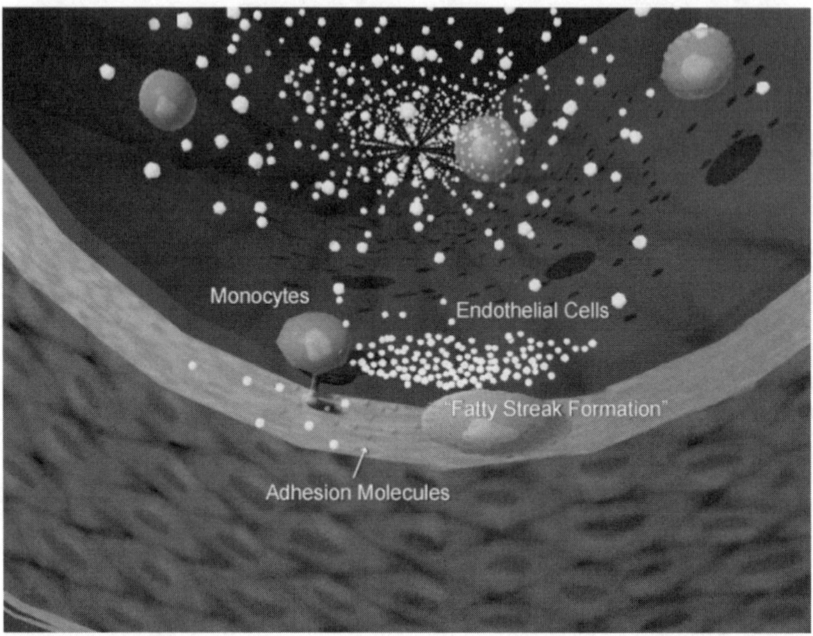

FIGURE 5.4
LDL oxidative modification and monocyte recruitment (fatty streak formation). The initial sign of atherogenic development is the formation of the fatty streak, underlying the endothelium of large arteries. The primary cellular events contributing to the fatty streak formation are the recruitment of monocytes which are converted to macrophages, which uptake LDL. Recruitment of monocytes to lesion probe areas is regulated by adhesion molecules that are expressed on the endothelium cell surface.

that hypercholesterolemia patients exhibit increased MCP-1 production.[81] Furthermore, disruption of MCP-1 and its receptor CCR2 genes was shown to reduce the development of atherosclerosis in mice.[81] Other chemokines such as interleukin-8 (IL-8), RANTES, and IP-10 have also been implicated in monocyte recruitment.[10] Current research in this area offers the potential for therapeutic use in deterring atherogenic processes by impairing leukocyte trafficking.

It has been speculated that macrophage-mediated uptake of modified LDL species may be an initial attempt to dampen the inflammatory environment produced by oxidative LDL species.[10] Ultimately, however, the response and uptake of oxidized LDL species leads to progressive inflammation and atherosclerotic lesions. The uptake of LDL occurs mainly via macrophage LDL receptors or by scavenger receptor-mediated uptake.[10] The mode of LDL uptake is determined by the nature of LDL modification. Studies show that while native LDL is normally endocytosed via specific LDL receptors, highly modified LDL, such as certain apolipoproteins, are not recognizable by the LDL receptors and are relegated to uptake by scavenger receptors. The latter is most associated with macrophage foam cell formation, a topic to be

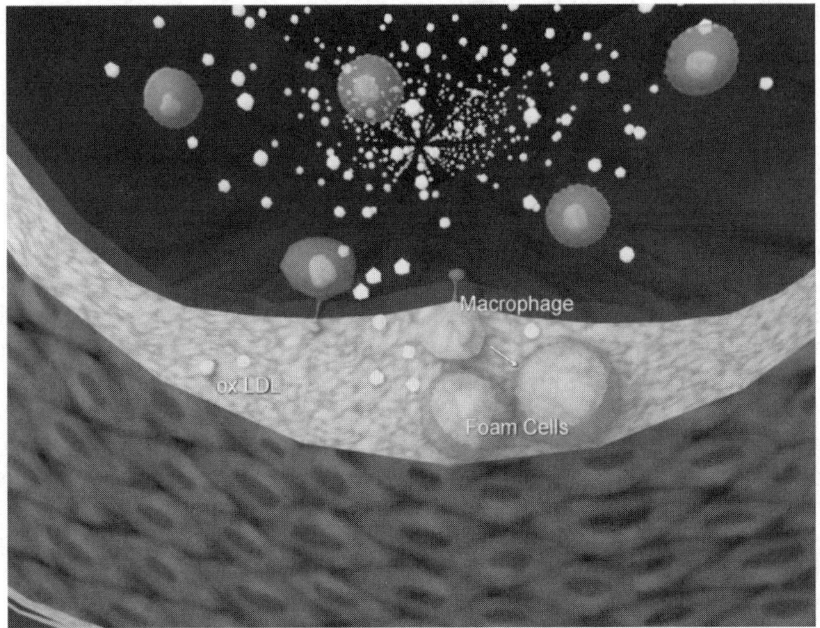

FIGURE 5.5
Foam cell formation (intracellular lipid accumulation) by macrophages. A hallmark of early atherosclerotic lesion development is conversion of the macrophage to foam cells that contain amounts of oxLDL, which is mediated primarily by scavenger receptors.

discussed in a subsequent section of this chapter. As a result of macrophage recruitment and uptake of LDL constituents, fatty streaks form and become what is the initial site of atherosclerotic lesions (Figure 5.5).

Another mechanism responsible for the initiation of atherosclerotic lesions is the increase in adhesion molecules present on endothelial cells. Under normal circumstances, the arterial endothelium is highly resistant toward cellular adhesion. However, studies have shown that hypercholesterolemia induces leukocyte adherence to the endothelium allowing diapedesis between the endothelial cell and entry into the lamina.[10] Several adhesion molecules have been implicated to significantly foster translocation of leukocytes across the endothelium. Vascular cell adhesion molecule-1 (VCAM-1), a member of the immunoglobulin superfamily, is expressed by endothelial cells and regulates the adherence of monocytes and T cells. VCAM-1 has been found to interact with very late antigen-4 (VLA-4) and influence monocyte adherence during the initial stages of atheroma formation.[82] Selectins P and E have also been implicated in monocyte adhesiveness to the endothelium. Quantitative decreases in atherosclerosis were shown in apo E mice lacking their respective genes.[83]

Foam Cell Formation (Intracellular Lipid Accumulation by Macrophages)

As mentioned in a previous section, macrophages play an important role in LDL metabolism by uptake of native LDL cholesterol and modified species of LDL via two major receptor mechanisms, LDL-specific receptor and scavenger receptor endocytosis, respectively. As the accumulation and modification of LDL ensues, macrophages within the subendothelium begin to incorporate large amounts of oxidized LDL species via scavenger receptor uptake, resulting in a phenotype given the term "foam cell" (Figure 5.5). The most notable scavenger receptors identified to date that have been demonstrated to have a significant impact on atherosclerotic development are the scavenger receptor A (SR-A) and the receptors of the cluster differentiation 36 surface molecules (CD36) receptors.[84] In particular, it was shown that in apo E-deficient murine models deficient in SR-A or CD36, gene receptor expression resulted in a significant reduction in lesion formation.[84,85]

As determined by the studies of Brown and colleagues, homeostatic control of cholesterol uptake is under strict mediation through LDL-specific receptor feedback mechanisms regulated by the SREBP transcription factors required for LDL receptor expression.[70] In the presence of elevated membrane-bound cholesterol, inactivation of SREBP occurs, inhibiting LDL receptor expression. In contrast, however, uptake of oxidative LDL species via scavenger receptors, SR-A or CD36 or by macrophage-mediated phagocytosis is not under such regulatory control. Instead, prevention of cholesterol intracellular overload is dependent on mechanisms of active efflux out of the cell. The vast majority of oxidized LDL entering macrophages via the scavenger receptors consists of free cholesterol or esterified cholesterol. There are several fates of native cholesterol metabolism, which include Acyl CoA esterification and the storage of lipid droplets containing cholesterol esters that characterize the phenotype of foam cells. Excretion of excess cholesterol by foam cells is believed to occur through processes that transform cholesterol into a more soluble form through enzymatic modifications.

A major pathway of cholesterol efflux is called the "reverse cholesterol transport" pathway that involves HDL as an acceptor molecule. The HDL-reverse cholesterol transport mechanism received much attention when studies found an inverse relationship between risk for atherosclerosis and HDL content.[86] A genetic basis for HDL-mediated cholesterol transport is shown in patients afflicted with Tangier disease, which is characterized by extremely low levels of HDL and accumulation of cholesterol within macrophages. Mutations in ABCA1, which encodes a member of the ATP binding cassette family of HDL transporters, were found to cause the genetic defect. Although the precise mechanism that is disrupted by this aberration is unclear, studies suggest that mutation in ABC A1 alters cholesterol transport to the HDL acceptor molecules.[87] Under normal conditions, HDL-cholesterol is esterified via lecithin-cholesterol acyltransferase (LCAT) or is directly transported to the liver via SR-B1 binding. Thus, it is clear that macrophages play a paramount role in cholesterol maintenance within its surrounding environment, but more important is its ability to control the fate of internalized cholesterol for self-preservation.

Immigration of Smooth Muscle Cells

A hallmark of advanced lesion development is the immigration of smooth muscles cells from the arterial wall into the subepithelial space (Figure 5.6). The factors that lead to the mobilization of smooth muscle cells are not well understood, but it is believed to be due to preexisting stimuli. For example, macrophages have been shown to secrete the chemokine platelet-derived growth factor (PDGF), which is a chemoattractant for smooth muscle.[88] In fact, studies have demonstrated PDGF expression to be elevated in individuals with atherosclerosis.[89] Smooth muscle cells found within the atherosclerotic region were found to have distinct characteristics from normal smooth muscle cells. These cells exhibit characteristics of clonal expansion. Studies have demonstrated that the slow but steady proliferation can be attributed

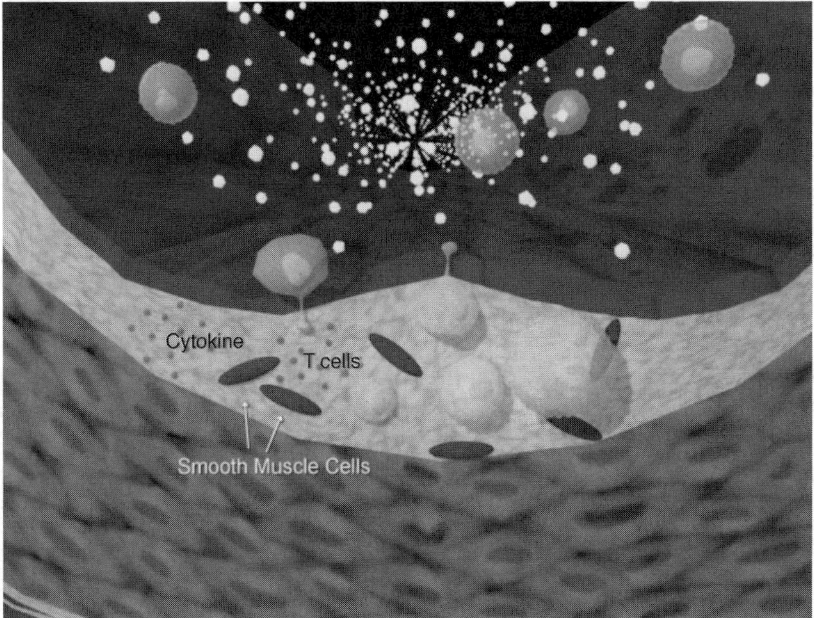

FIGURE 5.6
Immigration of smooth muscle cells and immune responsiveness during atherosclerotic development. A hallmark of advanced lesion development is the immigration of smooth muscle cells from the arterial wall into the subepithelial space, which may also contribute to foam cell development. As with many chronic inflammatory diseases, immune surveillance will ultimately make a significant contribution to the progression and disease outcome. Circulating leukocytes and lymphocytes of mainly T-cells respond to the site of injury.

to a single cell.[90] Smooth muscle cells in developing atheroma also are capable of taking up modified lipoproteins.[89] Not only does their proliferative capacity augment atheroma development, but apoptotic cell death of smooth muscle cells participates in lesion progression. Apoptosis of smooth muscle cells is believed to be associated with the presence of inflammatory cytokines at the lesion site.[91] Thus, smooth muscle cell immigration plays a significant role in progression of atheromas (Figure 5.6). Current research is aimed at developing molecular strategies targeting both proliferative and apoptotic pathways.

Immune Responsiveness during Atherosclerotic Development

With the exception of macrophage activation, lymphocyte activation does not appear to have a major impact on the initial stage of atherosclerotic formation. Studies using RAG-1 recombinase-deficient mice illustrated that the lack of functional B and T lymphocytes had no bearing on atherosclerotic development in the presence of elevated cholesterol.[92] However, as with many chronic inflammatory diseases, immune surveillance will ultimately make a significant contribution to the progression and outcome of disease. Circulating leukocytes and lymphocytes of mainly T lymphocytes respond to endothelial injury. At such stages of lesion development, a multitude of secreted and cell-associated mediators are accessible to lymphocyte recognition. For example, endothelial cell-associated adhesion molecules such as VCAM-1[93] can also increase the avidity for monocytes to enter lesion sites. Also, as previously mentioned, chemokines produced by activated macrophages can attract T-cells to the lesion site. As T-cells begin to accumulate in the surrounding lesion, they become activated and can modulate atherosclerotic development through the release of cytokines (Figure 5.7). Through the release of cytokines, T-cells can elicit both pro-atherogenic and anti-atherogenic responses. Such dichotomy is due to the presence of T subpopulations capable of secreting distinct cytokines that display opposing functionality. These populations of T-cells are commonly referred to as T-helper cells, subdivided into Th1 and Th2 subpopulations.[94] Th1 cells mainly secrete IL-2, interferon (IFN)-γ and tumor necrosis factor (TNF)-α. Th1-associated cytokines mediate pro-inflammatory responses and delayed hypersensitivity responses. On the other hand, the Th2 subpopulation preferentially secretes IL-4, IL-5, IL-6, IL-10 and IL-13.[94] Th2 cells function in anti-inflammatory responses and immune tolerance.

Studies that examined the role of Th1 versus Th2 cytokine responses in the progression of atherosclerosis have shown that T-helper cell cytokine mediation is not as clearly defined along the two divergent functions between Th1 and Th2. In fact, IFN-γ has been shown to suppress scavenger receptor expression and proliferation of smooth muscle cells, suggesting an anti-atherogenic potential.[10] On the other hand IFN-γ is capable of activating macrophages. In studies utilizing apo E-deficient mice that lacked a

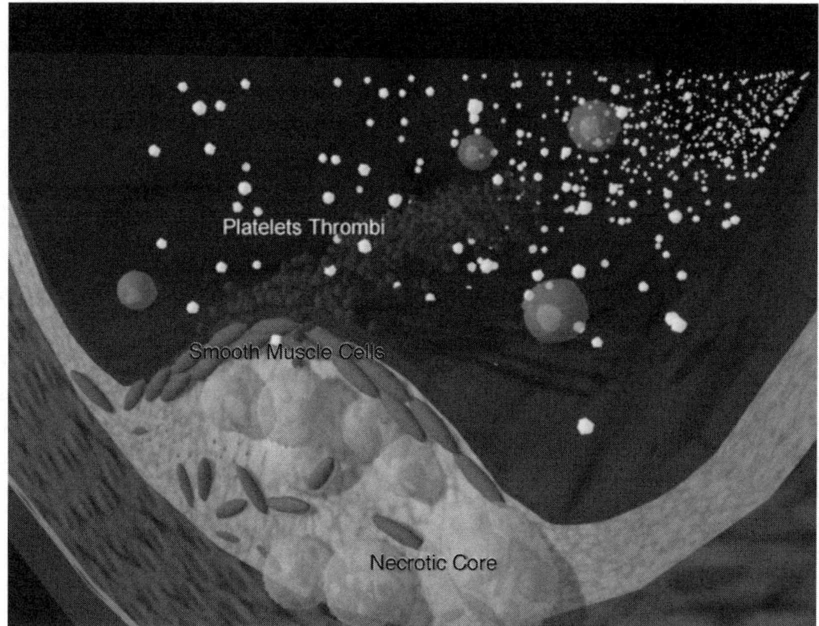

FIGURE 5.7
Plaque formation. Plaques develop from initial fatty streaks that progress into advanced lesions comprised of inflammatory cells, smooth muscle cells, extracellular lipids, and fibrous tissues. Their continued accumulation proliferation and activation within the lesion leads to plaque expansion. Consistent with the earlier events of atherosclerotic lesion development, plaque formation involves the participation of cytokines, chemokines, hydrolytic enzymes, and growth factors in this process. During the advanced stages of plaque formation, lipid moieties, leukocytes and necrotic materials are walled off by a fibrous cap. An accumulation of these cellular constituents and fibrotic tissues leads to further expansion and can lead to ischemic heart disease or stroke, which is due mainly to plaque rupture and thrombosis.

functional IFN-γ receptor, atherosclerosis was decreased as compared to normal mice.[95] The role of Th2 cytokine mediation is also very complex. While IL-4 cytokine production by Th2 cells acts antagonistically toward IFN-γ production, IL-4 has been shown to induce LDL oxidation through induction of 15-LO enzymatic activation.[10] IL-10 production by Th2 cells seems to be the most consistent in opposing pro-atherogenic processes such as macrophage deactivation[96,97] and plaque stability. Thus, the implication of T-cells' activation offers a complex environment in determination of their specific roles in atherosclerotic development and progression.

Plaque Formation

Plaques develop from initial fatty streaks that progress into advanced lesions comprised of inflammatory cells, extracellular lipid, and fibrous tissues (Figure 5.7). Their continued accumulation proliferation and activation within the lesion leads to plaque expansion. Consistent with the earlier events of atherosclerotic lesion development, plaque formation involves the participation of cytokines, chemokines, hydrolytic enzymes, and growth factors in this process.[98] During the advanced stages of plaque formation, lipid moieties, leukocytes and necrotic materials are walled off by a fibrous cap. An accumulation of these cellular constituents and fibrotic tissues leads to further expansion. At a particular threshold, the compensatory dilation of the artery is overcome by the intrusion of the lesion into the lumen resulting in eventual alterations in blood flow and plaque rupture.

While the initial events of atherogenesis involve mainly the disruption of the endothelia and leukocyte accumulation, the formation of the more advanced plaque includes smooth muscle cells (Figure 5.7). As mentioned previously, smooth muscle cells migrate via chemotactic regulation into the arterial intimal lesion site and become active participants in atheroma development. The smooth muscle cells involved in atheroma exhibit an altered phenotype in comparison to normal arterial tunica media smooth muscle cells. These smooth muscle cells proliferate at a higher rate within atherosclerotic plaques versus normal intimal regions of the aorta.[99] Further justification for the importance of smooth muscle cell proliferation demonstrated that clonal expansion of smooth muscle cells was likely and is the basis for lesion progression.[90] It is still unclear, however, what initiates medial smooth muscle proliferation versus normal smooth muscle cells. It is believed that growth factors in conjunction with additional stimuli promote the proliferative response by smooth muscle cells at the lesion site. For example, vascular smooth muscles cells (VSMCs) in the presence of serum show minimal mitogenic capacity.[100] Other studies substantiate this finding.[100,101] One possibility for the lack of mitogenicity could be due to the presence of suppressive factors. Based upon the evidence of this study it has been postulated that basement membrane constituents such as heparin can suppress smooth cell proliferation.[102,103] Thyberg, Hedin and colleagues also showed that the basement membrane component, laminin, inhibits while the interstitial matrix component, fibronectin, promotes phenotypic modulation of smooth muscle cells.[88,104] In contrast, the metalloproteinases that are induced by inflammatory cytokines[105,106] were found to induce smooth cell proliferation.[107] In addition to smooth muscle proliferation, the apoptosis of smooth muscle cells participates in advanced lesion development. Cell death may be the result of cytokine regulation present within the lesion site.[108] Also, interaction with *fas*-expressing T-cells can lead to cell death.[109] Therefore, understanding the regulation of smooth muscle expansion and depletion with regard to progression of plaque formation will likely have a great impact on the innovation of new therapies to combat atherosclerosis.

A large proportion of the developing atheroma includes connective tissue consisting of extracellular matrix macromolecules. Among the matrix proteins, the class collagens and proteoglycans are commonly associated with plaque development. Matrix proteins are produced by vascular smooth muscle cells and can accumulate within the developing plaque upon stimulation by transforming growth factor-β and platelet-derived growth factor.[110] Matrix molecules have an important regulatory function. For example, fibronectin and heparan sulfate are found to inhibit cell cycle and cell–matrix interactions and influence chemokine expression by macrophages.[111–114] Matrix accumulation within the intima is under control of matrix metalloproteinases (MMPs).[112] MMPs act in degradation of matrix molecules and therefore control lesion accumulation. Matrix molecules also contribute to the outward growth of the lumina. Thus, the extracellular matrix is a key component in plaque development.

Summary

Cardiovascular disease is the leading cause of mortality in the United States, Europe, and a vast majority of Asia and is likely to be the greatest threat to overall health worldwide. This chapter emphasizes the biological process of atherosclerosis and what is known about the cells and molecules that are associated with the evolution of this multifaceted disease. While evidence suggests that elevated lipids and endothelial dysfunction both play an important role in atherogenesis, more research is needed to determine the molecular and cellular interactions of these factors in promoting the pathogenesis of atherosclerosis. Whereas atherosclerosis has long been an area of significant biomedical, clinical, and epidemiological research emphasis, there is considerable evidence that the quantitative determinants of disease vulnerability must be identified.

Acknowledgments

Special thanks to Scott B. Robinson of scienceinflash.com for graphic illustrations. The authors express their deep appreciation to Drs. Samuel N. Cheuvront and Sangeeta Kaushik for reviewing the manuscript.

References

1. Yach D, Hawkes C, Gould CL, Hofman KJ. The global burden of chronic diseases: overcoming impediments to prevention and control. *JAMA* 2004;291(21):2616–2622.
2. Mitka M. Heart disease a global health threat. *JAMA* 2004;291(21):2533.

3. Rodenburg J, Vissers M, Wiegman A, Trip M, Bakker H, Kastelein JJ. Familial hypercholesterolemia in children. *Curr Opin Lipidol* 2004;15(4):405–411.
4. Enos WF, Holmes RH, Beyer J. Coronary disease among United States soldiers killed in action in Korea. *J Am Med Assoc* 1953;152:1090–1093.
5. Stary HC, Chandler AB, Glagov S, et al. A definition of initial, fatty streak, and intermediate lesions of atherosclerosis. A report from the Committee on Vascular Lesions of the Council on Arteriosclerosis, American Heart Association. *Circulation* 1994;89(5):2462–2478.
6. Adams GJ, Simoni DM, Bordelon CB Jr., et al. Bilateral symmetry of human carotid artery atherosclerosis. *Stroke* 2002;33(11):2575–2580.
7. McGill HC Jr., McMahan CA, Herderick EE, Malcom GT, Tracy RE, Strong JP. Origin of atherosclerosis in childhood and adolescence. *Am J Clin Nutr* 2000;72(5 Suppl):1307S–1315S.
8. Fuster V, Lewis A. Conner Memorial Lecture. Mechanisms leading to myocardial infarction: insights from studies of vascular biology. *Circulation* 1994;90(4):2126–2146.
9. Awareness of stroke warning signs — 17 states and the U.S. Virgin Islands, 2001. *MMWR Morbid Mortal Wkly Rep* 7 2004;53(17):359–362.
10. Glass CK, Witztum JL. Atherosclerosis: the road ahead. *Cell* 23 2001;104(4):503–516.
11. Mooteri SN, Petersen F, Dagubati R, Pai RG. Duration of residence in the United States as a new risk factor for coronary artery disease (the Konkani Heart Study). *Am J Cardiol* 2004;93(3):359–361.
12. Plutzky J. The vascular biology of atherosclerosis. *Am J Med* 2003;115(Suppl 8A):55S–61S.
13. Newby AC. An overview of the vascular response to injury: a tribute to the late Russell Ross. *Toxicol Lett* 2000;112–113:519–529.
14. Behrendt D, Ganz P. Endothelial function. From vascular biology to clinical applications. *Am J Cardiol* 2002;90(10C):40L–48L.
15. Cannon RO, 3rd. Role of nitric oxide in cardiovascular disease: focus on the endothelium. *Clin Chem* 1998;44(8 Pt 2):1809–1819.
16. Furchgott RF, Zawadzki JV. The obligatory role of endothelial cells in the relaxation of arterial smooth muscle by acetylcholine. *Nature* 1980; 288(5789):373–376.
17. Dimmeler S, Fleming I, Fisslthaler B, Hermann C, Busse R, Zeiher AM. Activation of nitric oxide synthase in endothelial cells by Akt-dependent phosphorylation. *Nature* 1999;399(6736):601–605.
18. Libby P. Vascular biology of atherosclerosis: overview and state of the art. *Am J Cardiol* 2003;91(3A):3A-6A.
19. O'Brien KD, Chait A. The biology of the artery wall in atherogenesis. *Med Clin North Am* 1994;78(1):41–67.
20. Flavahan NA. Atherosclerosis or lipoprotein-induced endothelial dysfunction. Potential mechanisms underlying reduction in EDRF/nitric oxide activity. *Circulation* 1992;85(5):1927–1938.
21. Weiss N, Keller C, Hoffmann U, Loscalzo J. Endothelial dysfunction and atherothrombosis in mild hyperhomocysteinemia. *Vasc Med* 2002;7(3):227–239.
22. Dandona P, Aljada A, Chaudhuri A, Mohanty P. Endothelial dysfunction, inflammation and diabetes. *Rev Endocr Metab Disord* 2004;5(3):189–197.
23. Landmesser U, Hornig B, Drexler H. Endothelial function: a critical determinant in atherosclerosis? *Circulation* 2004;109(21 Suppl 1):II27–II33.

24. Felmeden DC, Spencer CG, Chung NA, et al. Relation of thrombogenesis in systemic hypertension to angiogenesis and endothelial damage/dysfunction (a substudy of the Anglo-Scandinavian Cardiac Outcomes Trial [ASCOT]). *Am J Cardiol* 2003;92(4):400–405.
25. Libby P, Ridker PM, Maseri A. Inflammation and atherosclerosis. *Circulation* 2002;105(9):1135–1143.
26. Noll G. Pathogenesis of atherosclerosis: a possible relation to infection. *Atherosclerosis* 1998;140(Suppl 1):S3–S9.
27. Andel M, Tsevegjav A, Roubalova K, Hruba D, Dlouhy P, Kraml P. [Infectious and inflammatory factors in the etiology and pathogenesis of atherosclerosis.] *Vnitr Lek* 2003;49(12):960–966.
28. Viles-Gonzalez JF, Anand SX, Valdiviezo C, et al. Update in atherothrombotic disease. *Mt Sinai J Med* 2004;71(3):197–208.
29. Callow AD. Endothelial dysfunction in atherosclerosis. *Vascul Pharmacol* 2002;38(5):257–258.
30. Malek AM, Alper SL, Izumo S. Hemodynamic shear stress and its role in atherosclerosis. *JAMA* 1999;282(21):2035–2042.
31. Ludmer PL, Selwyn AP, Shook TL, et al. Paradoxical vasoconstriction induced by acetylcholine in atherosclerotic coronary arteries. *N Engl J Med* 1986;315(17):1046–1051.
32. Bae JH. Noninvasive evaluation of endothelial function. *J Cardiol* 2001;37 (Suppl 1):89–92.
33. Davignon J, Ganz P. Role of endothelial dysfunction in atherosclerosis. *Circulation* 2004;109(23 Suppl 1):III27–III32.
34. de las Heras N, Cediel E, Oubina MP, et al. Comparison between the effects of mixed dyslipidaemia and hypercholesterolaemia on endothelial function, atherosclerotic lesions and fibrinolysis in rabbits. *Clin Sci (Lond)* 2003; 104(4):357–365.
35. Komori K, Shimokawa H, Vanhoutte PM. Hypercholesterolemia impairs endothelium-dependent relaxations to aggregating platelets in porcine iliac arteries. *J Vasc Surg* 1989;10(3):318–325.
36. Sellke FW, Armstrong ML, Harrison DG. Endothelium-dependent vascular relaxation is abnormal in the coronary microcirculation of atherosclerotic primates. *Circulation* 1990;81(5):1586–1593.
37. Shimokawa H. Primary endothelial dysfunction: atherosclerosis. *J Mol Cell Cardiol* 1999;31(1):23–37.
38. Blankenberg S, Barbaux S, Tiret L. Adhesion molecules and atherosclerosis. *Atherosclerosis* 2003;170(2):191–203.
39. Blann AD, Nadar SK, Lip GY. The adhesion molecule P-selectin and cardiovascular disease. *Eur Heart J* 2003;24(24):2166–2179.
40. Huo Y, Ley K. Adhesion molecules and atherogenesis. *Acta Physiol Scand* 2001;173(1):35–43.
41. Walpola PL, Gotlieb AI, Cybulsky MI, Langille BL. Expression of ICAM-1 and VCAM-1 and monocyte adherence in arteries exposed to altered shear stress. *Arterioscler Thromb Vasc Biol* 1995;15(1):2–10.
42. Davies MJ, Gordon JL, Gearing AJ, et al. The expression of the adhesion molecules ICAM-1, VCAM-1, PECAM, and E-selectin in human atherosclerosis. *J Pathol* 1993;171(3):223–229.

43. Johnson-Tidey RR, McGregor JL, Taylor PR, Poston RN. Increase in the adhesion molecule P-selectin in endothelium overlying atherosclerotic plaques. Coexpression with intercellular adhesion molecule-1. *Am J Pathol* 1994; 144(5):952–961.
44. Johnson RC, Chapman SM, Dong ZM, et al. Absence of P-selectin delays fatty streak formation in mice. *J Clin Invest* 1997;99(5):1037–1043.
45. Dong ZM, Chapman SM, Brown AA, Frenette PS, Hynes RO, Wagner DD. The combined role of P- and E-selectins in atherosclerosis. *J Clin Invest* 1998;102(1):145–152.
46. Schober A, Manka D, von Hundelshausen P, et al. Deposition of platelet RANTES triggering monocyte recruitment requires P-selectin and is involved in neointima formation after arterial injury. *Circulation* 2002;106(12):1523–1529.
47. Libby P, Aikawa M. Mechanisms of plaque stabilization with statins. *Am J Cardiol* 2003;91(4A):4B–8B.
48. Corti R, Osende JI, Fallon JT, et al. The selective peroxisomal proliferator-activated receptor-gamma agonist has an additive effect on plaque regression in combination with simvastatin in experimental atherosclerosis: in vivo study by high-resolution magnetic resonance imaging. *J Am Coll Cardiol* 2004;43(3):464–473.
49. Bhakdi S. [An alternative hypothesis of the pathogenesis of atherosclerosis.] *Herz* 1998;23(3):163–167.
50. Bhakdi S. Pathogenesis of atherosclerosis: infectious versus immune pathogenesis. A new concept. *Herz* 2000;25(2):84–86.
51. Fan J, Watanabe T. Inflammatory reactions in the pathogenesis of atherosclerosis. *J Atheroscler Thromb* 2003;10(2):63–71.
52. Arakawa K, Urata H. Hypothesis regarding the pathophysiological role of alternative pathways of angiotensin II formation in atherosclerosis. *Hypertension* 2000;36(4):638–641.
53. Wilhelm MG, Cooper AD. Induction of atherosclerosis by human chylomicron remnants: a hypothesis. *J Atheroscler Thromb* 2003;10(3):132–139.
54. Ross R, Glomset JA. Atherosclerosis and the arterial smooth muscle cell: proliferation of smooth muscle is a key event in the genesis of the lesions of atherosclerosis. *Science* 1973;180(93):1332–1339.
55. Ross R. Rous-Whipple Award Lecture. Atherosclerosis: a defense mechanism gone awry. *Am J Pathol* 1993;143(4):987–1002.
56. Ross R. Atherosclerosis is an inflammatory disease. *Am Heart J* 1999;138(5 Pt 2):S419–S420.
57. Willis AI, Pierre-Paul D, Sumpio BE, Gahtan V. Vascular smooth muscle cell migration: current research and clinical implications. *Vasc Endovasc Surg* 2004;38(1):11–23.
58. Reape TJ, Groot PH. Chemokines and atherosclerosis. *Atherosclerosis* 1999;147(2):213–225.
59. Monaco C, Andreakos E, Kiriakidis S, Feldmann M, Paleolog E. T-cell-mediated signalling in immune, inflammatory and angiogenic processes: the cascade of events leading to inflammatory diseases. *Curr Drug Targets Inflamm Allergy* 2004;3(1):35–42.
60. Rosenfeld ME. Oxidized LDL affects multiple atherogenic cellular responses. *Circulation* 1991;83(6):2137–2140.

61. Masuda J, Ross R. Atherogenesis during low level hypercholesterolemia in the nonhuman primate. II. Fatty streak conversion to fibrous plaque. *Arteriosclerosis* 1990;10(2):178–187.
62. Masuda J, Ross R. Atherogenesis during low level hypercholesterolemia in the nonhuman primate. I. Fatty streak formation. *Arteriosclerosis* 1990; 10(2):164–177.
63. Kim DN, Schmee J, Lee KT, Thomas WA. Intimal cell masses in the abdominal aortas of swine fed a low-fat, low-cholesterol diet for up to twelve years of age. *Atherosclerosis* 1985;55(2):151–159.
64. Newby AC, Zaltsman AB. Fibrous cap formation or destruction–the critical importance of vascular smooth muscle cell proliferation, migration and matrix formation. *Cardiovasc Res* 1999;41(2):345–360.
65. Paul O. Background of the prevention of cardiovascular disease. II. Arteriosclerosis, hypertension, and selected risk factors. *Circulation* 1989;80(1):206–214.
66. Finking G, Hanke H. Nikolaj Nikolajewitsch Anitschkow (1885–1964) established the cholesterol-fed rabbit as a model for atherosclerosis research. *Atherosclerosis* 1997;135(1):1–7.
67. Asztalos BF. High-density lipoprotein metabolism and progression of atherosclerosis: new insights from the HDL Atherosclerosis Treatment Study. *Curr Opin Cardiol* 2004;19(4):385–391.
68. Witztum JL, Steinberg D. The oxidative modification hypothesis of atherosclerosis: does it hold for humans? *Trends Cardiovasc Med* 2001;11(3–4):93–102.
69. Stary HC, Chandler AB, Dinsmore RE. A definition of advanced types of atherosclerotic lesions and a histological classification of atherosclerosis. A report from the Committee on Vascular Lesions of the Council on Arteriosclerosis. 1995.
70. Brown MS, Herz J, Goldstein JL. LDL-receptor structure. Calcium cages, acid baths and recycling receptors. *Nature* 1997;388(6643):629–630.
71. Navab M, Berliner JA, Watson AD, et al. The yin and yang of oxidation in the development of the fatty streak. A review based on the 1994 George Lyman Duff Memorial Lecture. *Arterioscler Thromb Vasc Biol* 1996;16(7):831–842.
72. Heinecke JW. Oxidants and antioxidants in the pathogenesis of atherosclerosis: implications for the oxidized low-density lipoprotein hypothesis. *Atherosclerosis* 1998;141(1):1–15.
73. Knowles JW, Reddick RL, Jennette JC, Shesely EG, Smithies O, Maeda N. Enhanced atherosclerosis and kidney dysfunction in eNOS(−/−)Apoe(−/−) mice are ameliorated by enalapril treatment. *J Clin Invest* 2000;105(4):451–458.
74. Harats D, Shaish A, George J, et al. Overexpression of 15-lipoxygenase in vascular endothelium accelerates early atherosclerosis in LDL receptor-deficient mice. *Arterioscler Thromb Vasc Biol* 2000;20(9):2100–2105.
75. Cyrus T, Witztum JL, Rader DJ, et al. Disruption of the 12/15-lipoxygenase gene diminishes atherosclerosis in apo E-deficient mice. *J Clin Invest* 1999;103(11):1597–1604.
76. Detmers PA, Hernandez M, Mudgett J, et al. Deficiency in inducible nitric oxide synthase results in reduced atherosclerosis in apolipoprotein E-deficient mice. *J Immunol* 2000;165(6):3430–3435.
77. Yusuf S, Dagenais G, Pogue J, Bosch J, Sleight P. Vitamin E supplementation and cardiovascular events in high-risk patients. The Heart Outcomes Prevention Evaluation Study Investigators. *N Engl J Med* 2000;342(3):154–160.

78. Warmington KS, Boring L, Ruth JH, et al. Effect of C-C chemokine receptor 2 (CCR2) knockout on type-2 (schistosomal antigen-elicited) pulmonary granuloma formation: analysis of cellular recruitment and cytokine responses. *Am J Pathol* 1999;154(5):1407–1416.
79. Hogaboam CM, Steinhauser ML, Chensue SW, Kunkel SL. Novel roles for chemokines and fibroblasts in interstitial fibrosis. *Kidney Int* 1998; 54(6):2152–2159.
80. Hogaboam CM, Bone-Larson CL, Lipinski S, et al. Differential monocyte chemoattractant protein-1 and chemokine receptor 2 expression by murine lung fibroblasts derived from Th1- and Th2-type pulmonary granuloma models. *J Immunol* 1999;163(4):2193–2201.
81. Gosling J, Slaymaker S, Gu L, et al. MCP-1 deficiency reduces susceptibility to atherosclerosis in mice that overexpress human apolipoprotein B. *J Clin Invest* 1999;103(6):773–778.
82. Libby P. Molecular bases of the acute coronary syndromes. *Circulation.* 1995;91(11):2844–2850.
83. Dong ZM, Chapman SM, Brown AA, Frenette PS, Hynes RO, Wagner DD. The combined role of P- and E-selectins in atherosclerosis. *J Clin Invest* 1998;102(1):145–152.
84. Suzuki H, Kurihara Y, Takeya M, et al. A role for macrophage scavenger receptors in atherosclerosis and susceptibility to infection. *Nature* 20 1997;386(6622):292–296.
85. Febbraio M, Podrez EA, Smith JD, et al. Targeted disruption of the class B scavenger receptor CD36 protects against atherosclerotic lesion development in mice. *J Clin Invest* 2000;105(8):1049–1056.
86. Tall AR, Jiang X, Luo Y, Silver D. 1999 George Lyman Duff memorial lecture: lipid transfer proteins, HDL metabolism, and atherogenesis. *Arterioscler Thromb Vasc Biol* 2000;20(5):1185–1188.
87. Rust S, Rosier M, Funke H, et al. Tangier disease is caused by mutations in the gene encoding ATP-binding cassette transporter 1. *Nat Genet* 1999; 22(4):352–355.
88. Thyberg J. Differentiated properties and proliferation of arterial smooth muscle cells in culture. *Int Rev Cytol* 1996;169:183–265.
89. Ross R. The pathogenesis of atherosclerosis: a perspective for the 1990s. *Nature* 1993;362(6423):801–809.
90. Benditt EP, Benditt JM. Evidence for a monoclonal origin of human atherosclerotic plaques. *Proc Natl Acad Sci USA* 1973;70(6):1753–1756.
91. Stoneman VE, Bennett MR. Role of apoptosis in atherosclerosis and its therapeutic implications. *Clin Sci (Lond)* 2004.
92. Dansky HM, Charlton SA, Harper MM, Smith JD. T and B lymphocytes play a minor role in atherosclerotic plaque formation in the apolipoprotein E-deficient mouse. *Proc Natl Acad Sci USA* 1997;94(9):4642–4646.
93. Cybulsky MI, Gimbrone MA, Jr. Endothelial expression of a mononuclear leukocyte adhesion molecule during atherogenesis. *Science* 1991; 251(4995):788–791.
94. Mosmann TR, Coffman RL. TH1 and TH2 cells: different patterns of lymphokine secretion lead to different functional properties. *Ann Rev Immunol* 1989;7:145–173.

95. Gupta S, Pablo AM, Jiang X, Wang N, Tall AR, Schindler C. IFN-gamma potentiates atherosclerosis in ApoE knock-out mice. *J Clin Invest* 1997;99(11):2752–2761.
96. Mallat Z, Besnard S, Duriez M, et al. Protective role of interleukin-10 in atherosclerosis. *Circ Res* 1999;85(8):e17–e24.
97. Mallat Z, Heymes C, Ohan J, Faggin E, Leseche G, Tedgui A. Expression of interleukin-10 in advanced human atherosclerotic plaques: relation to inducible nitric oxide synthase expression and cell death. *Arterioscler Thromb Vasc Biol* 1999;19(3):611–616.
98. Falk E. [Plaque vulnerability and disruption.] *Rev Clin Esp* 1996;196(4 Monografico):6–12.
99. Orekhov AN, Andreeva ER, Krushinsky AV, et al. Intimal cells and atherosclerosis. Relationship between the number of intimal cells and major manifestations of atherosclerosis in the human aorta. *Am J Pathol* 1986;125(2):402–415.
100. Fingerle J, Kraft T. The induction of smooth muscle cell proliferation *in vitro* using an organ culture system. *Int Angiol* 1987;6(1):65–72.
101. Soyombo AA, Thurston VJ, Newby AC. Endothelial control of vascular smooth muscle proliferation in an organ culture of human saphenous vein. *Eur Heart J* 1993;14 (Suppl I):201–206.
102. Kuhn C, 3rd, Boldt J, King TE, Jr., Crouch E, Vartio T, McDonald JA. An immunohistochemical study of architectural remodeling and connective tissue synthesis in pulmonary fibrosis. *Am Rev Respir Dis* 1989;140(6):1693–1703.
103. Magil AB, Cohen AH. Monocytes and focal glomerulosclerosis. *Lab Invest* 1989;61(4):404–409.
104. Thyberg J, Hedin U, Sjolund M, Palmberg L, Bottger BA. Regulation of differentiated properties and proliferation of arterial smooth muscle cells. *Arteriosclerosis* 1990;10(6):966–990.
105. Galis ZS, Sukhova GK, Lark MW, Libby P. Increased expression of matrix metalloproteinases and matrix degrading activity in vulnerable regions of human atherosclerotic plaques. *J Clin Invest* 1994;94(6):2493–2503.
106. Galis ZS, Sukhova GK, Kranzhofer R, Clark S, Libby P. Macrophage foam cells from experimental atheroma constitutively produce matrix-degrading proteinases. *Proc Natl Acad Sci USA* 1995;92(2):402–406.
107. George SJ, Zaltsman AB, Newby AC. Surgical preparative injury and neointima formation increase MMP-9 expression and MMP-2 activation in human saphenous vein. *Cardiovasc Res* 1997;33(2):447–459.
108. Gibbons GH, Pratt RE, Dzau VJ. Vascular smooth muscle cell hypertrophy vs. hyperplasia. Autocrine transforming growth factor-beta 1 expression determines growth response to angiotensin II. *J Clin Invest* 1992;90(2):456–461.
109. Lacy F, O'Connor DT, Schmid-Schonbein GW. Plasma hydrogen peroxide production in hypertensives and normotensive subjects at genetic risk of hypertension. *J Hypertens* 1998;16(3):291–303.
110. Swei A, Lacy F, DeLano FA, Schmid-Schonbein GW. Oxidative stress in the Dahl hypertensive rat. *Hypertension* 1997;30(6):1628–1633.
111. Wesley RB, 2nd, Meng X, Godin D, Galis ZS. Extracellular matrix modulates macrophage functions characteristic to atheroma: collagen type I enhances acquisition of resident macrophage traits by human peripheral blood monocytes *in vitro*. *Arterioscler Thromb Vasc Biol* 1998;18(3):432–440.
112. Vanhoutte PM, Boulanger CM. Endothelium-dependent responses in hypertension. *Hypertens Res* 1995;18(2):87–98.

113. Mercurius KO, Morla AO. Inhibition of vascular smooth muscle cell growth by inhibition of fibronectin matrix assembly. *Circ Res* 1998;82(5):548–556.
114. Assoian RK, Marcantonio EE. The extracellular matrix as a cell cycle control element in atherosclerosis and restenosis. *J Clin Invest* 1996;98(11):2436–2439.

6

Exercise Training and Endothelial Function in Patients at Risk for and with Documented Coronary Artery Disease

Tom LaFontaine and Jeffrey L. Roitmann

CONTENTS

Introduction 85
Chronic Physical Activity, Exercise Training, and Reduced Morbidity and Mortality 87
Chronic Physical Activity: Enhanced Endothelial Function/Reversal of Endothelial Dysfunction 88
Overview of Animal Studies 88
Exercise Training and Endothelial Function in Humans 91
Correction of Endothelial Dysfunction in Youth 97
Mechanisms of Improved Endothelial Function Following Exercise Training 98
Case Study 102
Summary 104
References 106

Introduction

Numerous interventions, aside from exercise, have been shown to attenuate endothelial dysfunction in humans (see Table 6.1).[1] Several studies demonstrate improved endothelial function following lipid altering therapy.[2–6] A recent study demonstrated improved endothelial function in elderly Type 2 diabetes mellitus patients with just 3 days of cerivastatin therapy.[6] Other studies have shown improved endothelial function following LDL pheresis and antioxidant therapy with Vitamin C.[7,8] The data on Vitamin E is

TABLE 6.1

Important Vasoactive, Inflammatory, and Thromboactive Molecules Produced by the Intact Endothelium

Nitric oxide (NO)
Angiotensin II
Bradykinin
Endothelins
Prostacyclin
Anti-inflammatories
Monocyte chemotactic factor-1 (MCP-1)
Adhesion molecules (VCAM-1, selectins)
Interleukins 1, 6, & 18
Tumor necrosis factor
Tissue plasminogen activator
Plasminogen activator inhibitor-1 (PAI-1)
Prostaglandins
Von Willebrand's factor
Endothelial hyperpolarizing factor

equivocal although a recent report found that 2 weeks of Vitamin E therapy decreased P-selectin in dyslipidemic patients suggesting an improved environment favoring vasodilation.[9] However, recent studies have shown no benefit of antioxidant therapy on long-term morbidity and mortality among patients with or at risk for cardiovascular disease (CVD).[10] Several reports have shown that interventions, including ACE inhibitors, HMG-CoA reductase inhibitors, folic acid supplementation in hyperhomocysteinemic patients, grape juice, tea, dark chocolate, walnuts, L-arginine in high doses, iron chelation, tetrahydrobiopterin, and recently ACEII Receptor 1 blockers attenuate coronary endothelial dysfunction in patients with coronary artery disease (CAD).[2,11–16]

Exercise training, particularly in combination with comprehensive lifestyle changes, has been shown to reduce the risk for the development and progression of atherosclerosis and related manifestations, including sudden death and recurrent revascularizations.[17–22] Numerous studies have reported that physically active or fit persons have a significantly lower risk for cardiovascular morbidity and mortality even in the presence of major and traditional CAD risk factors.[23,24] However, the mechanism for these observed benefits is incompletely understood. Recent evidence has demonstrated that exercise training with or without diet and weight loss improves endothelial function among populations of children and adolescents with CAD risk factors and patients with long-standing diseases such as hypertension, dyslipidemia, diabetes, CAD, and congestive heart failure. This chapter discusses the particular role of exercise training in preserving normal endothelial function and in improving or reversing endothelial dysfunction in patients with or at risk for cardiovascular disease.

Chronic Physical Activity, Exercise Training, and Reduced Morbidity and Mortality

Wannamethee et al., in a prospective, 5-year cohort study, reported approximately a 50% reduction in CVD mortality and morbidity in patients with documented CAD who became or remained active compared with those who remained sedentary.[25] A recent 1-year follow-up investigation of post-CAD patients in cardiovascular rehabilitation (CVR) by Steffen-Batey et al. reported similar results.[26] The results of the ETICA study showed after 33 months of follow-up that 11.9% of patients who exercise trained (26% increase in VO_2 peak) after PTCA and/or stent implantation had a recurrent event compared with 32.2% among patients who did not exercise.[22]

Several meta-analyses have confirmed a 20–25% reduction in CVD mortality following participation in CVR.[27,28] Similar findings were reported in a recent meta-analysis that included data from trials for emergency thrombolysis and rescue percutaneous coronary interventions (PCI).[29]

In a single-center randomized trial in Finland, Hammalainen et al., after a 10-year follow-up of CVR following myocardial infarction, reported a 37% reduction in sudden death among patients participating in a multifactorial intervention program.[30] At 15 years, 16.5% of patients who were initially randomized to CVR experienced sudden death compared with 28.9% ($p < 0.006$) of patients randomized initially to the control group.[31] Coronary mortality was 47.9% and 58.5% ($p < 0.04$) in the CVR and control groups, respectively. Recently, Witt et al., in a study of community CVR following myocardial infarction, observed a 72% reduction in risk of mortality among participants versus non-participants in CVR.[32] Thus, it is clear that exercise training and comprehensive CVR in CAD patients improves mortality and, perhaps, morbidity. However, the mechanisms for these observed benefits have not been completely elucidated.

Numerous studies have shown that regular exercise training in patients at risk for or with CAD improves lipids, diabetes, hypertension, obesity, and thrombogenic risk factors.[33–35] However, the benefit of exercise on mortality and morbidity in CAD patients is independent of, and sometimes disproportionate to the effect on risk factors.[23,24] Exercise training improves myocardial perfusion, but has limited effect on the size and extent of atherosclerotic lesions.[17,21] Recent studies suggest that a mechanism by which exercise training in CAD patients reduces progression of atherosclerosis and risk for recurrent events is improvement in vascular tone and endothelial function.[36–45]

Chronic Physical Activity: Enhanced Endothelial Function/ Reversal of Endothelial Dysfunction

Overview of Animal Studies

The animal research provides substantial support for the beneficial influence of regular physical activity on endothelial function, particularly in the presence of established risk factors, endothelial dysfunction, and atherosclerosis. Numerous studies have shown that systematic exercise training can improve endothelium dependent vasodilation (EDD) in several animal species.[46–48] This section will provide a review of several pertinent investigations. For excellent and more comprehensive summaries of the basic animal research relating to exercise and its effect on endothelial and smooth muscle cellular function, the reader is referred to three excellent reviews.[46–48]

Muller and colleagues examined EDD in isolated arteries from the hearts of pigs and reported that arterioles and slightly larger resistance arteries from trained pigs showed significantly better EDD than the same arteries from untrained pigs.[49] These authors further demonstrated that this beneficial response was lost when endothelial nitric oxide synthase (eNOS) was blocked. Laughlin et al. and Woodman et al. also reported that exercise training increased mRNA for the eNOS gene in coronary arterioles and eNOS content in coronary arterioles and small resistance arteries.[50,51]

One hypothesis of the mechanism of how regular exercise improves EDD is through the effects of increased blood flow and shear stress acting on endothelial cells.[52] Results of studies in rats and dogs with an arterial-venous fistula that produced increased blood flow and shear stress demonstrated increased eNOS expression and improved endothelial function.[53,54] Woodman et al. reported that e-NOS expression is increased in isolated coronary arteries of pigs exposed to increased intraluminal flow for 4 h.[55] Other studies have shown that hindlimb unweighting of the rat soleus muscle for 2 weeks, a procedure that would reduce intraluminal blood flow and shear stress, resulted in decreased EDD in the feed arteries and 1A arterioles, but no change in 2A arterioles.[56–58]

Laughlin and colleagues addressed the non-uniformity across vascular beds in EDD and eNOS protein in response to exercise training.[47,59] In general it appeared that EDD was improved more in smaller coronary resistance than in larger conduit arteries, although eNOS protein content per gram of total protein was greater in the large coronary arteries.

Wang et al. reported that EDD was enhanced in large conduit coronary arteries but not in coronary resistance arteries of dogs.[60] In contrast, Laughlin and colleagues have reported increased EDD in coronary resistance arteries, but not in conduit arteries following longer-term training.[47] Laughlin et al. recently reported that short-term training (1 h 3.5 mph × 7 days) resulted in improved EDD in the conduit arteries of pigs, but not arterioles and that these short-term effects were not associated with changes in eNOS or superoxide dismutase (SOD-1).[61] These contrasting results suggested that the early adaptive response in the arterial tree may differ depending on the length of the exercise training period. Thus, EDD of conduit arteries appears to be enhanced early (7–10 days) in the adaptive process, but returns towards the pre-training state after several weeks of training. The responses in resistance or smaller order arterioles may involve a longer-term adaptation process. There also is the possibility of species differences. Perhaps with sustained training, EDD in conduit arteries normalizes as structural adaptations such as increased vessel diameter become manifest.

Laughlin and colleagues have reported improved EDD following exercise training in hypercholesterolemic pigs and in pigs subjected to progressive coronary artery occlusion and atherosclerosis induced by a high fat diet.[47,62–65] Henderson et al. hypothesized, for example, that exercise training would improve endothelial function of coronary arterioles of pigs in the early stages of coronary artery atherosclerosis induced by a high-fat, high-cholesterol diet.[66] Yucatan miniature swine were randomized to a normal fat diet (8% fat calories) or a high-fat diet (46% fat calories). Both groups were then subdivided into sedentary or exercise-trained groups. Responses to EDD induced by bradykinin, ADP, and increased blood flow were similar among groups after 20 weeks. However, EDD in response to aggregating platelets in the presence of indomethacin and ketanserin was attenuated in the high-fat sedentary animals whereas this attenuated response was prevented or reversed in the high-fat exercise trained animals. The mechanism of the observed improved EDD with exercise training may be related to increased eNOS expression and NO bioavailability, attenuation of a bradykinin induced release of an indomethacin-sensitive prostanoid constrictor, and/or decreased release of a vasoconstrictor substance produced by the action of the cyclooxygenase enzyme.[47]

Davis et al. demonstrated that 3 weeks of exercise training in c-SRC deficient mice resulted in no effect on either eNOS gene expression or the expression of SOD-1.[67] This finding further supported NO as the mediator of enhanced EDD. Graham and Rush recently reported that gp91phox-dependent oxidative stress and reduced antioxidant capacity contributed to impaired EDD in spontaneously hypertensive rats.[68] In contrast, exercise training reduced gp91phox-dependent oxidative stress, enhanced endothelial eNOS-derived NO and contributed to restored EDD. Yamashita et al. reported that exercise provided cardio-protection via activation of manganese SOD that decreases oxidative damage in endothelial cells.[69]

Several additional studies have shown that eNOS inhibition and decreased NO bioavailability promotes atherosclerosis.[70–75] Thus, one mechanism for how exercise training may prevent the development of atherosclerosis and/or retard its progression and prevent atherosclerotic events is through increasing NO bioavailability. Neibauer et al. investigated the effect of exercise in hypercholesterolemic, Apo-E deficient mice.[76] The mice were assigned to four groups: sedentary, exercise, sedentary plus eNOS inhibition, and exercise plus eNOS inhibition. The mice were trained on treadmills, 6 days per week, 2 h per day. Arteries of the sedentary, eNOS inhibited mice manifested a threefold greater atherosclerotic lesion formation compared with the exercise trained eNOS inhibited mice. In fact, there was no lesion formation in the exercise trained eNOS-inhibited animals, suggesting that regular exercise training completely counteracted the atherogenic effect of decreased NO bioavailability.

Fogarty et al. hypothesized that exercise training improves endothelial dysfunction by enhancing NO-mediated vasodilator responses to vascular endothelial growth factor (VEGF-165) in arteries exposed to chronic coronary occlusion.[77] Using female Yucatan miniswine, these investigators induced chronic proximal left circumflex occlusion with the ameroid occluder technique. Eight weeks post-surgery, the animals were randomized to either 14 weeks of inactivity or 5 days/week of exercise training on a treadmill. In non-occluded arteries, exercise training had no effect. However, exercise training markedly enhanced VEGF-165-induced vasodilation of collateral-dependent left circumflex arterioles. Furthermore, VEGF-165-induced vasodilation of the occluded left circumflex of exercise-trained swine exceeded that of non-occluded exercise-trained or sedentary left anterior descending artery (LAD) arterioles. Enhanced vasodilation of exercise-trained left circumflex arterioles was abolished by inhibition of eNOS. Combined inhibition of eNOS and cyclo-oxygenase decreased VEGF-165 induced vasodilation of all vessels. These results further support the conclusion that exercise-induced improvement in EDD is mediated via increased NO.

Laughlin et al. recently reported that sprint training (six bouts of treadmill running, 2.5 min at 60 m/min with 4.5 min rest periods, 5 days/week) improved ACH-induced vasodilation in rat white gastrocnemius second-order arterioles, but not in 2A or 3A arterioles in red muscle fibers.[78] This study suggested that training-specific effects may occur predominantly in white anaerobic versus red aerobic muscle fibers.

Several additional studies supported the role of exercise training in improving EDD via increasing eNOS and NO bioavailability. Tanabe et al. reported that exercise training of aging rats attenuated the aging-related decrease in eNOS and NO production and release in the aorta.[79] Regarding gender differences, Laughlin et al. found that baseline eNOS expression is greater in female compared with male pigs but that the increase in eNOS expression following exercise training is similar among genders.[80]

Recently, Suvorava et al. investigated the effects of physical inactivity on endothelial dysfunction in young healthy male mice.[81] The mice were randomized to either continue living in large groups of five in large cages where they were running, climbing, fighting, etc. or to live alone in small cages where they were primarily resting (sedentary). Aerobic capacity of skeletal muscle decreased significantly in the inactive mice ($p < 0.05$) as did EDD ($p < 0.001$) and eNOS protein expression ($p < 0.01$). These alterations in aerobic capacity, EDD, and vascular eNOS expression were completely reversible when the mice living alone underwent regular exercise training. This study nicely demonstrated in mice the dramatic negative effect of physical inactivity on vascular function and muscle aerobic capacity that is completely reversible by a short period of moderate exercise training.

In an interesting study, Hayward et al. investigated the effects of exercise training (30 min/day, for 8 weeks at a moderate to high intensity) in rats on endothelial function following exposure to the chemotherapeutic agent 5-fluorouracil (5-FU).[82] It had been demonstrated previously that 5-FU induces endothelial-independent vasoconstriction of vascular smooth muscle.[83] The results showed that exercise training enhanced EDD after 5-FU-induced vasoconstriction due, at least in part, to an increase in aortic eNOS protein content and activity.

Recently, an association between atherosclerosis, endothelial dysfunction, and low levels of bone marrow-derived endothelial progenitor cells (EPCs) has been reported.[84] Progenitor cells are primitive bone marrow cells that have the capacity to proliferate, migrate, and differentiate into various mature cell types including endothelial cells. EPCs may play a critical role in endothelial cell maintenance and repair and have been implicated in promoting both re-endothelialization and neovascularization.[85] Thus, EPCs may prevent endothelial dysfunction by contributing to the repair of damaged endothelial cells, maintaining vascular homeostasis, and promoting angiogenesis. One study of mice randomized to exercise training on running wheels or no running demonstrated that exercise training increases the production and circulating number of EPCs, inhibits neointimal formation after vascular injury, promotes angiogenesis, and decreases apoptosis of endothelial cells.[86] In addition, these authors also demonstrated increased circulating EPCs and reduced EPC apoptosis in the blood of exercise-trained humans with CAD.

Numerous additional studies in several species have demonstrated improved coronary and peripheral artery and arteriole EDD, increased expression of eNOS, increased NO bioavailability, and reduced oxidative stress following exercise training.[46–48,87,88] In conclusion, the animal evidence provides overwhelming support for the beneficial effects of exercise training on EDD in most vascular beds.

Exercise Training and Endothelial Function in Humans

Haskell et al. compared coronary vascular reactivity in ultra-distance runners and sedentary gender and age-matched men and women using quantitative angiography.[89] There was no significant difference among groups in basal diameter of epicardial coronary arteries. However, during angiography, when intravenous nitroglycerin, a stimulator of EDD was injected, the coronary arteries of the ultra-distance runners demonstrated a 200% greater increase in vasodilation than in the coronary arteries of sedentary men and women. This was one of the first studies to suggest improved endothelial function in highly physically active persons compared with sedentary peers. Kingwell et al. and others have reported improved EDD in healthy physically active subjects compared with sedentary young and middle-aged men and women and following aerobic exercise training in these same groups [90–93]

Cross-sectional studies show that age-related increases in arterial stiffness are attenuated in endurance-trained adults.[40,41] Tanaka et al. demonstrated that exercise training (walking/jogging, 40–45 min/session, 4–6 days/week at 70–75% of maximum heart rate) significantly improved arterial compliance.[40] These effects were independent of changes in body mass, adiposity, blood pressure, or peak oxygen uptake. In a second study, Tanaka and colleagues demonstrated that regular aerobic exercise for 3 months (primarily walking) restored age-related reductions in central arterial compliance in previously sedentary but healthy middle-aged and older men (18–77 years of age).[41] Clarkson et al. reported that a 10-week program of anaerobic and aerobic exercise in young military recruits resulted in improved EDD of the brachial artery as measured by flow mediated dilation (FMD) but there were no changes in endothelial-independent dilation (EID) assessed by nitroglycerine infusion.[91] DeSouza et al. found no age-related decline in EDD in response to acetylcholine in endurance-trained men.[42] In a sub-study of 13 middle-aged sedentary men who trained for 12 weeks, FMD increased 30% ($p < 0.01$) and was found to be similar to levels found in young adults and middle-aged and older endurance-trained men.

In another cross-sectional study, Taddei et al. reported that endurance training can prevent the age-associated endothelial dysfunction through the restoration of NO availability consequent to the prevention of oxidative stress.[43] These reports provided provocative evidence that endurance exercise training may prevent or attenuate the age-related decline in endothelium-dependent vasodilation and restore levels in previously sedentary middle-aged and older men.

Maiorana et al., in a randomized crossover study of combined aerobic and resistance training in healthy middle-aged men, found that exercise training did not affect either EDD or EID.[92] This is one of the few published studies that demonstrated no beneficial effect of exercise training on endothelial function and, according to Maiorana et al., raises the possibility that augmentation of endothelial function may occur more readily in patients with endothelial dysfunction.[46] In contrast, these same authors reported improved EDD and EID in CHF patients and EDD in Type 2 diabetes mellitus patients in response to combined aerobic and resistance training.[39,94]

Exercise training has been shown to improve insulin sensitivity and glycemic control in patients with diabetes mellitus and blood pressure in patients with Stages 1 and 2 hypertension.[34,35] Patients with diabetes, abnormal lipids, or hypertension or who are overweight, with or without central obesity, who are physically active and/or physically fit, have lower rates of CVD and all-cause mortality.[95,96] However, the mechanisms facilitating these benefits of exercise are incompletely understood. Recently, several groups have reported improved EDD following exercise training in patients with diabetes, hypertension, and documented coronary and/or peripheral atherosclerosis.

Higashi et al. studied the effects of exercise training on forearm blood flow in 17 patients with Stage 1 hypertension.[38] After 12 weeks, FMD during reactive hyperemia increased significantly ($p < 0.05$) in the exercise training group compared with the control group. There also was an increase in acetylcholine-stimulated NO release. This study also demonstrated improved EDD following exercise training in Stage 1 hypertensive patients that was mediated through increased endothelial release of NO. A study of combined aerobic and resistance exercise for 8 weeks in patients with Type 2 diabetes mellitus demonstrated enhanced EDD in conduit and resistance vessels.[39]

Guan-Da investigated the effects of aerobic exercise training (subjects progressed to 40–45 min of walking, 4–6 days per week at 70–75% of heart rate maximum) on EDD in 30 sedentary Chinese men with impaired fasting glucose (IFG) (mean age = 63 years).[97] After 6 months of training, EDD was significantly improved. Fuchsjager-Mayerl et al. reported similar findings in persons with Type 1 diabetes mellitus.[98] These authors exercise trained 26 persons with Type 1 diabetes mellitus with no evidence of overt angiopathy for 4 months. Peak oxygen uptake increased 27% and FMD was significantly enhanced. After 8 months of detraining, the vascular benefits were completely reversed. Lavrencic et al. also reported that physical training improves FMD in patients with the metabolic syndrome.[99]

Studies have shown that persons with high normal or Stage 1 hypertension who exhibit an exaggerated blood pressure response to aerobic exercise are at a significantly increased risk for worsening blood pressure.[100,101] Recently, Stewart et al. investigated the relationship between an exaggerated blood pressure response to exercise and EDD as assessed by FMD among 38 men and 44 women, 55–75 years of age with high normal blood pressure (prehypertension) or mild Stage 1 hypertension.[102] Overall, FMD accounted for 11% and 10%, respectively, of the variance in maximal SBP and maximal pulse pressure. The authors concluded that the results suggest that endothelial dysfunction may be a mechanism contributing to an exaggerated exercise blood pressure response and may be a link between exercise hypertension and worsening resting hypertension. Chang et al. reported similar findings in a study comparing 25 men and women with an exaggerated blood pressure response (defined as ≥ 210 mmHg in men and ≥ 190 mmHg in women) to 25 men and women with a normal blood pressure response during dynamic treadmill exercise testing.[103]

A recent study by Hambrecht et al. demonstrated improved vasodilatory capacity in the coronary arteries of patients with documented CAD and endothelial dysfunction.[44] Patients were randomized to an exercise training group and to a control group. Exercise training consisted of 4 weeks of 6 times/day, supervised 10-min exercise sessions on bicycle ergometers at 80% of peak heart rate. Paradoxical vasoconstriction of coronary arteries in response to acetylcholine infusion was reduced by 54% in the exercise group compared with the control group. Exercise training also resulted in significantly improved coronary blood-flow reserve ($p < 0.01$) and EDD ($p < 0.01$) compared with the control group. This study was the first to demonstrate improved endothelial function following aerobic exercise training in the coronary arteries of patients with CAD and documented endothelial dysfunction without evidence of CHF.

Linke et al. recently investigated the systemic effects of lower body exercise training on radial artery endothelial function.[45] Twenty-two male patients with CHF (left ventricular ejection fractions = 24 ± 2%) were randomized to either exercise training or an inactive control group. After 4 weeks, exercise trained patients demonstrated a significant increase in the baseline corrected internal diameter of the radial artery in response to acetylcholine infusion. In the training group, increases in agonist-mediated FMD correlated with changes in functional work capacity.

Hambrecht et al. also investigated the effects of 6 months of training on endothelial function in congestive heart failure (CHF) patients.[104] After training, EDD increased significantly ($p < 0.05$) in response to acetylcholine compared with the control group. Increased peak oxygen uptake was correlated with increased EDD. Hambrecht et al. reported similar findings in another study of CHF patients.[37] In this study, administration of L-arginine concurrent with exercise training further improved EDD. This suggested that an increase in NO bioavailability via supplementation with L-arginine, the substrate for NO formation, complemented the shear stress-induced increase in eNOS activity. Several other investigators have reported similar findings in CHF patients.[94,105,106]

An ongoing debate in CVR centers around the role of home-based compared with hospital or clinic-based programming. Gielen et al. recently investigated the effects of home-based versus hospital-based exercise training on coronary vasomotion.[107] Nineteen patients with CAD and documented coronary endothelial dysfunction were randomized to an in-hospital exercise training program ($n = 10$) for 4 weeks (60 min per day in 10–15-min sessions of bicycle ergometry) or a control group ($n = 9$). After 4 weeks, all training patients were enrolled in a 5-month home-based exercise program (20 min per day of bicycle ergometry plus one 60-min group session per week). Coronary artery endothelial function was assessed by ACH infusion and quantitative angiography at 4 weeks and 6 months. Endothelial dysfunction was significantly improved in the exercise training compared with the control group at 4 weeks and at 6 months. However, endothelial function was worse at 6 months compared with 4 weeks in the exercise-trained group. ACH-induced increases in coronary blood flow were also improved significantly at 4 weeks and 6 months but it was attenuated at the 6-month evaluation. Although this study did not directly compare a home-based (non-randomized and the home-based program involved a 1-hour session each week at the hospital) versus a hospital-based program, it suggested that there is a relation between daily training duration (60 min daily in the hospital-based versus 20 min daily in the home-based program) and improved coronary vasomotion.

An unresolved issue involves the systemic versus local nature of the effects of exercise training on endothelial function. Walsh et al. randomized ten persons with CAD in a crossover design to 8 weeks of combined lower body aerobic and resistance training.[108] FMD in response to reactive hyperemia was assessed before and after training. Baseline function in the exercise-trained group was compared with a convenience sample of ten controls without documented cardiovascular disease. Both EDD and EID of the brachial artery were impaired in untrained persons with CAD. Training significantly improved FMD, but not endothelial-independent vasodilation (EID). The effect of exercise training on EDD appeared to be generalized or systemic rather than limited to the exercise trained vascular beds.

In contrast, in patients with CHF, Kobayashi et al. recently reported that exercise training appeared to improve EDD only in the trained extremities.[109] These investigators randomized 28 persons with CHF to either a control group or an aerobic exercise training group that underwent 3 months of cycle ergometry. Walking performance, as assessed by the 6-min walk test, increased significantly only in the exercise group. FMD of the posterior tibial artery improved but there were no changes in the brachial artery in the exercise-trained group. Neither brachial nor posterior tibial artery EDD improved in the control group. Thus, exercise training appeared to correct endothelial dysfunction predominantly via a local effect in the trained limbs. Gokce et al. reported similar findings in a study of the effects of aerobic exercise on EDD in the peripheral circulation in 58 patients with CAD (mean age = 59 years).[110] FMD in response to reactive hyperemia and nitroglycerine-mediated vasodilation was assessed before and after 10 weeks of standard CVR (mostly lower limb exercise, 30 min, moderate intensity, 3 days/week) in 40 patients and 18 matched patients who remained sedentary. Exercise training resulted in a 29% increase in maximal METs and improved EDD in the leg, but not the arm vasculature. No changes occurred in nitroglycerine-mediated EID.

Edwards et al. recently reported the results of exercise training in a standard (upper and lower body aerobic exercise) CVR program on endothelial function in persons with documented CAD.[111] After 12 weeks, FMD of the brachial artery improved by 11.1%. Exercise training increased plasma nitrite and nitrate levels and SOD-1 activity and decreased oxidative stress. Belardinelli, in an excellent review of the role of vasomotor reactivity and the effects of exercise training on FMD in CVR patients, concluded that shear stress produced by pulsatile blood flow during exercise may be the most important factor inducing e-NOS activation, increased NO synthesis, and improved endothelial function.[112]

The benefits of exercise training on EDD are well documented. However, little is known about the optimal exercise intensity, frequency, duration, mode, volume, and other factors involved in an effective exercise prescription. Goto et al. recently investigated the effects of exercise intensity on EDD in 26 healthy, young men.[113] Subjects were randomized to 12 weeks of bicycle ergometry training, 30 min, 5–7 days/week at 25%, 50%, or 75% of maximal oxygen uptake. Forearm blood flow response to ACH (EDD) and isosorbide dinitrate (EID) was assessed before and after training. Only the group that exercised at 50% of maximal oxygen uptake demonstrated improved EDD. No group showed improved EID. The administration of L-NMMA (an inhibitor of eNOS) abolished the enhanced EDD in the 50% group. High intensity (75% of maximal oxygen uptake) appeared to increase, while moderate intensity (50% of maximal oxygen uptake) appeared to decrease oxidative stress. Mild exercise (25% of maximal oxygen uptake) did not alter any parameters. The finding that training at 75% of maximal oxygen uptake appeared to increase oxidative stress and did not improve endothelial function is provocative. Thus, intense exercise may impair EDD by increasing oxidative stress. However, Goto et al. were unable to demonstrate a relationship between EDD and oxidative stress in their healthy young subjects. Matsumoto et al. previously reported that NO increases with increasing intensity of exercise perhaps in response to the increased oxidative stress resulting in maintained endothelial function.[114] Although the Goto et al. study is provocative, further work with larger samples and in patients with risk factors and CAD is needed before reasonable conclusions may be drawn regarding the mode, frequency, intensity, duration, and volume of exercise necessary to enhance endothelial function.

Bergholm et al. reported that 3 months of high-intensity running (80% of maximal oxygen uptake, 1 h/session, 4 days/week) decreased circulating antioxidant levels resulting in impaired EDD, but not EID.[115] These authors postulated that high intensity training-induced decreases in circulating antioxidants may adversely affect EDD. It is also possible that these effects are transient, and that long-term (6–12 months or longer) exercise training may lead to increased antioxidative capacity and changes in vascular structure and function that facilitate improved blood flow to working muscles (i.e., increased vessel size and enhanced capillarization).

Previous studies investigated the effects of exercise training on endothelial function in stable CAD or CHF patients and in patients with CAD risk factors. Hosakawa et al. performed a non-randomized study of the effect of regular aerobic exercise training on endothelial function in 41 post-MI patients who also had undergone percutaneous coronary angioplasty (PTCA).[116] The investigators examined a non-infarct related coronary artery via ACH infusion at baseline and 6 months post-MI. Endothelial function was significantly improved in the regular exercise group ($n = 24$) compared with the non-exerciser group ($n = 17$). Regular exercise was the only significant predictor of improvement in endothelial function. Recently, Vona et al. examined the effects of 3 months of moderate aerobic training (40 min of cycle ergometry, 3 days/week, at 75% of peak exercise heart rate or ~ 60% of maximal oxygen uptake) in 54 patients with documented CAD and a recent MI.[117] Compliance to the training program was 88%. FMD of the brachial artery was significantly impaired at 3 weeks post MI. After excluding patients on statins or ACE inhibitors that have documented beneficial effects on endothelial function, patients with classic risk factors known to impair endothelial function, and patients with left ventricular dysfunction, only 54 of 968 patients (5.6%) were randomized to the exercise or the control group. This study therefore allowed for an independent evaluation of the effects of exercise training on endothelial dysfunction in patients with a recent MI. The results showed that FMD significantly improved in the trained compared with the control group. In addition, FMD was correlated with increased maximal oxygen uptake, as has been demonstrated in other studies.[93,104,118]

Although this review has focused on NO and enhanced endothelial vasodilatory capacity, exercise may also improve EDD via mechanisms related to reduced vasoconstrictive factors. Endothelin-1 (ET-1) and angiotensin II are the primary endothelial-derived substances that induce vasoconstriction.[18,119] Therefore, lower levels of ET-1 are associated with less vasoconstrictive tone and a greater capacity for unopposed vasodilation. Maeda and colleagues have reported significantly higher ET-1 concentration in young athletic humans after 30 min of cycle ergometry above (130%) and below (90%) the ventilatory threshold and that aerobic exercise training results in decreased ET-1 concentration in healthy, young adults.[119,120] In a recent study of healthy older women (61–69 years of age), 3 months of aerobic exercise training using bicycle ergometers at 80% of ventilatory threshold for 30 min, 5 days/week significantly decreased plasma ET-1.[121] This reduction in ET-1 may have beneficial effects on EDD and may contribute to the prevention of hypertension and the development and progression of atherosclerosis. Callaerta-Vegh et al. reported no change in ET-1 in CHF patients after myocardial infarction following 8 weeks of exercise training.[122] In addition, nitrate elimination which mirrors NO production was decreased over 2 months following myocardial infarction. However, exercise training reversed this trend suggesting increased NO bioavailability. Maeda and colleagues interestingly have reported an increase in ET-1 production in inactive muscles of humans during exercise and also a reduction in the magnitude of the decrease in blood flow to the splanchnic bed after ET-1 blockade in rats.[123,124] It is beyond the scope of this chapter to thoroughly discuss the effect of exercise training on ET-1. For more information we recommend reviewing the articles by Maeda et al.[119,120]

Correction of Endothelial Dysfunction in Youth

Atherosclerosis often begins in childhood and endothelial dysfunction appears to be a necessary stage in the transition from normal vascular structure and function to plaque formation and obstructive atherosclerotic disease. Consistent with the recognition of the role of endothelial dysfunction in the early onset of atherosclerotic vascular disease, several studies have shown that overweight and obese children and adolescents demonstrate impaired endothelial function as assessed by FMD.[125,126] Three recent studies demonstrate that exercise training improves endothelial dysfunction in overweight and obese children and adolescents.[127–130]

Watts et al. studied the influence of aerobic exercise on endothelial function in 14 obese children (8.9 ± 0.4 years of age).[127] All subjects initially demonstrated impaired FMD. After 8 weeks of exercise training, FMD significantly improved in the obese children compared with a matched non-exercise trained control group. In another study of 19 obese adolescents, mean age of 14.3 years, with impaired endothelial function, Watts et al. reported that 8 weeks of circuit training (combined aerobic and resistance training) normalized FMD.[128] Finally, Woo et al. reported that diet and exercise training in 82 9–12-year-old obese children with impaired endothelial function resulted in improved FMD at 6 weeks and a reduction in carotid intima-media thickness at 1 year.[129,130]

Mechanisms of Improved Endothelial Function Following Exercise Training

Although the literature clearly supports a direct effect of exercise training in both animals and humans on improving endothelial function, particularly in the presence of impaired EDD, the mechanisms of this benefit are incompletely understood. Numerous investigators have examined the role of several observed vascular adaptations to exercise training that may explain the exercise training-induced improvements in EDD.

Exercise training has been repeatedly shown to improve myocardial perfusion in CAD and CHF patients and to reduce clinical events.[17–22,26–33] Hambrecht suggests that four mechanisms are important mediators of the observed reduction in morbidity and mortality with exercise training and CVR: improved endothelial function, reduced progression of coronary lesions, reduced thrombogenic risk, and improved coronary collateral circulation.[131]

Regression of coronary atherosclerotic lesions has been reported following high-volume exercise training, particularly when combined with low-fat diet, lipid-lowering medications, and other lifestyle changes such as tobacco cessation.[17–19,21] However, the magnitude of the change in coronary stenoses is small (~ 41–37% after 1 year, for example in the Lifestyle Heart Trial).[17] It is unlikely that this degree of change can explain the observed improvement in myocardial perfusion and reduction in clinical events following sustained exercise training.

Studies have shown that coronary diameter increases with exercise training but again this cannot adequately explain the improved myocardial perfusion following exercise training.[89] Additionally, human studies do not document any significant increases in coronary collateral circulation in response to exercise training.[132]

The vascular endothelium releases tissue-type plasminogen activator (t-PA) that is critical for effective endogenous fibrinolysis. A recent study of 62 men, aged 22–35 or 50–75 years, who were either sedentary or endurance exercise trained, found that net t-PA release was significantly blunted in the older men.[133] At the highest dose of bradykinin, the increase in t-PA release was 35% less in the older, sedentary men compared with the younger sedentary men. In contrast, the endurance trained older men did not demonstrate an age-related decline in net t-PA release and activity. In a subgroup of sedentary older men who completed 3 months of endurance exercise training, the capacity of the endothelium to release t-PA increased 55% over baseline and was comparable with that observed in younger sedentary men. This study suggests that other aspects of endothelial function such as antithrombotic functions can also be enhanced with regular endurance exercise and may be partially responsible for the reduction in cardiovascular mortality and morbidity observed in physically active and fit individuals.

Thus, improvement in endothelial function favoring vasodilation, fibrinolysis, less oxidative stress, and reduced arterial inflammation may explain observed improvements in myocardial perfusion and reduced clinical events following a regular aerobic exercise program. It also is possible that the shear stress associated with increased blood flow during exercise results in vascular remodeling leading to an increased heart and skeletal muscle capillarity (angiogenesis) and enlargement of conduit vessels (arteriogenesis).[134,135] However, the following discussion will focus on factors which result in improved endothelial function, particularly EDD as a mechanism for reduction in risk of clinical cardiovascular disease and events.

Cell culture studies and animal experiments suggest that shear stress increases endothelial L-arginine uptake and enhances eNOS activity and expression. These changes result in increased NO bioavailability, as well as increased activity of SOD-1 thus preventing premature NO breakdown.[136,137]

Maiorana et al. and Green et al., in excellent review articles cited earlier, concluded that the animal literature suggests that initially (1–4 weeks) exercise training enhances eNOS expression and NO bioavailability in order to buffer the increased shear stress associated with exercise hyperemia.[46,48] With prolonged training of greater than 4 weeks, structural adaptations become manifest resulting in increased lumen diameter, thus normalizing shear stress. Endothelial-derived NO then returns towards baseline. In support of this hypothesis, Oltman et al. reported that after 16 weeks of training (pigs) that vasodilator response to adenosine in large epicardial arteries remains augmented even after the endothelium was removed.[138]

Fukai et al. and Gielen both conclude that exercise training may improve EDD and myocardial perfusion by increasing eNOS and SOD-1 expression and NO bioavailability.[139,140] Gielen speculated that these changes occur rapidly after initiating an exercise program and that, if prospective studies confirm that endothelial function is an independent prognostic marker of future CVD events, exercise training would be a key intervention to treat symptomatic atherosclerosis and an important preventive strategy with both short- and long-term prognostic benefits.[141] In a recent review on the effect of exercise training on endothelial function in cardiovascular diseases in humans, Walther et al. concluded that exercise training through repetitive increases in laminar shear stress leads to an increase of NO bioavailability via increased NO production and a reduction in NO inactivation through reduced reactive oxygen species.[142]

Kemi et al. recently examined the effect of 13 weeks of high intensity training followed by 4 weeks of detraining on cardiomyocyte contractile activity and endothelial function in adult rats.[143] Multiple regression analysis revealed that cell length, relaxation, and calcium decay were the main explanatory variables related to increased maximal oxygen uptake ($r^2 = 0.87$, $p < 0.02$). With detraining, maximal oxygen uptake decreased 50% at 2 weeks and stabilized at 5% above baseline at 4 weeks. Cardiomyocyte size regressed in parallel with the increase in maximal oxygen uptake and remained 9% greater than control at 4 weeks. Cardiomyocyte shortening, calcium transit time course, cardiomyocyte contraction/relaxation, and EDD regressed completely within 2–4 weeks of detraining. Multiple regression analysis identified cardiomyocyte length and vasorelaxation as the main determinants of regression of maximal oxygen uptake during detraining ($r^2 = 0.76$, $p < 0.02$). EDD and enhanced vascular sensitivity to NO returned to baseline within 2 weeks of detraining. Although the time course of the onset of enhanced EDD could not be measured in this study, the authors speculate that improvements in endothelial function occur rapidly with training in parallel to the return to baseline following detraining.

There is little work in humans elucidating the time course of the improvement of EDD. A recent, non-randomized small study suggested that exercise acutely improves FMD.[144] In part one of this study, brachial artery FMD was assessed during exercise to exhaustion on five consecutive days. FMD improved daily, was significantly improved by day 3 ($p = 0.012$), reached maximal improvement on day 6 and returned to baseline by day 9. In the second part of this study, 17 subjects (38 ± 2 years of age) trained for 4 weeks, 30 min/session, 3 days/week at 70% of maximal heart rate, on bicycle ergometers. FMD improved significantly ($p = 0.028$) post-training, but returned to baseline following 2 weeks of detraining. The results suggested that the beneficial effects of aerobic exercise training on endothelial function are rapid but short-lived. This study, however, was non-randomized, involved a small number of male subjects, and was short-term, thus great care must be used in interpreting these data. Longer (6–12 months), randomized, and well-controlled studies with larger samples in clinical populations are required before conclusions can be drawn regarding the frequency, duration, and intensity of exercise necessary to induce and sustain improvements in endothelial function.

Hambrecht et al. investigated the molecular mechanisms mediating the observed exercise training-induced improvements in EDD.[145] Using left internal mammary artery (LIMA) tissue harvested during coronary artery bypass surgery of 17 exercise-trained (ET) and 18 control (C) patients, eNOS expression and content of phospho eNOS–Ser[1177], AKT, and phospho-AKT were determined. EDD improved 56% in response to ACH in the ET group after 4 weeks. There were no changes in the control patients. The improvement in ACH-induced vasodilation of the LIMA was closely related to a shear stress-induced AKT-dependent phosphorylation of eNOS on Ser[1177].

Recently, Erbs et al. examined the effects of polymorphisms in the promoter (T-786c) and exon 7 (G894T) of the eNOS gene on endothelial function and, more specifically, on the endothelial response to physical training in patients with CAD.[146] Both of these polymorphisms have been shown to be associated with reduced vascular NO production and/or proteolytic cleavage of eNOS. The results of this study suggested that patients with either the promoter or exon 7 polymorphism of the eNOS gene demonstrate attenuated EDD, but only the promoter polymorphism attenuated the training-induced improvement in EDD.

The anti-inflammatory effects of exercise training represent another possible mechanism that may partially explain how regular exercise training improves endothelial dysfunction. Hingorani et al. reported that systemic inflammation promotes endothelial dysfunction and others have reported that hsCRP, a marker of systemic arterial inflammation, directly contributes to endothelial dysfunction.[147–149] Several recent studies have shown that aerobic exercise training exerts anti-inflammatory effects in older healthy adults and in patients with the metabolic syndrome, risk factors for CVD, and CHF.[150–154]

As indicated earlier in this chapter, a recent area of interest has been the discovery of endothelial progenitor cells (EPCs). Progenitor cells are primitive bone marrow cells that have the capacity to proliferate, migrate, and differentiate into various mature cells.[84–86] For example, EPCs have the ability to mature into cells that line the lumen of blood vessels or the endothelium. In adult humans, EPCs primarily appear to contribute to rapid re-endothelialization at sites of endothelial cell damage to prevent migration of leukocytes and other cells into the intima, and de novo formation of blood vessels and promotion of angiogenesis.[84–86]

Studies demonstrate an inverse correlation between CAD risk factors and the number and migratory activity of EPCs.[155,156] Smoking seems to be the major independent predictor of reduced EPC levels while impairment of EPC migration was most influenced by hypertension. The level and migratory activity of EPCs may serve as surrogate biological markers for vascular function and cumulative CVD risk.[84] Rauscher and colleagues also demonstrated that chronic treatment with bone marrow-derived progenitor cells from young mice without atherosclerosis prevented atherosclerosis progression in older mice despite persistent high fat diet-induced hypercholesterolemia.[157] Treatment with cells from older mice with atherosclerosis was much less effective. These authors concluded that a progressive decline in progenitor cells may contribute to the development of atherosclerosis. These findings suggest that interventions to increase EPCs may prove beneficial in preventing the development and progression of atherosclerosis.

Recently, acute exercise has been shown to increase circulating levels of EPCs in humans.[158,159] Rehman et al. investigated whether a single episode of exercise acutely increases the number of EPCs and cultured/circulating angiogenic cells (CACs).[158] Twenty-two middle-aged (mean age = 54 years) men and women without known CAD underwent exhaustive dynamic exercise on a bicycle ergometer. The results indicate that circulating EPCs increase fourfold in peripheral blood and circulating CACs increase 2.5-fold. Adams et al. studied whether a maximal stress test in patients with known CAD (n = 28) and in healthy subjects (n = 11) acutely increases the number of circulating EPCs.[159] Sixteen of the CAD patients had exercise-induced ischemia. Circulating EPCs were monitored for 144 h post-exercise. EPCs increased only in the ischemic patients. This was in contrast to the study by Rehman et al., which showed an increase in EPCs in patients without evidence of exercise-induced ischemia. However, these studies suggested, given the ability of EPCs to promote angiogenesis and vascular repair that exercise-induced increases in EPCs may serve as a physiological repair or compensation mechanism that may partially explain the preventive effects of exercise on atherosclerosis development and progression.

Case Study

A 50-year-old man presented to the Emergency Room (ER) with a recent 30–60 min history of substernal chest pain radiating to the left shoulder and scapula precipitated by exertion. He rated the pain 3–4 on a 0–10 scale. He has had several of these episodes in the past 3–4 months that usually resolved after a few minutes of rest. However, this episode was persistent. He denied nausea, dyspnea, or diaphoresis. He had become progressively more anxious about these episodes, which together with the persistence of this episode brought him to the ER. A resting ECG showed mild ST elevation with T-wave inversion in anterior leads. Troponin and CKMB band were mildly elevated, suggesting a possible evolving myocardial infarction. He reported a history of untreated dyslipidemia, pre-hypertensive blood pressure of 134/88 mmHg, and lack of regular physical exercise.

A lipid profile at the time of the presentation revealed a total cholesterol of 221 mg/dl, triglycerides of 211 mg/dl, high-density lipoprotein of 39 mg/dl, and low-density lipoprotein of 140 mg/dl. Homocysteine (8 mg/dl) and lipoprotein (a) [Lp(a)] (15 mg/dl) were within normal limits. Highly sensitive C-reactive protein (hsCRP) was slightly elevated at 3.4 mg/L. Body mass index was 28.2 with a waist circumference of 40.25 inches. His father had died of a myocardial infarction at age 58 years and his mother, who is alive, had a transient ischemic attack (TIA) at age 72 years. His only sibling, a 48-year-old brother, has a history of dyslipidemia, hypertension, and is overweight and physically inactive.

A cardiac catheterization was done within 90 min of the onset of chest pain that revealed an 85% proximal left anterior descending stenosis with irregularities distal to the lesion, and two areas of 20–30% narrowing in the right and left circumflex coronary arteries. Left ventricular ejection fraction was 58%.

A percutaneous coronary angioplasty with implantation of a sirolimus eluting stent was performed across the LAD lesion. The patient tolerated this procedure without complications and was discharged after 48 h of observation. Prior to discharge, a sestamibi exercise test was administered to 85% of maximal predicted heart rate. Results showed a 55% left ventricular ejection fraction and mild reversible perfusion abnormalities in the anterior and inferior walls. Medically, the patient was placed on Atenolol, 25 mg BID, Ramipril, 10 mg QD, 81 mg ASA QD, and Zocor, 20 mg QD. He was advised to take a daily multivitamin with 400 μg of folic acid and no iron, 200 IU Vitamin E, 250 mg Vitamin C, and 100 μg selenium. He was referred to Outpatient Cardiovascular Rehabilitation (CVR) to start within 1 week of discharge.

On entry into the CVR program, he underwent cardiopulmonary exercise testing and a prescription was prepared based on the heart rate at the ventilatory threshold. He was advised to consume an anti-atherogenic diet consisting of 20–25% fat, < 7% saturated fat, < 150 mg/day cholesterol, 25–40 g fiber/day, and < 2000 mg/day sodium. He also was advised to consume more coldwater fish and foods rich in monounsaturated and omega-3 fatty acids such as olives, olive oil, canola oil, flaxseed, avocados, walnuts, almonds, peanuts, peanut butter and other nut butters.

During the first exercise session, he experienced mild substernal chest pain rated 1 on a 0–4 pain scale, which was similar to his historical pain. The patient was hemodynamically stable and the pain resolved with rest. He was referred to Cardiology and a repeat sestamibi exercise test was administered which was similar to the post-discharge test. The patient was referred back to CVR and advised to exercise within tolerance for chest pain (not > 1–1.5 on a 0–4 scale). Support for reentering CVR in the presence of mild but stable ischemia comes from a recent report by Hambrecht et al. that showed, in stable patients with documented CAD, 1-year outcomes superior in patients randomized to CVR compared with those under PTCA with stent implantation.[20] He was advised to continue to aggressively manage risk factors for atherosclerotic progression.

This case illustrates a relatively common scenario in CVR programs. One explanation for the persistent, though less severe symptoms in light of an apparent successful revascularization procedure, is endothelial dysfunction. The patient has several risk factors for endothelial dysfunction including dyslipidemia, upper normal blood pressure, slightly high hsCRP level, positive family history, high-fat diet, overweight, known CAD, and sedentary lifestyle. As discussed previously, studies in patients with single-vessel, occlusive disease demonstrate paradoxical coronary vasoconstriction in response to intracoronary injection of vasodilators such as acetylcholine in epicardial arteries with "visually" normal lumens.[160]

Further support for the role of endothelial dysfunction in recurrent ischemia following a successful percutaneous intervention (PCI) comes from a report by Caramori et al.[161] It is well documented that catheter-based coronary interventions are associated with extensive arterial injury resulting in endothelial dysfunction. Caramori et al. performed intracoronary acetylcholine infusion in 39 CAD patients treated with a PCI for a LAD stenosis 6 months earlier. Twelve had received a PTCA with stent implantation, 15 had PTCA only, and 12 had directional coronary atherectomy. The results showed that although all patients demonstrated some degree of endothelial dysfunction, the LAD constricted more in response to acetylcholine in the stented patients, suggesting that stenting may be associated with more residual endothelial impairment. Monnink et al. also recently demonstrated that exercise-induced ischemia after a successful PCI was due to endothelial dysfunction distal to the interventional site.[162]

Summary

The growing knowledge that the luminal diameter of coronary epicardial and resistance vessels and major peripheral arteries is highly dynamic in response to flow-mediated (shear stress) and agonist-mediated (nitric oxide and endothelin-1) factors has greatly advanced the understanding of atherosclerosis. Ludmer et al. first observed a paradoxical vasoconstriction of atherosclerotic segments of coronary arteries in response to the infusion of acetylcholine.[160] This paradoxical vasoconstriction was observed in angiographically "normal" arteries. It is also known that a large portion of the control of luminal diameter resides in the endothelium, the single cell lining of the vascular system.

In addition, it has been observed that persons with major coronary risk factors often demonstrate endothelial dysfunction even before anatomical atherosclerotic lesions are observed.[163–169] Thus, it appears that endothelial dysfunction is a key pathological feature in the early stages of atherosclerosis. Additionally, endothelial dysfunction also plays a significant role in acute coronary syndrome (ACS), by the relative inability of the vascular surface to inhibit platelet aggregation and the increased endothelial permeability to influx of cellular material leading to both ACS and/or progression of atherosclerotic lesions. This dysfunction may also contribute to plaque rupture as the initiating event in ACS. Recent studies demonstrate that treatment and management of major risk factors improves endothelial function. This has been observed for dyslipidemia, weight loss, hypertension, enhanced management of diabetes mellitus, and smoking cessation. Statins, ACE inhibitors, purple grape juice, folic acid, L-arginine, dark chocolate, and other

TABLE 6.2

Risk Factors Documented to Be Associated with Endothelial Dysfunction

Presence of oxidized LDLs	Post-menopausal state
Presence of small, dense LDLs	Insulin resistance/diabetes mellitus
Hypertension	Impaired fasting glucose
Type 1 and 2 diabetes mellitus	Acute postprandial hypertriglyceridemia
Hyperhomocysteinemia	Active and passive smoking
Elevated lipoprotein (a)	Psychosocial stress
Low HDLs	Aging
Overweight and obesity	Physical Inactivity
Impaired glucose tolerance	Inflammation (hsCRP)
Lipoprotein remnant particles	Metabolic syndrome

TABLE 6.3

Interventions Demonstrated to Improve Endothelial Dysfunction

LDL lowering by statins	Purple grape juice
LDL lowering by low-fat diet	Iron chelation
ACE/ACE II receptor inhibitors	Black and green tea
L-Arginine	High monounsaturated diet
Moderate alcohol intake	Smoking cessation
Premenopausal status	Anti-oxidant therapy
Exercise training	Weight loss and loss of central body fat
Increasing HDL	Dark chocolate
LDL lowering with pheresis	Thermal therapy

substances have been shown to correct or improve impaired endothelial function (Tables 6.2 and 6.3).

Exercise training has been shown to improve endothelial function in patients with congestive heart failure, hypertension, diabetes mellitus, and CAD. Hambrecht et al. were the first to demonstrate that just 4 weeks of daily moderate intensity endurance exercise training in patients with CAD attenuates paradoxical coronary vasoconstriction in response to acetylcholine.[44] Linke et al. demonstrated that the enhanced endothelial function following exercise training in CHF patients is systemic in nature, although other studies failed to substantiate this finding.[45,108–111] These data provide compelling support for an important mechanism by which regular exercise may improve endothelial function, enhance coronary blood flow in patients with or at risk for CAD, and reduce the risk for progression of atherosclerosis and recurrent events.

Hambrecht et al. recently reported that regular physical activity improves endothelial function in persons with CAD by increasing the phosphorylation of nitric oxide synthase.[145] Erbs et al. have shown that the improvement in EDD following 4 weeks of exercise training in stable CAD patients is attenuated in the presence of the promoter polymorphism of the eNOS gene, but not in patients with the wild-type or the exon 7 (G894T) polymorphisms.[146]

In addition, it has been shown that EPCs, which can differentiate into endothelial cells and may also be involved in vascular repair and angiogenesis, increase with acute exercise in humans and with short-term exercise training in animals.[84–86, 155–159]

It has been consistently demonstrated that both acute exercise and exercise training enhance endothelial function in animals and humans. Exercise clearly improves endothelial function in arteries that are dysfunctional secondary to the presence of risk factors or atherosclerotic vascular disease or other mechanisms (e.g., aging). Endothelial function (EDD and FMD) is enhanced in fit and/or physically active compared with unfit and/or physically inactive populations, and exercise may potentiate the effects of other agents that enhance endothelial function.

At this time the appropriate intensity, duration, and frequency of exercise to optimize enhancement of endothelial function are unknown. Goto et al. suggested that moderate-intensity exercise improves EDD whereas higher-intensity exercise may impair EDD, but more work is necessary to determine the generalizability of this finding.[113] More studies with larger sample sizes including women, middle-aged and older adults and persons with CAD and CVD are necessary before definitive recommendations can be made. The few studies that have been completed suggest that a common prescription of 30–45 min of moderate intensity (50–75% of maximal oxygen uptake reserve or heart rate reserve), 4–5 days per week is effective. This exercise should be coupled with other daily activity, because the benefits of exercise on the endothelium may be acute and related to recent exercise.

References

1. Davignon J, Ganz P. Role of endothelial dysfunction in atherosclerosis, *Circulation*, 109(Suppl), III-27, 2004.
2. Gokce N, Vita JA. Clinical manifestations of endothelial dysfunction. In: Loscalzo J, Schafer AJ, editors. *Thrombosis and Hemmorhage*. Lippincott-Williams & Wilkins, Philadelphia, pp 685–706, 2003.
3. Treasure CB, Klein JL, Weintraub WS, et al. Beneficial effects of cholesterol-lowering therapy on the coronary endothelium in patients with coronary artery disease, *N Engl J Med*, 332, 481, 1995.
4. Anderson TJ, Meredith IT, Yeung AC, et al. The effect of cholesterol-lowering and antioxidant therapy n endothelial-dependent coronary vasomotion, *N Engl J Med*, 332, 488, 1995.
5. O'Driscoll G, Green D, Taylor RR, et al. Simvastatin, an HMG-coenzyme A reductase inhibitor, improves endothelial function within 1 month, *Circulation*, 95, 1126, 1997.
6. Tsunekawa T, Hayashi T, Kano H, et al. Cerivastatin, a hydroxymethylglutaryl coenzyme A reductase inhibitor, improves endothelial function in elderly diabetic patients within 3 days, *Circulation*, 104, 376, 2001.

7. Tamai O, Matsuoka H, Itabe H, et al. Single LDL apheresis improves endothelium-dependent vasodilation in hypercholesterolemic humans, *Circulation*, 95, 76, 1997.
8. Solzbach U, Hornig B, Jeserich M, et al. Vitamin C improves endothelial dysfunction of epicardial coronary arteries in hypertensive patients, *Circulation*, 96, 1513, 1997.
9. Davi G, Romano M, Mezzetti A, et al. Increased levels of soluble P-selectin in hypercholesterolemic patients, *Circulation*, 97, 953, 1998.
10. Hasnain BI, Mooradian AD. Recent trials of antioxidant therapy: what should we be telling our patients, *Cleve Clin J Med*, 71, 327, 2004.
11. Mancini GBJ, Henry GC, Macaya C, et al. Angiotensin converting enzyme inhibition with quinapril improves endothelial vasomotor dysfunction in patients with coronary artery disease: The TREND study, *Circulation*, 94, 258, 1996.
12. Wilson SH, Simari RD, Best PJ, et al. Simvastatin preserves coronary endothelial function in hypercholesterolemia in the absence of lipid lowering, *Arterioscler Thromb Vasc Biol*, 21, 122, 2001.
13. Holven KB, Holm T, Aukrust P, et al. Effect of folic acid treatment on endothelium-dependent vasodilation and nitric oxide-derived end products in hyperhomocysteinemic subjects, *Am J Med*, 110, 536, 2001.91.
14. Prasad A., Halcox JP, Waclawiw MA, et al. Angiotensin type 1 receptor antagonism reverses abnormal coronary vasomotion in atherosclerosis, *J Am Coll Cardiol*, 38, 1089, 2001.
15. Engler MB, Engler MM, Chen CY, et al. Flavonoid-rich dark chocolate improves endothelial function and increases plasma epicatechin concentrations in healthy adults, *J Am Coll Nutr*, 23, 197, 2004.
16. Ros E, Nunez I, Perez-Heras A, et al. A walnut diet improves endothelial dysfunction in hypercholesterolemic subjects: A randomized crossover trial, *Circulation*, 109, 1609, 2004.
17. Ornish D, Scherwitz LD, Billings JH, et al. Intensive lifestyle changes for reversal of coronary heart disease, *JAMA*, 280, 2001, 1998.
18. Haskell WL, Alderman EL, Fair JM, et al. Effects of intensive multiple risk factor reduction on coronary atherosclerosis and clinical cardiac events in men and women with coronary artery disease: The Stanford Coronary Risk Intervention Project (SCRIP), *Circulation*, 89, 975, 1994.
19. Niebauer J, Hambrecht R, Velich T, et al. Attenuated progression of coronary artery disease after 6 years of multifactorial risk intervention: Role of physical exercise, *Circulation*, 96, 2534, 1997.
20. Hambrecht R, Walther C, Mobius-Winkler S, et al. Percutaneous coronary angioplasty compared with exercise training in patients with stable coronary artery disease: A randomized trial, *Circulation*, 109, 1371, 2004.
21. Sdringola S, Nakagawa K, Nakagawa Y, et al. Combined intense lifestyle and pharmacologic lipid treatment further reduce coronary events and myocardial perfusion abnormalities compared with usual care cholesterol-lowering drugs in coronary artery disease, *J Am Coll Cardiol*, 41, 263, 2003.
22. Belardinelli R., Paolini I, Cianci G, et al. Exercise training after coronary angioplasty: The ETICA Trial, *J Am Coll Cardiol*, 37, 1891, 2001.
23. Blair SN, Kampert JB, Kohl HW 3rd, et al. Influences of cardiorespiratory fitness and other precursors on cardiovascular disease and all-cause mortality, *JAMA*, 276, 205, 1996.

24. Myers J, Prakash M, Froelicher V, et al. Exercise capacity and mortality among men referred for exercise testing, *N Engl J Med*, 346, 793, 2002.
25. Wannamethee SG, Shaper AG, Walker M. Physical activity and mortality in older men with diagnosed coronary heart disease, *Circulation*, 102, 1358, 2000.
26. Steffen-Batey L, Nichaman MZ, Goff DC Jr, et al. Change in level of physical activity and risk of all-cause mortality or reinfarction: The Corpus Christi Heart Project, *Circulation*, 102, 2204, 2000.
27. Oldridge NB, Guyatt GH, Fischer ME, et al. Cardiac rehabilitation after myocardial infarction: Combined experience of randomized clinical trials, *JAMA*, 260, 945, 1988.
28. O'Connor G, Buring JE, Yusuf S, et al. An overview of randomized trials of rehabilitation with exercise after myocardial infarction, *Circulation*, 80, 234, 1989.
29. Taylor RS, Brown A, Ebrahim S, et al. Exercise-based rehabilitation for patients with coronary heart disease: Systematic review and meta-analysis of randomized controlled trials, *Am J Med*, 116, 682, 2004.
30. Hammalainen H., Luurila OJ, Kallio V, et al. Long-term reduction in sudden deaths after a multifactorial intervention program in patients with myocardial infarction: 10-year results of a controlled investigation, *Eur Heart J*, 10, 55, 1989.
31. Hammalainen, H, Luurila CJ, Kallio V. Reduction in sudden deaths and coronary mortality in myocardial infarction patients after rehabilitation. 15-year follow-up study, *Eur Heart J*, 16, 1839, 1995.
32. Witt BJ, Jacobsen SJ, Weston SA. Cardiac rehabilitation after myocardial infarction in the community, *J Am Coll Cardiol*. 44, 988, 2004.
33. Shephard RJ, Balady GJ. Exercise as cardiovascular therapy, *Circulation*, 99, 963, 1999.
34. Boule NG, Haddad E, Kenny GP, et al. Effects of exercise on glycemic control and body mass in type 2 diabetes mellitus: A metaanalysis of controlled clinical trials, *JAMA*, 286, 1218, 2001.
35. Pescatello LS, Franklin BA, Fagard R, et al. Exercise and hypertension, *Med Sci Sports Exerc*, 36, 533, 2004.
36. Moyna NM, Thompson PD. The effect of physical activity on endothelial function in man, *Acta Physiol Scand*, 180, 113, 2004.
37. Hambrecht R, Hilbrich L, Erbs S, et al. Correction of endothelial dysfunction in chronic heart failure: Additional effects of exercise training and oral L-arginine supplementation, *J Am Coll Cardiol*, 35, 706, 2000.
38. Higashi Y, Sasaki S, Kurisu S, et al. Regular aerobic exercise augments endothelium-dependent vascular relaxation in normotensive as well as hypertensive subjects, *Circulation*, 100, 1194, 1999.
39. Maiorana A, O'Driscoll G, Cheetham C, et al. The effect of combined aerobic and resistance training on vascular function in type 2 diabetes, *J Am Coll Cardiol*, 38, 860, 2001.
40. Tanaka H, DeSouza CA, Seals DR. Absence of age-related increase in central arterial stiffness in physically active women, *Aterioscler Thromb Vasc Biol*, 18, 127, 1998.
41. Tanaka H, Dinenno FA, Monahan KD, et al. Aging, habitual exercise, and dynamic arterial compliance, *Circulation*, 109, 1270, 2000.
42. DeSouza CA, Shapiro LF, Clevenger CM, et al. Regular aerobic exercise prevents and restores age-related declines in endothelium-dependent vasodilation in healthy men, *Circulation*, 102, 1351, 2000.

43. Taddei S, Galetta F, Virdis A, et al. Physical activity prevents age related impairment in nitric oxide availability in elderly athletes, *Circulation,* 101, 2896, 2000.
44. Hambrecht R, Wolf A, Geilen S, et al. Effect of exercise on coronary endothelial function in patients with coronary artery disease, *N Engl J Med,* 342, 454, 2000.
45. Linke A, Schoene N, Gielen, et al. Endothelial dysfunction in patients with chronic heart failure: Systemic effects of lower-limb exercise training, *J Am Coll Cardiol,* 37, 392, 2001.
46. Maiorana A, O'Driscoll G, Taylor R, et al. Exercise and the nitric oxide vasodilator system, *Sports Med,* 33, 1013, 2003.
47. Laughlin MH. Physical activity in prevention and treatment of coronary disease: The battle line is in exercise cell biology, *Med Sci Sports Exerc,* 36, 352, 2004.
48. Green DJ, Maiorana AJ, O'Driscoll G, et al. Effect of exercise training on endothelium-derived nitric oxide function in humans, *J Physiol,* Sept. 16 (preprint published electronically).
49. Muller JM, Myers PR, Laughlin MH. Vasodilator responses of coronary resistance arteries of exercise trained pigs, *Circulation,* 89, 2308, 1994.
50. Laughlin, MH, Pollock JS, Amann JF, et al. Training induces non-uniform increases in eNOS content along the coronary arterial tree, *J Appl Physiol,* 90, 501, 2001.
51. Woodman CR, Muller JM, Laughlin MH, et al. Induction of nitric oxide synthase mRNA in coronary resistance arteries isolated from exercise-trained pigs, *Am J Physiol,* 276, H2575, 1997.
52. Neibauer J, Cooke JP. Cardiovascular effects of exercise: Role of endothelial shear stress, *J Am Coll Cardiol,* 28, 1652, 1996.
53. Miller VM, Vanhoutte PM. Enhanced release of endothelial-derived factors by chronic increases in blood flow, *Am J Physiol,* 255, 446, 1998.
54. Nadaud S, Philippe M, Arnal JF, et al. Sustained increase in aortic endothelial nitric oxide synthase expression *in vivo* in a model of chronic high blood flow, *Circ Res,* 79, 857, 1996.
55. Woodman CR, Muller JM, Rush JR, et al. Flow regulation of eNOS and Cu/Zn SOD mRNA expression in porcine coronary arterioles, *Am J Physiol,* 276, H1058, 1999.
56. Jasperse JL, Laughlin MH. Vasomotor responses of soleus feed arteries from sedentary and exercise trained rats. *J Appl Physiol,* 86, 441, 1999.
57. Schrage WG, Woodman CR, Laughlin MH. Mechanism of flow and ACH-induced dilation in rat soleus arterioles are altered by hindlimb unweighting, *J Appl Physiol,* 91, 901, 2002.
58. Schrage WG, Woodman CR, Laughlin MH. Hindlimb unweighting alters endothelial-dependent vasodilation and eNOS expression in soleus arterioles, *J Appl Physiol,* 89, 1483, 2000.
59. Laughlin, MH, Turk JR, Schrage WG, et al. Influence of coronary artery diameter on eNOS protein content, *Am J Physiol Heart Circ Physiol,* 284, H1307, 2003.
60. Wang J, Wolin MS, Hintze TH. Chronic exercise enhances endothelium-mediated dilation of epicardial coronary artery in conscious dogs, *Circ Res,* 73, 829, 1993.
61. Laughlin, MH, Rubin LJ, Rush JW, et al. Short-term training enhances endothelial-dependent dilation in coronary arteries not arterioles, *J Appl Physiol,* 94, 234, 2003.

62. Woodman, CR, Turk JR, Williams DP, et al. Exercise training preserves endothelial-dependent dilation in the brachial artery of hyperlipidemic pigs, *J Appl Physiol*, 94, 2017, 2003.
63. Thompson, MA, Henderson KK, Woodman CR, et al. Exercise preserves endothelium-dependent relaxation in coronary arteries of hypercholesterolemic male pigs, *J Appl Physiol*, 96, 1114, 2004.
64. Woodman, CR, Turk JR, Rush JW, et al. Exercise attenuates the effects of hypercholesterolemia on endothelium-dependent relaxation in coronary arteries from adult female pigs, *J Appl Physiol*, 96, 1105, 2004.
65. Henderson KK, Turk JR, Rush JW, et al. Endothelial function in coronary arterioles from pigs with early-stage coronary disease induced by high-fat, high-cholesterol diet: Effects of exercise, *J Appl Physiol*, 97, 1159, 2004.
66. Henderson KK, Turk JR, Rush JW, et al. Endothelial function in coronary arterioles from pigs with early stage coronary disease induced by high fat/ high cholesterol diet: Effects of exercise, *J Appl Physiol*, 96, 2004 (preprint published electronically).
67. Davis ME, Cai H, McCann L, et al. Role of c-SRC in the regulation of eNOS expression during exercise training, *Am J Physiol: Heart Circ Physiol*, 284, H1449, 2003.
68. Graham DA, Rush JWE. Exercise training improves endothelial-dependent vasorelaxation and determinants of NO bioavailability in spontaneously hypertensive rats, *J Appl Physiol*, 96, 2088, 2004.
69. Yamashita N, Hoshida S, Otsu K, et al. Exercise provides direct biphasic cardioprotection via manganese SOD activation, *J Exp Med*, 189, 1699, 1999.
70. Landmesser U, Hornig B, Drexler H. Endothelial function: A critical determinant of atherosclerosis, *Circulation*, 109(Suppl II), II-27, 2004.
71. Kuhlencordt PJ, Gyurko R, Han F, et al. Accelerated atherosclerosis, aortic aneurysm formation, and ischemic heart disease in apolipoprotein E/endothelial nitric oxide synthase double-knockout mice, *Circulation*, 104, 448, 2001.
72. Verma S, Wang CH, Li SH, et al. A self-fulfilling prophecy: C-reactive protein attenuates nitric oxide production and inhibits angiogenesis, *Circulation*, 106, 913, 2002.
73. Venugopal SK, Devaraj S, Yuhanna I, et al. Demonstration that C-reactive decreases eNOS expression and bioactivity in human aortic endothelial cells, *Circulation*, 106, 1439, 2002.
74. Russo G, Leopold JA, Loscalzo J., Vasoactive substances: Nitric oxide and endothelial dysfunction in atherosclerosis, *Vasc Pharmacol*, 38, 259, 2002.
75. Napoli, C, Nitric oxide and atherosclerotic lesion progression: An overview. *J Card Surg*, 17, 355, 2002.
76. Neibauer J, Maxwell AJ, Lin PS, NO inhibition accelerates atherosclerosis: Reversed by exercise. *Am J Physiol: Heart Circ Physiol*, 285, H535, 2003.
77. Fogarty, JA, Muller-Delp JM, Delp MD, et al. Exercise training enhances vasodilation responses to vascular endothelial growth factor in porcine coronary arterioles exposed to chronic coronary occlusion, *Circulation*, 109, 664, 2004.
78. Laughlin MH, Woodman CR, Schrage WG, et al. Interval sprint training enhances endothelial function and eNOS content in some arteries that perfuse white gastrocnemius muscle, *J Appl Physiol*, 96, 233, 2004.
79. Tanabe T, Maeda S, Miyauchi T, et al. Exercise training improves ageing-induced decreases in eNOS expression of the aorta, *Acta Physiol Scand*, 178, 3, 2003.

80. Laughlin, MH, Welshons WV, Sturek M, et al. Gender, exercise training, and eNOS expression in porcine skeletal muscle arteries, *J Appl Physiol*, 95, 250, 2003.
81. Suvorava T, Lauer N, Kojda G. Physical inactivity causes endothelial dysfunction in healthy young mice, *J Am Coll Cardiol*, 44, 1320, 2004.
82. Hayward, R, Ruangthai R, Schneider CM, et al. Training enhances vascular relaxation after chemotherapy-induced vasoconstriction, *Med Sci Sports Exerc*, 36, 428, 2004.
83. Mosseri MHJ, Fingert HJ, Varticovski S, et al. In vitro evidence that myocardial ischemia resulting from 5-fluorouracil chemotherapy is due to protein kinase C-mediated vasoconstriction of vascular smooth muscle, *Cancer Res*, 53, 3028, 1993.
84. Hill, JM, Zalos G, Halcox JP, et al. Circulating endothelial progenitor cells as novel biological determinants of vascular function and risk, *N Engl J Med*, 348, 593, 2003.
85. Szmitko PE, Fedak PW, Weisel RD, et al. Endothelial progenitor cells: New hope for a broken heart, *Circulation*, 107, 3093, 2003.
86. Laufs, W, Werner N, Link A, et al. Physical training increases endothelial progenitor cells, inhibits neointima formation, and enhances angiogenesis, *Circulation*, 109, 220, 2004.
87. Yang AL, Tsai SJ, Jiang MJ, et al. Chronic exercise increases both inducible and endothelial nitric oxide synthase expression in endothelial cells of rats aorta, *J Biomed Sci*, 9, 145, 2002.
88. Yen MH, Yang JH, Sheu JR, et al. Chronic exercise enhances endothelium-mediated dilation in spontaneously hypertensive rats, *Life Sci*, 57, 2205, 1995.
89. Haskell WL, Sims C, Myll J, et al. Coronary artery size and dilating capacity in ultradistance runners, *Circulation*, 87, 1076, 1993.
90. Kingwell, BA, Sherrard B, Jennings GL, et al. Four weeks of cycle training increases basal production of nitric oxide from the forearm, *Am J Physiol*, 272, H1070, 1997.
91. Clarkson, P, Montgomery HE, Mullen MJ, et al. Exercise training enhances endothelial function in young men, *J Am Coll Cardiol*, 33, 1379, 1999.
92. Maiorana A, O'Driscoll G, Dembo L, et al. Exercise training, vascular function, and functional capacity in middle-aged subjects, *Med Sci Sports Exerc*, 33, 2022, 2001.
93. Rozanski A, Qureshi E, Bauman M, et al. Peripheral arterial responses to treadmill exercise among healthy subjects and atherosclerotic patients, *Circulation*, 103, 2084, 2001.
94. Maiorana A, O'Driscoll G, Dembo L, et al. Effects of aerobic and resistance exercise training on vascular function in heart failure, *Am J Physiol Heart Circ Physiol*, 279, H1999, 2000.
95. U.S. Surgeon General. Physical Activity and Health: A Report of the Surgeon General. Atlanta: US Dept of Health and Human Services, Centers for Disease Control and Prevention, National Center for Chronic Disease Prevention and Health Promotion. S/N 017-023-00196-5, 1996.
96. Hu G, Eriksson J, Barengo NC, et al. Occupational, commuting, and leisure-time physical activity in relation to total and cardiovascular mortality among Finnish subjects with type 2 diabetes, *Circulation*, 110, 666, 2004.
97. Guan-Da X, Wang Y, Regular aerobic exercise training improves endothelial-dependent arterial dilation in patients with impaired fasting glucose, *Diabetes Care*, 27, 801, 2004.

98. Fuchsjager-Mayerl G, Pleiner J, Wiesinger GF, et al. Exercise training improves vascular endothelial function in patients with type 1 diabetes, *Diabetes Care,* 25, 1795, 2002.
99. Lavrencic A, Salobir BG, Keber I., Physical training improves flow-mediated dilation in patients with the polymetabolic syndrome, *Arterioscler Thromb Vasc Biol,* 20, 551, 2000.
100. Matthews CE, Pate RR, Jackson KL, et al. Exaggerated blood pressure response to dynamic exercise and risk of future hypertension, *J Clin Epidemiol,* 51, 29, 1998.
101. Miyai N, Arita M, Morioka I, et al. Exercise BP response in subjects with high-normal BP: Exaggerated blood pressure response to exercise and risk of future hypertension in subjects with high-normal blood pressure, *J Am Coll Cardiol,* 36, 1626, 2000.
102. Stewart KJ, Sung J, Silber HA, et al. Exaggerated exercise blood pressure is related to impaired endothelial vasodilator function, *Am J Hypertens,* 17, 314, 2004.
103. Chang HJ, Chung J, Choi SV, et al. Endothelial dysfunction in patients with exaggerated blood pressure response during treadmill test, *Clin Cardiol,* 27, 421, 2004.
104. Hambrecht R, Fiehn E, Weigl C, et al. Regular physical exercise corrects endothelial dysfunction and improves exercise capacity in patients with chronic heart failure, *Circulation,* 98, 2709, 1998.
105. Hornig B, Maier V, Drexler H. Physical training improves endothelial function in patients with chronic heart failure, *Circulation,* 93, 210, 1996.
106. Katz SD, Yuen J, Bijou R, et al. Training improves endothelium-dependent vasodilation in resistance vessels of patients with heart failure, *J Appl Physiol,* 82, 1488, 1997.
107. Gielen S, Erbs S, Linke A, et al. Home-based versus hospital-based exercise program in patients with CAD: Effects on vasomotion, *Am Heart J,* 145, E3, 2003.
108. Walsh JH, Bilsborough W, Maiorana A, et al. Exercise training improves conduit vessel function in patients with coronary artery disease, *J Appl Physiol,* 95, 20, 2003.
109. Kobayashi N, Tsuruya Y, Iwasawa T, et al. Exercise training in patients with chronic heart failure improves endothelial function predominantly in the trained extremities, *Circ J,* 505, 2003.
110. Gokce N, Vita J, Bader D, et al. Effect of exercise on upper and lower extremity endothelial function in patients with coronary artery disease, *Am J Cardiol,* 90, 124, 2002.
111. Edwards DG, Schofield RS, Lennon SL, et al. Effect of exercise training on endothelial function in men with coronary artery disease, *Am J Cardiol,* 93, 617, 2004.
112. Belardinelli R, Perna GP. Vasomotor reactivity evaluation in cardiac rehabilitation, *Mondaldi Arch Chest Dis,* 58, 79, 2002.
113. Goto C, Higashi Y, Kimura M, et al. Effect of different intensities of exercise on endothelium-dependent vasodilation in humans: Role of endothelium dependent nitric oxide and oxidative stress, *Circulation,* 10, 1161, 2003.
114. Matsumoto A, Hirata Y, Momomura S, et al. Increased nitric oxide production during exercise, *Lancet,* 343, 849, 1994.

115. Bergholm, R, Makimattila S, Valkonen N, et al. Intense physical training decreases circulating antioxidants and endothelium-dependent vasodilation *in vivo*, *Atherosclerosis*, 145, 141, 1999.
116. Hosakawa, S, Hiasa Y, Takahashi T, et al. Effects of regular exercise on coronary endothelial function in patients with a recent MI, *Circ J*, 67, 221, 2003.
117. Vona M, Rossi A, Capodaglio P, et al. Impact of physical training and detraining on endothelium-dependent vasodilation in patients with recent acute myocardial infarction, *Am Heart J*, 147, 1039, 2004.
118. Hambrecht R, Gielen S, Linke A, et al. Effects of exercise training on left ventricular function and peripheral resistance in patients with chronic heart failure: A randomized trial, *JAMA*, 283, 3095, 2000.
119. Maeda S, et al. Alteration of plasma endothelin-1 by exercise above and below the ventilatory threshold, *J Appl Physiol*, 77, 1399, 1994.
120. Maeda S, Miyauchi T, Kakiyama T, et al. Effects of exercise training of 8 weeks and detraining on plasma levels of endothelium-derived factors, endothelin-1, and nitric oxide in healthy young humans, *Life Sci*, 69, 1005, 2001.
121. Maeda S, Tanabe T, Miyauchi T, et al. Aerobic exercise training reduces plasma endothelin-1 concentration in older women, *J Appl Physiol*, 95, 336, 2003.
122. Callaerta-Vegh Z, Wenk M, Goebbels U, et al. Influence of intensive physical training on urinary nitrate elimination and plasma endothelin-1 levels in patients with congestive heart failure, *J Cardiopulm Rehabil*, 18, 450, 1998.
123. Maeda S, Miyauchi T, Sakano M, et al. Does endothelin-1 participate in the exercise-induced changes of blood flow distribution of muscles in humans?, *J Appl Physiol*, 82, 1107, 1997.
124. Maeda S, Miyauchi T, Kobayashi T, et al. Exercise causes tissue-specific enhancement of endothelin-1 mRNA expression in internal organs, *J Appl Physiol*, 85, 425, 1998.
125. Tounian P, Aggoun Y, Dubern B, et al. Presence of increased stiffness of the common carotid artery and endothelial dysfunction in severely obese children: A prospective study, *Lancet*, 358, 1400, 2001.
126. Woo KS, Chook P, Yu CW, et al. Overweight in children is associated with arterial dysfunction and intima-media thickening, *Int J Obesity Related Metab Disord*, 28, 852, 2004.
127. Watts K, Beye P, Siafarikas A, et al. Effects of exercise training on vascular function in obese children, *J Pediatr*, 144, 620, 2004.
128. Watts K, Beye P, Siafarikas A, et al. Exercise training normalizes vascular dysfunction and improves central adiposity in obese adolescents, *J Am Coll Cardiol*, 43, 1823, 2004.
129. Gielen, S, Hambrecht R., The childhood obesity epidemic: Impact on endothelial function, *Circulation*, 109, 1911, 2004.
130. Woo KS, Chook P, Yu CW, et al. Effects of diet and exercise on obesity-related vascular dysfunction in children, *Circulation*, 109, 1981, 2004.
131. Hambrecht R, Physical exercise as treatment strategy, *Herz*, 29, 381, 2004.
132. Niebauer J, Hambrecht R, Marburger C, et al. Impact of intensive exercise and low-fat diet on collateral vessel formation in stable angina pectoris and angiographically confirmed coronary artery disease, *Am J Cardiol*, 76, 771, 1995.
133. Smith DT, Hoetzer GL, Greiner JJ, et al. Effects of ageing and regular aerobic exercise on endothelial fibrinolytic capacity in humans, *J Physiol*, 546(Pt 1), 289, 2003.

134. Hudlicka OM, Brown D, Silgram H, Angiogenesis in skeletal and heart muscle, *Physiol Rev*, 72, 369, 1992.
135. Prior BM, Lloyd PG, Yang HT, et al. Exercise-induced vascular remodeling, *Exerc Sports Sci Rev*, 31, 26, 2003.
136. Sessa WC, Pritchard K, Seyedi N, et al. Chronic exercise in dogs increases coronary vascular nitric oxide production and endothelial cell nitric oxide synthase gene expression, *Circ Res*, 74, 349, 1994.
137. Gielen S, Erbs S, Schuler G, et al. Exercise training and endothelial dysfunction in CAD and CHF: From molecular biology to clinical benefits, *Minerva Cardioangiol*, 50, 95, 2002.
138. Oltman C, Parker JL, Adams HR, et al. Effect of exercise training on vasomotor reactivity of porcine coronary arteries, *Am J Physiol*, 263, H72, 1992.
139. Fukai T, Siegfried MR, Ushio-Fukai M, et al. Regulation of the vascular extracellular superoxide dismutase by nitric oxide and exercise training, *J Clin Invest*, 105, 1631, 2000.
140. Gielen S, Hambrecht R., Effects of exercise training on vascular function and myocardial perfusion, *Cardiol Clin*, 19, 357, 2001.
141. Gielen, S, Schuler G, Hambrecht R., Exercise training and coronary vasomotion, *Circulation*, 103, E1, 2001.
142. Walther C, Gielen S, Hambrecht R. The effect of exercise training on endothelial function in cardiovascular diseases in humans, *Exerc Sport Sci Rev*, 32, 129, 2004.
143. Kemi OJ, Haram PM, Wisloff U, et al. Aerobic fitness is associated with cardiomyocyte contractile capacity and endothelial function in exercise training and detraining, *Circulation*, 19, 2897, 2004.
144. Pullin CH, Bellamy MF, Bailey D, et al. Time course of changes in endothelial function following exercise in habitually sedentary men, *J Exerc Physiol* (online), 7, 14, 2004.
145. Hambrecht R, Adams V, Erbs S, et al. Regular physical activity improves endothelial function in patients with coronary artery disease by increasing phosphorylation of endothelial nitric oxide synthase, *Circulation*, 107, 3118, 2003.
146. Erbs S, Baither Y, Linke A, et al. Promoter but not exon-7 polymorphism of the eNOS gene affects training-induced correction of endothelial dysfunction, *Arterioscler Thromb Vasc Biol*, 23, 1841, 2003.
147. Hingorani AD, Cross J, Kharbanda RK, et al. Acute systemic inflammation impairs endothelium-dependent dilatation in humans, *Circulation*, 102, 994, 2000.
148. Fichtlscherer S, Rosenberger G, Walter DH, et al. Elevated C-reactive protein levels and impaired endothelial vasoreactivity in patients with coronary artery disease, *Circulation*, 102, 1000, 2000.
149. Pasceri V, Willerson JT, Yeh ETH. Direct proinflammatory effect of C-reactive protein on human endothelial cells, *Circulation*, 102, 2165, 2000.
150. Rauramaa R, Halonen P, Valsanen SB, et al. Effects of aerobic physical exercise on inflammation and atherosclerosis in men: The DNASCO study, *Ann Intern Med*, 140, 1007, 2004.
151. Gielen S, Adams V, Mobius-Winkler S, et al. Anti-inflammatory effects of exercise training in the skeletal muscle of patients with chronic heart failure, *J Am Coll Cardiol*, 42, 861, 2003.
152. Smith JK, Dykes R, Douglas JE, et al. Long-term exercise and atherogenic activity of blood mononuclear cells in persons at risk for developing ischemic heart disease, *JAMA*, 281, 1722, 1999.

153. Troseid M, Lappegard KT, Claudi T., Exercise reduces plasma levels of chemokines MCP-1 and IL-8 in subjects with the metabolic syndrome, *Eur Heart J*, 25, 349, 2004.
154. Jankford R, Jemiolo B., Influence of physical activity on serum IL-6 and IL-10 levels in healthy older men, *Med Sci Sports Exerc*, 36, 960, 2004.
155. Luttum A, Carmeliet G, Carmeliet P., Vascular progenitor cells: From biology to treatment, *Trends Cardiovasc Med*, 12, 88, 2002.
156. Vasa M, Fichtlscherer S, Aicher A, et al. Number and migratory activity of circulation EPCs inversely correlate with risk factors for CAD, *Circ Res*, 89, e1, 2001.
157. Rauscher FM, Goldschmidt-Clermont PJ, et al. Aging, progenitor cell exhaustion, and atherosclerosis, *Circulation*, 108, 457, 2003.
158. Rehman J, Li J, Parvathaneni L, et al. Exercise acutely increases circulating endothelial progenitor cells and monocyte/macrophage-derived angiogenic cells, *J Am Coll Cardiol*, 43, 2314, 2004.
159. Adams V, Lenk K, Linke A, et al. Increase of circulating endothelial progenitor cells in patients with coronary artery disease after exercise-induced ischemia, *Arterioscler Thromb Vasc Biol*, 24, 684, 2004.
160. Ludmer PL, Selwyn AP, Shook TL, et al. Paradoxical vasoconstriction induced by acetylcholine in atherosclerotic coronary arteries, *N Engl J Med*, 315, 1046, 1986.
161. Caramori PR, Lima VC, Seidelin PH, et al. Long-term endothelial dysfunction after coronary artery stenting, *J Am Coll Cardiol*, 34, 1675, 1999.
162. Monnink SH. Exercise-induced ischemia after successful PTCA is related to distal endothelial dysfunction, *J Inves Med*, 51, 221, 2003.
163. Tuzcu EM, Kapadia SR, Tutar E, et al. High prevalence of coronary atherosclerosis in asymptomatic teenagers and adults: Evidence from intravascular ultrasound, *Circulation*, 103, 2705, 2001.
164. Quinones MJ, Hernandez-Pampaloni M, Schelbert H, et al. Coronary vasomotor abnormalities in insulin-resistant individuals, *Ann Intern Med*, 140, 700, 2004.
165. Reddy KG, Nair RN, Sheehan HM, et al. Evidence that selective endothelial dysfunction may occur in the absence of angiographic or ultrasound atherosclerosis in patients with risk factors for atherosclerosis, *J Am Coll Cardiol*, 23, 833, 1994.
166. McGill HC, McMahan CA, Zieske AW, et al. Associations of coronary heart disease risk factors with the immediate lesion of atherosclerosis in youth: The Pathological Determinants of Atherosclerosis in Youth (PDAY) Research Group, *Arterioscler Thromb Vasc Biol*, 20, 1998, 2000.
167. Berenson GS, Wattigney WA, Tracy RE, et al. Atherosclerosis of the aorta and coronary arteries and cardiovascular risk factors in persons aged 6 to 30 years and studied at necropsy (the Bogalusa Heart Study), *Am J Cardiol*, 70A, 851, 1992.
168. McLenachan JM, Vita JA, Fish DR, et al. Early evidence of endothelial vasodilator dysfunction at coronary branch points, *Circulation*, 82, 1169, 1990.
169. von Mering GO, Arant CB, Wessel TR, et al. Abnormal coronary vasomotion as a prognostic indicator of cardiovascular events in women: Results from the National Heart, Lung, and Blood Institute-sponsored Women's Ischemia Syndrome Evaluation (WISE), *Circulation*, 109, 722, 2004.

7

Essential Laboratory Methods for Blood Lipid and Lipoprotein Analysis

Peter W. Grandjean and Sofiya Alhassan

CONTENTS

Introduction 118
Plasma and Serum Preparation 119
Quantifying Blood Lipid Concentrations 120
  Materials 121
  General Procedures 121
Quantifying Apolipoprotein Concentrations 123
  Materials 123
  General Procedures 123
Methods for Isolating Lipoproteins 123
  Sequential Ultracentrifugation 124
    Materials 124
    General Procedures 124
    Calculating the Plasma Density 125
    Calculating the NaBr Needed to Adjust Plasma Density 126
  Lipoprotein Precipitation 126
    Materials 127
    General Procedures 127
    Solutions 127
  Lipoprotein Separation 128
  Gel Electrophoresis 128
    Materials 129
    General Procedures 129
    Solutions 129
  Pre-Electrophoresis Procedures 130
  Lipoprotein Isolation 131
  Lipoprotein Analysis 132
Analyses of Intravascular Enzyme and Transfer Protein Activities 133
  Lipoprotein Lipase and Hepatic Lipase Activities 133

Materials 134
General Procedures 135
Solutions 135
Preparation 136
Preliminary Procedures 136
Final Preparations 137
Assay Procedures 137
Calculations 138
Example Calculation 138
Estimating the Rate of Cholesterol Ester Exchange 139
Materials 139
General Procedures 139
Preliminary Procedures (Determining Assay Linearity) 140
Developing the Standard Curve (Determining Neutral Lipid from Fluorescence Intensity) 140
Assay Procedure 141
Calculations 141
Summary 142
References 142

Introduction

Contemporary blood lipid and lipoprotein analytical techniques were born largely from early observations that these blood constituents were strongly related to the development of cardiovascular diseases and the need to standardize analytical methods so that population standards could be established.[1,2] The methodologies described in this chapter are employed in clinical settings or may be found cited in the scientific literature describing different facets of blood lipid transport in humans.

Obviously, the full array of analytical methods available to lipid researchers and complete descriptions of each analytical method are well beyond the scope of this chapter. We will outline the essential and most common methods for determining blood lipid and apolipoprotein concentrations, lipoprotein size and densities, and activities of intravascular enzymes and transfer proteins in human blood. We will explain the underlying principles, identify the necessary instrumentation and supplies, and describe a general approach for each technique. Thus, the purpose of this chapter is to provide information that is essential for establishing these methods in your laboratory. Readers are encouraged to access additional resources for more specific information on these and other analytical techniques.[1,3,4]

Plasma and Serum Preparation

Daily variation in blood cholesterol concentrations can range from 5% to 10% and may be attributed to such factors as dietary intake, alcohol consumption, menstrual cycle fluctuations, recent physical exertion, hydration status, illness and acute inflammation.[5–7] Even greater variation (5–25%) is observed for triglyceride concentrations.[6] Therefore, these factors should be taken into consideration when interpreting blood lipid data and, certainly, every effort should be made to control or account for these factors if serial samples are being obtained from an individual for comparison or monitoring purposes. To reduce measurement variation due to environmental influences, blood samples for routine blood lipid analyses should be obtained after an 8- to 12-hour fast. The fasting blood samples should also be obtained at the same time of day in order to encourage consistent conditions under which serial blood samples are obtained.

Most assay procedures for lipid and apolipoprotein concentrations recommend the use of serum, although plasma may be used in some assays with similar results.[8–11] Likewise, plasma or serum may be used when isolating lipoproteins for particle size and density determination.[3] When quantifying the activities of intravascular lipases, the methods employed for obtaining the blood samples dictate that plasma samples be utilized.[12,13] In all instances, it is recommended that the collection tubes be chilled either in a refrigerator at 4°C or on ice for several minutes prior to blood collection. Serum from fasting blood samples can be obtained from collection tubes containing no additive. Immediately after collection, the blood samples should once again be stored on ice and allowed to clot prior to centrifugation. If plasma samples are desired, the use of Na^+–EDTA collection tubes are generally recommended because heparin additive in collection tubes will interfere with lipoprotein isolation techniques such as gel electrophoresis.[14,15] The collection tubes are then chilled immediately after blood sampling and prior to undergoing centrifugation. The use of Na^+–heparin collection tubes, however, is recommended when the purpose of the blood sampling is to determine lipase activities.[13]

The collection tubes are centrifuged at 1500–3000 × g for 15–30 min at 4°C and serum or plasma is obtained by pipette. Serum samples obtained for measuring lipid and apolipoprotein concentrations can be aliquoted and frozen prior to analyses. Serum that will be used for high-density lipoprotein (HDL) separation by precipitation can be stored at 4°C for up to 72 h after blood sampling and should not be frozen until after completing the separation procedures. Likewise, plasma obtained for lipoprotein isolation should not be frozen.[16]

Blood lipid transport is a dynamic process, involving lipid and apoprotein exchanges between lipoprotein fractions as well as lipoprotein, apoprotein and lipid modifications. These exchanges and modifications continue in the blood after collection. Therefore, in addition to maintaining chilled collection tubes throughout the blood sampling process, preservatives may be introduced to the serum or plasma prior to storage.[17] Protease activity can be inhibited by the addition of phenylmethylsulfonylfluoride (PMSF) at a final sample concentration of 0.015%. Sodium azide (NaN_3) may be added to the plasma or serum at a final concentration of 0.04% to inhibit bacterial decomposition. Ethylenediaminetetraacetic acid (EDTA) can be added to the samples at a final concentration of 0.4% to prevent oxidation and bacterial phospholipase activity.[3,17]

Under all circumstances it is important to establish a plan for blood collection, processing and storage so that samples are handled consistently. Sample analyses should be carried out as soon after collection as possible. However, in longitudinal research, multiple serum or plasma samples are collected from an individual over a period of time. In these research settings, a common practice is to collect all blood samples from an individual prior to lipid and lipoprotein analyses. As the samples are collected and processed, they are stored frozen at –20 to –70°C and all samples from an individual are assayed in a single run in order to avoid inter-assay variation.

Quantifying Blood Lipid Concentrations

Enzymatic procedures are the most commonly employed method for estimating cholesterol and triacylglycerol concentrations in plasma or serum. The enzymatic reagents can be prepared by the researcher as previously described;[8,10] however, these reagents are produced commercially, are fairly inexpensive and, once reconstituted, have a shelf life of up 30 days.

The cholesterol reagent contains three enzymes, and the dye necessary for the indirect quantification of cholesterol concentration. These enzymes are: *cholesterol esterase, cholesterol oxidase,* and *peroxidase.* The enzymatic reactions that take place in the serum–reagent mixture generally occur as follows: (1) cholesterol esters are hydrolyzed by *cholesterol esterase* to free cholesterol and fatty acids; (2) free cholesterol is oxidized by *cholesterol oxidase* to cholest-4-en-3-one and hydrogen peroxide; (3) a quinoneimine dye is produced when hydrogen peroxide oxidizes *p*-hydroxybenzenesulfonate and 4-aminoantipyrine in the presence of *peroxidase.* The dye has a maximum absorbance in the visible light spectrum at approximately 500 nm. Cholesterol is indirectly quantified by reading the sample absorbance using a spectrophotometer. The intensity of the color produced by these reactions is proportional to the total cholesterol concentration.

The contemporary enzymatic method for estimating serum triacylglycerol concentration actually employs a series of reactions designed to quantify the glycerol concentration in the serum.[10] Thus, triacylglycerol concentrations are determined indirectly using a reagent containing four enzymes. The enzymes in the reagent are: *lipoprotein lipase, glycerol kinase, glycerol phosphate oxidase*, and *peroxidase*. The enzymatic reactions occur as follows: (1) triglycerides are hydrolyzed by *lipoprotein lipase* into fatty acids and glycerol; (2) through the action of *glycerol kinase*, glycerol is phosphorylated to glycerol-1-phosphate and adenosine-5-diphosphate (ADP); (3) *glycerol phosphate oxidase* oxidizes G-1-P to dihydroxyacetone phosphate and hydrogen peroxide and; (4) a quinoneimine dye is formed when the hydrogen peroxide reacts with 4-amino-antipyrine and 5-dichloro-2-hydroxybenzene sulfonate. The dye has an optimal absorbance in the visible light spectrum at 540 nm. As with cholesterol, triacylglycerol is indirectly quantified by reading the sample absorbance since the intensity of the color produced by these reactions is proportional to the total triacylglycerol concentration.

As with cholesterol and triacylglycerol concentrations, there are several methods that may be employed for determining plasma free fatty acids.[3] The enzymatic approach for determining free fatty acid concentration is generally recommended due to the reduced cost — in terms of time and necessary equipment — and comparable precision and accuracy versus gas chromatography.[18] The reagents for determining free fatty acid concentrations are available commercially, and the approach is similar to that described for cholesterol and triglyceride.[19]

Materials

Constant temperature incubator, spectrophotometer, pipettes with volumes from 10 to 100 μl and from 100 to 1000 μl, stopwatch or timing mechanism, matched cuvettes suitable for wavelength analysis in the visible light spectrum, lipid reagent, calibrator standard serum with known concentration values, control and test sera are needed.

General Procedures

It is important to collect blood samples according to the manufacturer's recommendations in order to avoid contaminants and substances that may interfere with the enzymatic reagents. The procedures described in the package inserts should be followed so as to minimize technician error and sample variability. Reagents should be prepared and stored according to manufacturer instructions in order to optimize the performance and shelf life. Assay reliability should be quantified by including control serum at several intervals within a single assay run.

Prior to each assay, the reagent is removed from refrigerated storage and allowed to warm to room temperature. Matched cuvettes are labeled in duplicate and a temperature-controlled incubator is set at 30 or 37°C. The reagent is then introduced into each cuvette. Next, distilled water, control serum or test serum is introduced into appropriately labeled cuvettes (usually in a 1:100 ratio with the reagent), gently mixed by inversion and placed in the incubator at regularly timed intervals (30-s to 1-min intervals are often used). The cuvettes remain in the incubator for the specified time (e.g., 10 min at 37°C or 15 min at 30°C) and are removed from the incubator and read in the spectrophotometer in keeping with the timed intervals.

The cuvettes containing reagent and distilled water are used as "blanks" and read first in order to "zero" the absorbance reading in the spectrophotometer. Duplicate cuvettes containing control serum are placed at the beginning, middle and end of each assay run. For quality control measures, the duplicate control and test sample absorbances should be within 0.01 of each other. Duplicate samples that meet this criterion are averaged and the lipid concentration is determined against calibrator standard values.

The lipid concentrations may be determined from a single calibrator standard or a regression equation developed from several levels of calibrator standards. If a regression equation is developed, the range of calibrator standard values should encompass all test serum values. If a single calibrator standard is used, the lipid concentration may be determined as follows:

$$\left(\frac{\text{Test Sample absorbance}}{\text{Calibrator Standard absorbance}}\right) * \text{Known Lipid Concentration Value of the Calibrator Standard}$$

Reference ranges for assessing lipid concentrations, comparing lipid concentrations to population-based standards and determining level of cardiovascular disease risk have undergone considerable revision in recent years.[20,21] Table 7.1 provides a summary of the most recent classification for blood lipids as established by the report from the National Cholesterol Education Program Adult Treatment Panel III.[21]

TABLE 7.1

National Cholesterol Education Program: Adult Treatment Panel Recommendations for Blood Lipid Levels

Total Cholesterol		LDL-C		TG		HDL-C	
		Optimal	< 100			Low[a]	< 40
Desirable	< 200	Near optimal	100–129	Normal	< 150		
Borderline high	200–239	Borderline high	130–159	Borderline high	150–199		
High	≥ 240	High	160–189	High	200–499	High	60
		Very high	≥ 190	Very high	≥ 500		

LDL-C, low-density lipoprotein cholesterol; TG, triglyceride; HDL-C, high-density lipoprotein cholesterol. All lipid concentrations are given in mg/dl.

[a] HDL-C less than 40 mg/dl is considered low for men. HDL-C of 50 mg/dl is considered low for women.

Source: National Cholesterol Education Program. *J.A.M.A.*, 285, 2486, 2001. Visit http://www.nhlbi.nih.gov/guidelines/cholesterol for the most recent report from the National Cholesterol Education Program's Adult Treatment Panel III.

Quantifying Apolipoprotein Concentrations

Apolipoprotein concentrations are commonly determined using various immunoassay techniques. Radioimmunoassay, radial immunodiffusion, enzyme-linked immunosorbent assay, fluorescence immunoassay, nephelometric immunoassay, electroimmunoassay, and immunoturbidimetric assays have each been employed with a different degrees of sensitivity and specificity for apolipoproteins A-I, A-II, B, C-III, E and lipoprotein (a).[22–26] Of these methods, immunoturbidimetric assays are probably the most widely used procedures for quantifying apolipoproteins due to the technical simplicity, robust results for serum and plasma specimens, and high degree of reliability.[27] Population-based reference values remain dependent on the method for quantifying apolipoproteins.[28]

Materials

Auto-analyzer, commercially available reagents, apolipoprotein calibrators, control plasma or serum, test plasma or serum samples are needed.

General Procedures

Test plasma or serum is introduced into the reagent containing anti-human apolipoprotein antibodies. The antibodies bind the apolipoproteins in the sample causing an insoluble aggregate. The degree of turbidity that results in the sample is proportional to the specific apolipoprotein concentration and may be determined spectrophotometrically at ~ 700 nm.[26,27]

Methods for Isolating Lipoproteins

A number of analytical techniques may be used for isolating lipoproteins. The most common approaches for isolating lipoprotein classes include various ultracentrifugation techniques, precipitation and gel electrophoresis.[3,4] Recent advances in lipoprotein separation by nuclear magnetic resonance (NMR) spectroscopy provide more comprehensive lipoprotein and lipid information than can be obtained from any of the methods described here, and show tremendous promise for clinical and research purposes.[29,30] Although the methods for NMR spectroscopy have been described, the means of completing such analysis are beyond the scope and resources for most laboratories. Currently, lipoprotein and lipid profiles can be obtained by NMR through commercial contract (www.liposcience.com).

Sequential Ultracentrifugation

Sequential ultracentrifugation, first described by Havel et al.[31] in the 1950s, is a principal method for characterizing lipoproteins. Lipoproteins can be separated by ultracentrifugation because these macromolecules have lower hydrated densities than other plasma proteins and because of differences in the relative percentages of lipids and proteins among the lipoprotein classes.[16] Lipoprotein isolation by ultracentrifugation is a relatively slow and labor-intensive process. Moreover, it is recognized that apolipoproteins redistribute among lipoproteins and lipid peroxidation may occur during these procedures.[16] However, the major lipoprotein fractions as we describe them today — very low-density, intermediate-density, low-density and high-density lipoprotein classes — were first described by ultracentrifugation separation techniques. Today, a variety of ultracentrifugation procedures exist, some of which reduce the time and effort required by earlier methods.[16,32]

Materials

Ultracentrifuge and appropriate rotor(s), weight scale sensitive to 0.0000 g, balance scales for determining plasma densities, wax paper or disposable weighing trays (for weighing solutes), glass containers for mixing and storing the prepared solutions, capped ultracentrifuge tubes, tube racks (capable of holding sample preparation tubes), pin light or small flashlight, syringes or capillary pipette for removing top lipoprotein fractions, NaN_3 and PMSF solutions, NaBr are needed.

General Procedures

Plasma samples are obtained and the total volume and density of the samples are determined. Additives, as described previously, are introduced to preserve the plasma sample. Next, a volume of sodium bromide (NaBr) is added to the plasma sample in order to adjust the sample to the appropriate density (g/ml) and the sample is mixed thoroughly (see Table 7.2). After eliminating trapped air in the plasma while it is under a light vacuum, aliquot the adjusted plasma into ultracentrifuge tubes and tightly cap each tube. The tubes undergo ultracentrifugation at constant temperature and speed for 18–24 h.[3] The top plasma fraction is then removed by capillary pipette. This process is repeated in order to isolate each lipoprotein class from the lowest to the highest densities. A thorough description of the equipment, materials and procedures required for sequential ultracentrifugation is provided by Schumaker and Puppione.[16] The general steps and calculations for determining the density of plasma and the NaBr needed to adjust plasma density is explained below.

TABLE 7.2

Characteristics of Major Lipoprotein Classes in Human Plasma

Lipoprotein Class	Electrophoretic Class	Density Range (g/ml)	Lipoprotein Size (nm)	Concentration Range (mg/dl)	
				Males	Females
Chylomicron	Origin	< 0.940	80–500	12 ± 13	2 ± 3
VLDL	Pre-β	0.940–1.006	30–80	129 ± 122	59 ± 63
IDL	Pre-β & β	1.006–1.019	25–30	40 ± 23	24 ± 14
LDL	β	1.019–1.063	16–25	399 ± 81	365 ± 56
HDL	α	1.063–1.210	9–13	300 ± 83	457 ± 115

VLDL, very low-density lipoprotein; IDL, intermediate-density lipoprotein; LDL, low-density lipoprotein; HDL, high-density lipoprotein.

Source: Adapted from Schumaker, V.N., Puppione, D.L., in *Methods in Enzymology Vol. 128*, Albers, J., Segrest, J., Eds., Academic Press, Philadelphia, 1986, p. 155.

Calculating the Plasma Density

First, determine the weight of a volume of water (pipette 600–700 µl of water into a capillary tube and cap the tube. Place the capillary tube on the ultra-sensitive scale and tare the weight so that the display reads 0.0000 g. Next, withdraw 100 µl of water and return the capillary tube to the scale. Allow the display to stabilize, and record the weight. Tare the scales again so that the display reads 0.0000 g. Repeat the weight measurements at least five times, making sure there is no more than 0.05% error in the weights. Use the average of the five measurements as the weight of water.

Second, determine the weight of an equal volume of plasma. (Repeat the same procedure outlined above.) The density of the plasma sample may now be calculated as follows:

$$d\,\text{pl} = \frac{w\,\text{pl} * d\,\text{H}_2\text{O}}{w\,\text{H}_2\text{O}}$$

where $d$pl = density of the plasma (g/ml); dH_2O = density of water (specific for temperature); $w$pl = determined weight of the plasma (g); wH_2O = determined weight of water (g). For example: If the water temperature is 24°C, the water density is 0.997327 g/ml.

If the average weight of water was determined to be 0.10027 g and the average weight of plasma was determined to be 0.10413 g, then:

$$d\,\text{pl} = \frac{0.10413\,\text{g} * 0.997327\,\text{g/ml}}{0.10027\,\text{g}} = 1.0357\,\text{g/ml}$$

Calculating the NaBr Needed to Adjust Plasma Density

First, calculate the volume of NaBr needed to adjust the plasma to the desired density as follows:

$$V\,\text{NaBr} = V\,\text{pl} \times \frac{d\,\text{desired} - d\,\text{pl}}{d\,\text{NaBr} - d\,\text{desired}}$$

where: *V*NaBr = volume of NaBr; *V* pl = volume of plasma sample; *d*desired = desired density of the plasma; *d*NaBr = density of solid sodium bromide = 3.21 g/ml.

For example, if the volume of our plasma sample is 90 ml and the current plasma density is 1.0357 g/ml (from above), the volume of NaBr required to achieve a desired density of 1.063 g/ml is calculated as:

$$V\,\text{NaBr} = 90\text{ ml} \times \frac{1.063 - 1.0357}{3.21 - 1.063}$$

$$= 90\text{ ml} \times 0.012715$$

$$= 1.1444$$

After determining the volume of NaBr, we must calculate the weight of NaBr needed to adjust the plasma sample to the desired density as follows:

$$w\,\text{NaBr} = V\,\text{NaBr} \times \text{mol.wt.NaBr}$$

$$= 1.444 \times 3.21\text{ g/ ml}$$

$$= 3.6735\text{ g}$$

Lipoprotein Precipitation

Precipitation methods for separating plasma lipoproteins were first introduced in the 1970s[33] and have since been refined so that lipoprotein fractions can be isolated in just a few hours of obtaining blood samples.[34] Precipitation methods for isolating high-density lipoproteins have shown good correlation with the more time-consuming and labor-intensive benchmark technique, preparative ultracentrifugation.[34,35] In addition, these methods are compatible with the enzymatic procedures for cholesterol determination.[3] As such, precipitation methods are commonly employed in both clinical and research laboratories for quantifying high-density lipoproteins and subfractions of this lipoprotein class.

Although a number of precipitating agents for apolipoprotein B (apo B)-containing lipoproteins exist, there are two commonly used precipitation procedures for obtaining high-density lipoproteins: the use of heparin/manganese or magnesium/phosphotungstic acid solutions.[36] Of note, the heparin/manganese-chloride ($MnCl_2$) method is recommended by the International Federation of Clinical Chemistry and was the methodology used in the Lipid Research Clinic Prevalence Study.[1]

Both methods work by precipitating apo B-containing lipoproteins from the whole plasma or serum. The precipitate forms a pellet in the bottom of the reaction tube after addition of these solutions and subsequent centrifugation. High-density lipoproteins remain in the supernatant or soluble fraction for lipoprotein or cholesterol quantification. If the heparin/$MnCl_2$ solution is used, a second precipitation step involving dextran/sulfate may be employed to precipitate the larger high-density lipoproteins (HDL_2 fraction). The dextran/sulfate precipitates the larger high-density lipoproteins by polyanion precipitation, leaving HDL_3 lipoproteins in the soluble fraction.[34]

The high-density lipoprotein cholesterol values obtained from the precipitation procedures may be influenced by the blood samples (pH, the final concentration of EDTA in collection tubes), characteristics of the lipoproteins (protein–lipid ratios), and the presence of heparin and $MnCl_2$ in the supernatant.[36] HDL-cholesterol concentrations are systematically about 10% lower when precipitation is carried out using the $MgCl_2$/phosphotungstic acid solution as compared with heparin and $MnCl_2$.[36] Nonetheless, cholesterol concentrations obtained by precipitation are in close agreement with those obtained by preparative ultracentrifugation.[34,35] The double-precipitation procedures, using heparin/$MnCl_2$ and dextran sulfate, are outlined below. These procedures have been described previously by Gidez et al.[34] and Warnick and Albers,[37] and the outside influences on the methodological results have been discussed in detail.[36]

Materials

Refrigerated centrifuge, pipettes with volumes from 10 to 100 μl and from 100 to 1000 μl, weight scale sensitive to 0.0000 g, wax paper or disposable weighing trays (for weighing solutes), magnetic stir plate and stir bars, glass containers for mixing and for storing the prepared solutions, ice trays for sample tubes, polypropylene sample tubes (12 × 75 mm), distilled water, heparin (from porcine intestinal mucosa — 170 USP units/mg), $MnCl_2 \cdot 4H_2O$, dextran sulfate (M_r 15,000) are needed.

General Procedures

Solutions

A. Heparin–$MnCl_2$ Solution: Add 20.0 g $MnCl_2 \cdot 4H_2O$ to distilled water and dissolve completely using a magnetic plate and stir bar. Dilute the solution to 100 ml with water. Next, dissolve 81.6 mg of heparin in 5.0 ml of 1.01 M $MnCl_2$.

B. Dextran/Sulfate Reagent: Prepare 500 ml of 0.15 M NaCl solution by adding 4.383 g NaCl to distilled water and diluting to 500 ml. Next, dissolve 0.143 g (143 mg) of dextran sulfate in 10 ml of 0.15 M NaCl solution.

Lipoprotein Separation

Plasma or serum samples are obtained as described previously. If plasma samples are obtained from EDTA collection tubes, make sure that the tubes were filled to capacity during collection so that the final concentration of EDTA is proper and consistent throughout all samples.[36] If plasma or serum samples appear turbid, as occurs with elevated triglyceride concentrations, the triglyceride-rich lipoproteins must be removed by ultracentrifugation at *d* 1.006 g/ml before undergoing precipitation. Otherwise, incomplete precipitation will result and HDL-cholesterol values may be greatly overestimated.[36]

Place all samples and solutions on ice and maintain them on ice during the separation procedure. Introduce a volume of plasma or serum into the appropriately labeled reaction tubes (usually 3.0 ml). Next, add one-tenth volume (0.3 ml or 300 μl) of the heparin-$MnCl_2$ solution. Mix thoroughly and let the tubes stand at room temperature for 20 min. Centrifuge the tubes at 1500 × *g* in a clinical centrifuge for 1 h at 4°C.

After centrifugation, withdraw the supernatant immediately. The supernatant will be used to determine total HDL-cholesterol and, if so desired, to precipitate HDL_2. Therefore, dispense the supernatant into a tube marked for HDL-cholesterol analysis. (Use 2.0 ml of the supernatant for HDL_2 precipitation and retain the remainder of the supernatant for the subsequent HDL-cholesterol determination.)

The HDL_2 subfraction can be precipitated by adding one volume (usually 2.0 ml) of the supernatant obtained above to an appropriately marked reaction tube. Add one-tenth volume (usually 0.2 ml or 200 μl) of the dextran sulfate solution. Mix thoroughly and allow the tubes to stand at room temperature for 20 min. Next, centrifuge as before for 30 min at 4°C (or you may centrifuge in a refrigerated super-speed centrifuge at 10,000 rpm at 4°C for 10 min). Remove the supernatant immediately after centrifugation and transfer into a storage tube marked for HDL_3-cholesterol analysis.

If the cholesterol analysis is to be performed within a few days, samples can be refrigerated at 4°C. If the analysis is to be performed within a few months, samples should be frozen at –20 to –70°C. Cholesterol concentrations may be determined using the enzymatic procedures described previously.

Gel Electrophoresis

Differences in size and electrical charge among lipoprotein classes and subclasses allow them to be separated by electrophoresis.[14,15,38] Separation of lipoproteins by polyacrylamide gradient gel electrophoresis (PAGE) yields distinct regions in which very low-density, low-density, and high-density lipoproteins and their subclasses can be resolved. In the past, different polyacrylamide gradient gels were used for low-density lipoprotein subclasses and high-density lipoproteins. However, the introduction of composite gels allows electrophoretic separation of low- and high-density lipoprotein subclasses in the same gel.[39] PAGE has also shown great utility in identifying different apolipoproteins from delipidated lipoprotein samples.[3] A thorough discussion of the methodology and common variations in electrophoresis procedures for separating lipoprotein classes have been published elsewhere.[14]

Materials

Fume hood for mixing solutions, cold room or refrigerator (capable of temperatures < 10°C), gel chamber and constant voltage power source, pipettes (0.5–10 μl, 10–100 μl, 100–1000 μl), gel staining trays, digital camera, flatbed scanner and gel-scanning software or densitometer, microcentrifuge tubes, polyacrylamide gradient gels (these may be prepared or purchased commercially), Sudan black B stain (lipid stain), colloidal Coomassie blue (protein stain), bromophenol blue (0.2% w/v bromophenol blue, 40% w/v sucrose) tracking dye, high molecular weight (HMW) standard and latex microspheres of known diameter (25–30 nm) are needed.

General Procedures

Serum or plasma samples are applied to a polyacrylamide gradient gel and electrophoresed at a constant voltage. Lipoproteins in the sample migrate through the gel according to electrical charge until reaching gel pores that are smaller than the lipoprotein particle diameter. After electrophoresis, the gel is stained with a lipid- or protein-specific stain. The stained lipoprotein bands that result can be quantified by densitometry. When lipid stain is used, the integrated optical density obtained for each lipoprotein band is directly related to the cholesterol ester and triglyceride contained in the lipoproteins.[14] The procedures described below are for commercially available composite gels. These procedures may vary, depending on the gels, electrophoresis equipment and laboratory preference; however, the general electrophoretic approach to identifying specific lipoprotein classes and subclasses remain similar.

Solutions

A. TBE Running Buffer: Add 250 ml of stock Tris Borate EDTA (TBE) solution to 2.25 L of deionized water and mix thoroughly. The stock TBE solution (90 mM Tris-Base, 80 mM boric acid, 2.5 mM Na_2–EDTA; pH 8.3) is prepared by adding 109 g Tris, 49.5 g boric acid, 9.3 g Na_2EDTA into 1 L deionized water and stirring to mix.

Adjust the pH of the solution to 8.35 with HCl or K_2CO_3. The stock TBE solution can be stored indefinitely at room temperature. The TBE running buffer should be stored at 40°C.

B. 50% Ethylene Glycol Monoethyl Ether (Cellosolve) Solution: Mix Cellosolve with deionized water in a 1:1 ratio (500 ml of Cellosolve and 500 ml of deionized water) and invert to mix. This stock solution will be used to prepare the Sudan black B post-stain and will serve as the de-staining solution.

C. Sudan Black B Post-Stain: First, combine 8.0 g zinc acetate with 400 ml of deionized water and heat to ~ 100°C for 30 min with slow stirring until the zinc acetate is dissolved. Next, add 200 ml of Cellosolve and maintain the preparation temperature for an additional 30 min. Add another 200 ml of Cellosolve while continuing to stir the solution at 100°C. Slowly add 5.0 g of Sudan black B when the total volume is reduced to ~ 700 ml and continue to stir and maintain temperature until the final volume reaches ~ 450 ml. Filter the solution while it is hot using medium pore quantitative grade filter paper. Repeat the filtering process after the solution has cooled to room temperature. Maintain this as the Sudan black B stock solution. Prepare the final post-stain solution by diluting 20 ml of the Sudan black B stock solution with 80 ml of 50% Cellosolve solution. Mix by gentle inversion and store at room temperature.

D. Coomassie Blue Post-Stain & De-Stain: Add 40 ml methanol and 10 ml glacial acetic acid to 50 ml deionized water and mix by slow stirring. Next, add 7.5 mg Coomassie Blue and stir to dissolve. The de-stain solution is prepared by adding 100 ml methanol and 15 ml glacial acetic acid to 85 ml of deionized water and mixing by slow stirring.

E. Fixing Solution (10% trichloroacetic acid): Add 10 g trichloroacetic acid to 100 ml deionized water and mix by stirring until dissolved.

Pre-Electrophoresis Procedures

Prepare the electrophoresis chamber in the cold room or refrigerator and add chilled TBE running buffer to the lower reservoir. Position the gels appropriately, fill the top reservoir and clear the top of the gels of trapped air bubbles with the TBE running buffer. The gels are then pre-electrophoresed for a period (10–60 min) at 100–120 V.

The test and control samples are prepared by mixing 15 µl of bromophenol blue tracking dye and 10 µl of sample. Plasma or serum samples may be used for PAGE. (Avoid heparinized plasma, as the heparin activates lipoprotein lipase and modifies the lipid content in the lipoprotein fractions. Thus, heparinized plasma interferes with lipoprotein migration and will result in streaks and non-specific bands forming in the sample lanes.)

Reconstitute the HMW standard with 100 μl of TBE running buffer and then combine 60 μl of bromophenol blue tracking dye with 40 μl of reconstituted HMW standard. Prepare the latex beads by adding 10 μl of the latex beads to 90 μl of bromophenol blue tracking dye.

Lipoprotein Isolation

Again, clear any trapped air bubbles from the top of the gels with the TBE running buffer and then carefully pipette the plasma samples into designated gel lanes. Prepare a separate gel for the HMW standards and latex beads. Introduce only the HMW standard to each lane at this time. Electrophorese the gels progressively (15 V for 15 min, 70 V for 20 min) and then achieve a constant voltage for ~ 3000 volt-hours (e.g., 120 V for 24 h). Introduce 10 μl of latex bead mixture to the HMW standard lanes after approximately 3 h of electrophoresis. This insures that the HMW proteins do not combine with the beads prior to migrating down the gel lanes.

Once electrophoresis is completed, carefully remove the gels and place them in a tray containing enough deionized water to cover the gel and provide occasional gentle shaking for 1 h. Decant the water and add 50 ml of 10% trichloroacetic acid. Again, provide occasional gentle shaking for 1 h and then decant and rinse the gel with deionized water. Next, place the gel into 50% Cellosolve solution for 1 h with gentle shaking. Discard the solution, introduce fresh Cellosolve solution and repeat shaking for an additional hour. Remove the gel and place it in a new tray with enough Sudan black B post-stain to completely immerse the gel. Stain the gel overnight (~ 18 h). The gel with the HMW standards undergoes the same procedures, except that this gel is placed in a tray containing the Coomassie blue stain and stained for 1.5–2 h.

After staining, decant the post-stain and rinse the gel several times with deionized water. Next, add the Cellosolve solution and de-stain for 1 h with gentle shaking. Decant and add new Cellosolve solution and repeat the de-staining each hour for an additional 3 h. De-staining takes approximately 4 h in total; however, if bands are not distinguishable from the gel background or the gel background is not clear after 3–4 changes of de-staining solution, then the gel may continue to undergo de-staining overnight. The gel with the HMW standards is placed immediately in the de-stain solution (prepared as described for solutions in the section *Quantifying Apolipoprotein Concentrations*).

After de-staining, rinse all gels several times with deionized water until the acid smell from the de-staining solution is no longer evident on the gels. Place the gels in a new tray with TBE running buffer and provide gentle shaking until the gels regain their original shape. The gels may be stored in TBE running buffer indefinitely in sealed trays (see Figures 7.1 and 7.2).

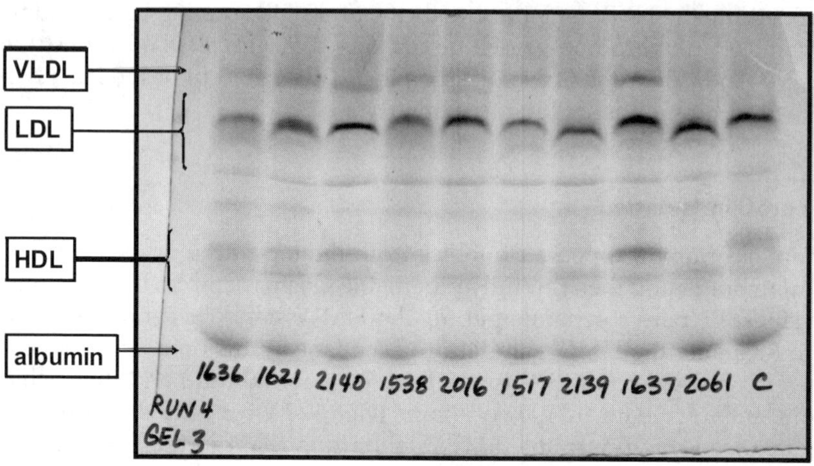

FIGURE 7.1
Whole plasma was introduced into pre-cast gradient gels (2–27% polyacrylamide) and underwent electrophoresis at constant voltage. Gels were stained with Sudan black B, photographed and scanned for further analysis.

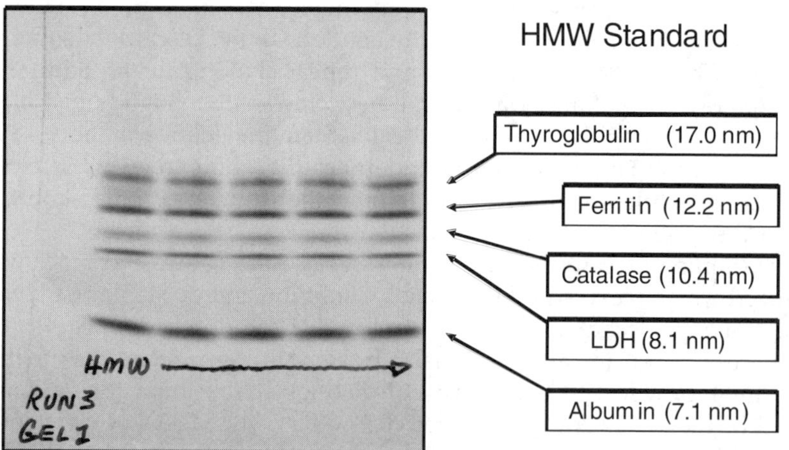

FIGURE 7.2
A HMW standard was introduced to multiple lanes of a single pre-cast gradient gel (2–27% polyacrylamide) and underwent electrophoresis at constant voltage. Gels were stained with Coomassie blue, photographed and scanned for further analysis.

Lipoprotein Analysis

Quantitation of gel bands may be carried out with a densitometer or photo system equipped with a background light source. If the latter technique is employed, digital photos are either scanned electronically or by flatbed

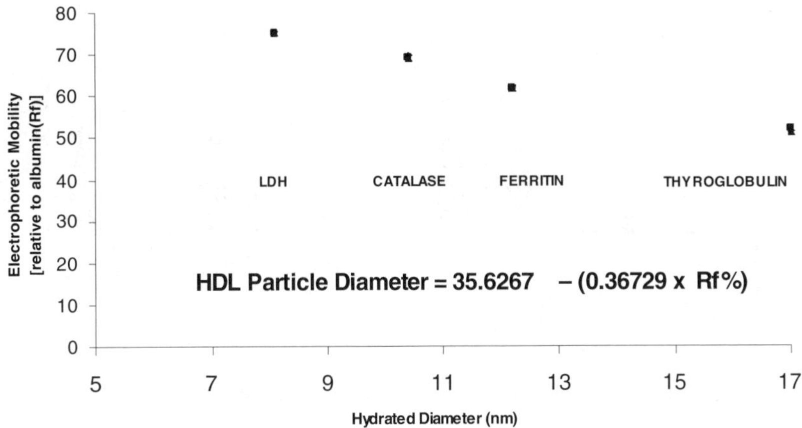

FIGURE 7.3
Relationship between hydrated diameter (nm) and electrophoretic mobility relative to albumin (R_f) was determined using an HMW standard containing protein with known hydrated diameters (bovine serum albumin 7.1 nm, lactate dehydrogenase 8.1 nm, catalase 10.4 nm, ferritin 12.2 nm, and thyroglobulin 17.0 nm) (#17-0445-01, Amersham Pharmacia Biotech).

scanner and imported into gel-scanning software. The resulting scans are typically analyzed by determining the area under the curve or the peaks for each of the bands. Particle size determination is carried out by plotting the relative migration of the HMW standards and latex beads against the known hydrated diameters for each of the proteins in the standard (see Figure 7.3). Since albumin in the plasma or serum will have the smallest particle diameter, the migration of albumin is typically designated as 100% migration and all lipoproteins will migrate as a percentage of the albumin. The resulting regression equation is then used to estimate lipoprotein particle sizes from the known relative migration for each of the lipoprotein band peaks (see Figure 7.4). Additional information for quantifying lipoprotein bands is available.[40]

Analyses of Intravascular Enzyme and Transfer Protein Activities

Lipoprotein Lipase and Hepatic Lipase Activities

Both hepatic lipase and endothelial-bound lipase hydrolyze triglyceride from triglyceride-rich lipoproteins. The hydrolysis of triglyceride is important physiologically for the uptake and subsequent metabolism of free fatty acids. The remnant material generated from this hydrolysis is integral for the intravascular formation of HDL precursors and the transformation of HDL_3 to HDL_2.[41,42] Post-heparin plasma contains endothelial-bound lipase derived

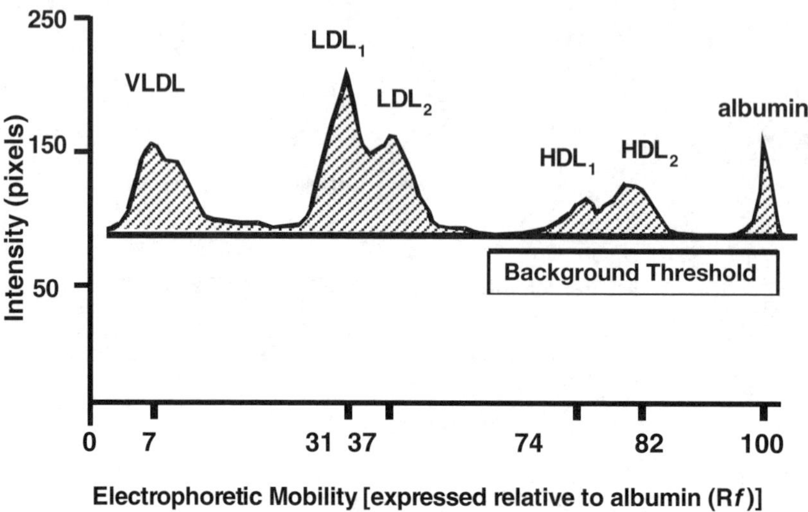

FIGURE 7.4
Representative analysis of a single lane in a composite gel (2–27% polyacrylamide). Lipoprotein particle diameter peaks were quantified on the basis of their electrophoretic mobility (R_f) relative to albumin. HDL particle profile scores were calculated using the R_f and the intensity (as a multiple of the threshold intensity [represented by the trace]) of each HDL peak.

from adipose tissue, muscle tissue, the liver (hepatic triglyceride lipase), and phospholipid lipase.[43]

The plasma protein concentrations of lipoprotein lipase are determined using immunoassays that are similar in approach to those described previously for apolipoproteins.[27,44] Plasma lipase activities are generally quantified by incorporating a radioactive or fluorescence label in a triglyceride substrate and measuring the label remaining after exposure to the lipase in a test sample.[43,45–49] Today, versions of the fluorescence techniques for quantifying lipase protein concentrations and lipase activities may be carried out using commercially available kits. Here we outline procedures for estimating plasma lipase activity using radio-labeled substrate and post-heparin plasma samples.[43,49]

Materials

Weight scale sensitive to 0.0000 g, magnetic stir plate and magnetic stir bars, pH meter, sonicator, cell disruptor, water bath with metabolic shaker, refrigerated super-speed centrifuge, scintillation counter, fume hood (for storage and equipped with nitrogen gas and multiple sample lines), adjustable pipettes (10–100 µl, 100–1000 µl, and 1–5 ml), 2 ml cryovials with rubber o-ring seal (sample and label storage), 15 ml polypropylene reaction tubes, bullet tubes with snap cap, tube racks (capable of holding 15 ml conical reaction tubes), 20 ml scintillation vials with foil-lined caps, scintillation cocktail, absorbent paper, radioactive detergent, various sizes of cylindrical beakers from 25 ml to 2 L capacities, stoppered glass containers (250 ml to 1 L in size), Tris(hydroxymethyl aminomethane), NaCl, heparin (grade 1A from porcine intestinal mucosa), K_2CO_3 (potassium carbonate, anhydrous ACS reagent), H_3BO_3 (boric acid), HCl (hydrochloric acid) and KOH (potassium hydroxide) for pH adjustment of solutions, MeOH (methanol, research grade), $CHCl_3$ (chloroform, research grade), pH calibrators (pH 7.0 and pH 10.0), C_7H_{14} (heptane, research grade), Triton X-100, triolein, phosphatidylcholine (L-α lecithin from egg yolk), FA-free albumin, [^{3}H]triolein (glycerol tri[9,10(n)-^{3}H]oleate in toluene solution) (1 ml = 5 μCi), toluene, plasma or serum in at least 1-ml aliquots for the apolipoprotein CII source are needed.

General Procedures

In the presence of ^{3}H-labeled lipid substrate and supplied apolipoprotein CII (as a cofactor), the rate of hydrolysis of the labeled substrate is measured in a timed assay at physiologic temperature.[43,49] The reaction is immediately stopped by denaturing the plasma lipase proteins and the labeled free fatty acids are partitioned from the mono-, di-, and triglycerides.[50] The radioactivity of the labeled free fatty acids is then measured in a liquid scintillation counter. Distinction of total triglyceride lipase activity is determined in low sodium buffer, while only hepatic triglyceride lipase is active in a high sodium buffer.[43] Thus, the activity of endothelial-bound lipase can be calculated as the difference between the determined total lipase activity and that of hepatic triglyceride lipase.

Solutions

A. Buffer 1; used for post-heparin lipase activity (PHLA): Add 2.35 g Tris, 1.11 g NaCl, and 0.015 g (15 mg) heparin to 75 ml of distilled water while stirring. Adjust the pH to 8.6 with concentrated HCl and bring to a final volume of 100 ml (0.194 M Tris–HCl buffer, pH 8.6, containing 0.19 M NaCl and heparin).

B. Buffer 2; used for hepatic triglyceride lipase activity (HTGLA): Add 2.35 g Tris, 13.5 g NaCl, and 0.015 g (15 mg) heparin to 75 ml of distilled water while stirring. Adjust the pH to 8.6 with concentrated HCl and bring to a final volume of 100 ml (0.194 M Tris–HCl buffer, pH 8.6, containing 2.31 M NaCl and heparin).

C. Buffer 3; used for substrate and diluent preparation: Add 2.35 g Tris and 0.88 g NaCl to 75 ml of distilled water while stirring. Adjust the pH to 8.6 with concentrated HCl and bring to a final volume of 100 ml (0.194 M Tris–HCl buffer, pH 8.6, containing 0.15 M NaCl).

D. Solution 4; Triton X-100 for substrate: Add 1 ml of Triton X-100 to 100 ml of distilled water and place in a sonicator until dissolved completely. Avoid shaking or allowing this solution to foam. [1% (v/v) aqueous solution of Triton X-100].

E. Solution 5; Lipid solvent: Under a fume hood, combine 282 ml MeOH (methanol), 250 ml $CHCl_3$ (chloroform) and 200 ml C_7H_{14} (heptane). Mix by gentle swirling.
F. Solution 6; FFA extraction: Add 13.8 g K_2CO_3 to 1 L of distilled water while stirring. In a separate container, add 3.1 g H_3BO_3 to 500 ml of distilled water while stirring. Next, add 200 ml of the 0.1 M H_3BO_3 solution to 800 ml of the 0.1 M K_2CO_3 solution while stirring (0.1 M K_2CO_3–H_3BO_3 buffer, pH 10.5).

All solutions should be stored in glass containers. Solutions 1 and 2 should be stored at 4°C. Other solutions can be stored at room temperature.

Preparation

Post-heparin blood samples should be drawn into Na^+–heparin tubes and placed on ice, centrifuged cold, and the plasma is either analyzed immediately or placed at –70°C until analysis.

Obtain approximately 20 ml of plasma from a single donor for the apolipoprotein CII source. Allocate the plasma into 1.1-ml aliquots and store at –70°C.

Aliquot 15 µl of the labeled triolein into cryovials for storage at –20°C immediately after receiving the ^{3}H-labeled triolein. Only one 15-µl aliquot will be used for each substrate preparation.

Preliminary Procedures

Heat a water bath to 56°C. A separate water bath with metabolic shaker should be heated to 37°C. Reconstitute the 15 µl of the labeled triolein with 300 µl of toluene and vortex vigorously for 5 min. The vortexing is repeated two more times at 30-min intervals.

Remove the test plasma samples from cold storage and place on ice for slow thawing. Remove one of the plasma samples to be used as the apo CII source from cold storage and allow it to thaw on ice. Label 15 ml conical reaction tubes in duplicate for total (PHLA) and hepatic lipase activity (HTGLA) and the test sample identification. (Four reaction tubes, two for PHLA and two for HTGLA will be labeled for each of the test samples.) Label blanks for total (BT) and hepatic activities (BH) in triplicate. Also label microcentrifuge tubes for each subject and/or time point.

Prepare the plasma sample diluent by adding 5 ml of buffer #3 (0.194 M Tris–HCl buffer, pH 8.6, containing 0.15 M NaCl) into a 15-ml container. While stirring, add 0.3 g of fatty acid-free albumin. After the solution is homogenous, place the diluent on ice.

Aliquot 10 ml of scintillation fluid into 20-ml scintillation vials. Prepare a scintillation vial for each of the reaction tubes prepared for test samples and blanks.

The substrate is prepared by separately preparing aqueous and lipid portions. Prepare the aqueous portion as follows: Add 10 ml of buffer #3 (0.194 M Tris–HCl buffer, pH 8.6, containing 0.15 M NaCl) into a 25-ml glass container. While stirring, add 0.6 g of fatty acid-free albumin. After solution is homogeneous, place on ice. Next, place the plasma apo CII source in the water bath at 56°C for 10 min. Withdraw 1.0 ml from the aqueous solution and introduce 1.0 ml of the heat-deactivated plasma into the aqueous solution while stirring. Replace the aqueous solution on ice.

Prepare the lipid portion of the substrate solution by pipetting 206 µl of unlabeled triolein, 8 µl of phosphatidylcholine (lecithin) and 125–130 µl of the ^{3}H-labeled triolein into a 20-ml scintillation vial. Evaporate the lipid solvents under N_2 gas. (The solvents are evaporated when the contents of the scintillation vial are odorless.) Add 600 µl of the 1% (v/v) solution of Triton X-100 to the scintillation vial.

The final substrate solution is prepared by adding the aqueous portion to the lipid portion in the scintillation vial. Cap the solution and vortex vigorously. Emulsify the contents of the substrate solution by placing the probe from the cell disruptor into the substrate solution for 1 min. (The setting on the cell disruptor should be set at a moderate energy level.) Remove the substrate for 30 s and then repeat the emulsification for an additional minute. Place the substrate emulsion on ice until proceeding with the assay. The substrate is stable for approximately 6 h after emulsification.

Final Preparations

Pipette 100 µl of the diluent and 50 µl of plasma sample into the appropriately labeled microcentrifuge tubes. Cap the tubes, vortex and place on ice.

Into the appropriately labeled 15-ml reaction tubes, pipette 80 µl of buffer #1 (0.194 M Tris–HCl buffer, pH 8.6, containing 0.19 M NaCl and heparin) into tubes marked for PHLA. Pipette 80 µl of buffer #2 (0.194 M Tris–HCl buffer, pH 8.6, containing 2.31 M NaCl and heparin) into tubes marked for HTGLA. Next, add 20 µl of the 3:1 diluted sample from the bullet tubes into appropriately labeled reaction tubes. Add 20 µl of distilled water to the blank tubes (BT and BH). Place all tubes on ice. Finally, pipette 20 µl of the substrate into 20-ml scintillation vials (in triplicate) for determining the total activity of the ^{3}H-labeled substrate.

Assay Procedures

Turn on the metabolic shaker in the water bath heated to 37°C. Pipette 100 µl of substrate into each reaction tube at 30-s intervals. After introducing the substrate, gently vortex the tube and place it in the water bath for 45 min. Following the 45-min incubation, remove the reaction tubes in keeping with the 30-s intervals. As the reaction tubes are removed, introduce 3.25 ml of solution # 5 (methanol: chloroform: heptane) immediately followed by 1.05

ml of solution #6 (potassium carbonate: borate). Vortex the tubes and place them on ice until all reaction tubes have been removed from the water bath.

Centrifuge the reaction tubes at 2500 × *g* and 4°C for 15 min. A liquid (alkaline methanol–water): liquid (chloroform–heptane organic phase) partition should be visible after centrifugation. Withdraw 1 ml of the top phase (alkaline methanol–water phase) from each sample and introduce into the appropriately labeled 20-ml scintillation vials. Cap the vials and vortex vigorously. The scintillation vials should be placed in a dark place overnight (6 h). Count the activity of each sample (cpm) in the scintillation counter for 10 min.

Calculations

A. Average the total counts of the three substrate vials and the blanks (BT and BH). Do the same for each of the duplicate total lipase and hepatic lipase sample vials.
B. Adjust the sample cpm by subtracting the background cpm from each of the sample averages (sample cpm - blank cpm). BT counts are subtracted from PHLA sample counts and BH counts are subtracted from HTGLA sample counts.
C. Calculate the lipase activity: (Adjusted sample cpm/Substrate cpm) × (1/incubation time) × (1/specific activity of the substrate) × volume of the organic phase × (1/partition coefficient) × (1/volume of the plasma analyzed), where: (1/incubation time) is = 1/0.75 h; (1/specific activity) = (3.0817 μmol free fatty acid/substrate cpm × 5); volume of the organic phase = 2.45 ml; (1/partition coefficient) = 1/0.76 h;(1/plasma volume) = 1/0.02. Each of the terms above may be combined (3.0817 μmol free fatty acid × 2.45 ml)/(5 × 0.75 h × 0.76 × 0.02 ml). Thus, the ratio of the adjusted sample counts to the substrate counts is multiplied by the constant, 132.4275.
D. Multiply both PHLA and HTGLA results by 3.
E. Subtract HTGLA from PHLA to estimate the endothelial-bound lipase activity LPLA.

Example Calculation

In this example, substrate average = 50,000 cpm; PHLA sample average = 3000 cpm; HTGLA sample average = 2000 cpm; BT average = 150 cpm; BH average = 100 cpm.

PHLA = (3000 – 150)/50,000 × 132.4275 = 7.5484
7.5484 × 3 = 22.65 μmol FFA/ml/h
HTGLA = (2000–100)/50,000 × 132.4275 = 5.0322
5.0322 × 3 = 15.10 μmol FFA/ml/h
LPLA = 22.65 – 15.10 = 7.55 μmol FFA/ml/h

Estimating the Rate of Cholesterol Ester Exchange

Cholesterol ester transfer protein (CETP) is one of several lipid transfer proteins that have been isolated in human plasma.[51–53] CETP is of particular interest to those studying reverse cholesterol transport because it facilitates the exchange of triglycerides and cholesterol esters between lipoproteins.[53,54] Both CETP activity — the CETP-mediated transfer of lipids among lipoproteins — and CETP protein concentrations have been measured previously. CETP concentrations, which correlate well with CETP activity, are commonly measured by radioimmunoassay and ELISA techniques.[55–57] CETP-mediated transfer of lipids is estimated by quantifying the lipid exchange between donor (HDL) and acceptor (VLDL and LDL) lipoprotein fractions.[55] Previous methodology for measuring CETP activity required the isolation of donor and acceptor lipoprotein fractions by sequential ultracentrifugation, radiolabeled cholesterol to be esterified and incorporated into the donor lipoprotein fraction, the determination of an optimal donor:acceptor mass ratio and an optimal incubation time for the linear rate of cholesterol ester exchange between donor and acceptor lipoproteins.[54,55,58] CETP activity was then measured as the transfer of ^{3}H-HDL$_3$–cholesterol ester to the $d < 1.063$ g/ml lipoproteins [VLDL + LDL (V + LDL)] during incubation at 37°C. The donor (^{3}H-HDL$_3$) and acceptor lipoproteins (V + LDL) were separated by lipoprotein precipitation and the radioactivity in the HDL$_3$-containing supernatant was determined. A recently developed method for quantifying CETP activity is available as a commercial kit.[59] Lipid transfer between donor and acceptor is quantified by fluorescence, the donor and acceptor sources are not influenced by variations in endogenous lipoproteins and the specific activity of the donor is not influenced by HDL concentrations. The procedures, described below, require less preparatory time and exhibit improved reliability and specificity over previous methodology.

Materials

Fluorescence spectrophotometer, multi-channel pipette (10–100 μl), multi-channel sample loading tray, 96-well black microplate, 12 × 75 mm culture tubes, book tape, microcentrifuge tubes, 15 ml reaction tubes, 50 ml sample tubes, parafilm, CETP Activity Kit (Roar Biomedical Inc., No. RB-CETP), isopropanol, Tris-Base (hydroxymethyl aminomethane), Na$_2$EDTA (ethylenediaminetetraacetic acid, disodium salt dihydrate), NaCl, pooled plasma samples (from at least three different individuals to use as control) are needed.

General Procedures

The optimal incubation time and donor acceptor ratio for the test kit is determined and a standard curve is developed for calculating CETP activity from the measured fluorescence. CETP activity is determined by incubating the test sample with donor and acceptor particles resulting in the transfer of fluorescent-neutral lipid from donor to acceptor particles. The CETP activity is then measured as the increase in fluorescence intensity as the fluorescent-neutral lipid is exchanged from the donor to the acceptor fraction.[59]

Preliminary Procedures (Determining Assay Linearity)

Each of the three pooled "control" plasma samples are combined with buffer (included in the CETP Activity Kit) in microcentrifuge tubes by pipetting 90 μl of buffer and 10 μl of plasma, capping the tube and mixing by gentle vortex.

Assign microplate wells in triplicate for progressively greater volumes of each diluted plasma sample. For example, assign wells A1 to A3 as "blank wells" for control plasma 1. Assign wells A5 to A7 for 2 μl, A9 to A11 for 5 μl, B1 to B3 for 8 μl, B5 to B7 for 10 μl of diluted plasma. Assign microplate wells D and E for control plasma 2 and G and H for control plasma 3 in the same manner. (Skip a row of wells in the microplate between the assigned rows for each of the diluted control plasmas.)

Prepare a mixture of the buffer, donor and acceptor by combining 204 μl of donor, 204 μl of acceptor and 4.692 ml of buffer in a 15 ml reaction tube. Mix the solution by gentle vortex.

Using a multi-channel pipette, introduce into the appropriately assigned microplate wells the following contents so that the total assay volume for each well is 200 μl. Diluted control plasma sample 1:

Microplate Well Assignment	Buffer (μl)	Diluted Control Plasma (μl)	Buffer + Donor + Acceptor Mixture (μl)
A1 to A3	10	0	190
A5 to A7	8.0	2.0	190
A9 to A11	5.0	5.0	190
B1 to B3	2.0	8.0	190
B5 to B7	0	10	190

Repeat the same procedure for each of the diluted control plasma samples. After the microplate wells have been prepared, cover the microplate with book tape and incubate for 1–3 h at 37°C in a water bath. Fluorescence intensities will be read each hour of the incubation in order to determine optimal assay linearity for time and concentration. Fluorescence intensity is read at an excitation of 465 nm and an emission of 535 nm. The book tape is removed prior to reading the fluorescence and new book tape is used to cover the plate prior to re-incubation.

Developing the Standard Curve (Determining Neutral Lipid from Fluorescence Intensity)

Label 12 × 75-mm culture tubes from T0 to T5. Add 1 ml of isopropanol to each tube. Next, add an additional 1 ml of isopropanol and 5 μl of donor into the tube marked T5, cover with parafilm and mix by gentle inversion. Remove 1 ml of solution from T5 and add to the tube marked T4, cover with parafilm and mix by gentle inversion. Repeat the process by removing solution from T4 and adding to the tube marked T3, from T3 to T2 and T2 to T1.

Assign microplate wells in triplicate for each of the T tubes (T0 through T5), skipping a well between each. For example, assign wells A1 to A3 for T0, A5 to A7 for T1, etc. Next, pipette 200 µl of solution from each tube into the appropriately assigned microplate wells. Cover the microplate with book tape and place on ice until reading. The book tape is removed prior to reading and the fluorescence intensity is read at an excitation of 465 nm and an emission of 535 nm. The book tape is removed prior to reading the fluorescence.

A standard curve is developed by plotting the fluorescence intensity against the fluorescent donor substrate in ρmoles (which is dispersed proportionally in isopropanol).

Assay Procedure

Add 90 µl buffer and 10 µl test plasma into appropriately labeled microcentrifuge tubes, cap the tubes and mix by gentle vortex. Prepare the buffer–donor–acceptor solution by adding 4 µl of donor, 4 µl of acceptor and 92 µl of buffer for each of the test samples, controls and blanks into a 15-ml reaction tube. Assign microplate wells in triplicate for each of the test samples, controls and blanks as before. All test samples from an individual should be determined on the same microplate due to variations in the fluorescence intensity that may occur between different microplates.

Into each of the appropriately labeled microplate wells, pipette 95 µl of buffer and 5 µl of buffer (for blanks) or diluted plasma sample (for tests). Next, introduce 100 µl of the buffer–donor–acceptor solution into each well for a final well volume of 200 µl. Cover the plate with book tape, incubate in a water bath at 37°C for 3 h and read the fluorescence intensity as before after 3 h of incubation.

Calculations

A. Average the test and blank fluorescence intensity units (FIU) from the triplicate measures of each.
B. Subtract the blank FIU from the test sample FIU.
C. Use the standard curve (described previously) to determine the remaining neutral lipid in the donor fraction of the test sample.
D. Calculate the CETP activity in ρmol cholesterol ester transferred/µl plasma/hr as follows:

CETP Activity (µmol/µl/h) =
$[(m \times (\text{sample FIU} - \text{blank FIU})) + b)/0.5\ \mu\text{l plasma}/3\ \text{h})$

where: m = slope; b = intercept; 0.5 µl = diluted sample volume; 3 h = incubation time.

Summary

It is our hope that the assays outlined in this chapter are helpful for establishing these methods and procedures in your laboratory. Although these methods have been employed in our laboratories as described, we recognize that variations in our procedures may be incorporated in other laboratories with equal success. We encourage readers to review other resources on these and other analytical techniques for researching lipid and lipoprotein metabolism.[3,4]

References

1. National Institutes of Health. *Lipid & Lipoprotein Analysis. Lipid Research Clinics Manual of Laboratory Operations 1*. HEW Publication No. NIH 75-628, U.S. Government Printing Office, Washington, DC, 1974.
2. National Institutes of Health. Current status of blood cholesterol measurement in clinical laboratories in the U.S.: A report from the Laboratory Standardization Panel of the National Cholesterol Education Program. *Clin. Chem.*, 34, 193, 1988.
3. Converse, C., Skinner, E.R., *Lipoprotein Analysis: A Practical Approach*, 1st ed., Oxford University Press, New York, 1992.
4. Rifai, N., Warnick, G.R., *Laboratory Measurements of Lipids, Lipoproteins and Apolipoproteins*, AACC Press, Washington, DC, 1994.
5. Hegsted, D.M., Nicolosi, R.J., Individual variation in serum cholesterol levels. *Proc. Natl. Acad. Sci. USA*, 84, 6259, 1987.
6. Durrington, P., Biological variation in serum lipid concentrations. *Scand. J. Lab. Invest.*, 198, 86, 1990.
7. Hammond, J., et al., Daily variation of lipids and hormones in sera of healthy subjects. *Clin. Chim. Acta*, 73, 347, 1976.
8. Allain, C., et al., Enzymatic determination of total cholesterol. *Clin. Chem.*, 20, 470, 1974.
9. Grande, F., Amatuzio, D.S., Wada, S., Cholesterol measurement in serum and plasma. *Clin. Chem.*, 10, 619, 1964.
10. Bucolo, G., David, H., Quantitative determination of serum triglycerides by the use of enzymes. *Clin. Chem.*, 19, 476, 1973.
11. Kahn, S., et al., Multicenter evaluation of automated immunoturbidimetric assays for measurement of apolipoproteins A-I and B in serum and plasma. *Clin. Chem.*, 40, 1722, 1994.
12. Krauss, R., et al., Heparin-released plasma lipase activities and lipoprotein levels in distance runners. *Circulation*, 6 (Suppl. II), 73, 1979.
13. Thompson, P., et al., Postheparin plasma lipolytic activities in physically active and sedentary men after varying and repeated doses of intravenous heparin. *Metabolism*, 35, 999, 1986.
14. Rainwater, D.L., Electrophoretic separation of LDL and HDL subclasses, in *Methods in Molecular Biology, Vol. 110*, Ordovas, J., Ed., Humana Press, Totowa, NJ, 1998, p. 137.

15. Krauss, R.M., Burke, D.J., Identification of multiple subclasses of plasma low density lipoproteins in normal humans. *J. Lipid Res.*, 23, 97, 1982.
16. Schumaker, V.N., Puppione, D.L. Sequential flotation ultracentrifugation, in *Methods in Enzymology, Vol. 128,* Albers, J., Segrest, J., Eds., Academic Press, Philadelphia, 1986, p. 155.
17. Edelstein, C., Scanu, A.M., Precautionary measures for collecting blood destined for lipoprotein isolation, in *Methods in Enzymology, Vol. 128,* Albers, J., Segrest, J., Eds., Academic Press, Philadelphia, 1986, p. 151.
18. Mulder, C., Schouten, J.A., Popp-Snijders, C., Determination of free fatty acids: A comparative study of the enzymatic versus the gas chromatographic and the colorimetric method. *J. Clin. Chem. Clin. Biochem.*, 21, 823, 1983.
19. Mizuno, K., et al., A new enzymatic method for colorimetric determination of free fatty acids. *Anal. Biochem.*, 108, 6, 1980.
20. National Cholesterol Education Program. Third Report of the National Cholesterol Education Program (NCEP) Expert Panel on Detection, Evaluation and Treatment of High Cholesterol in Adults (Adult Treatment Panel III) Final Report. *Circulation,* 106, 3143, 2002.
21. Grundy, S.M., et al., Implications of recent clinical trials for the National Cholesterol Education Program Adult Treatment Panel III Guidelines. *Circulation,* 110, 227, 2004.
22. Cheung, M., Albers, J., The measurement of apolipoproteins A-I and A-II levels in men and women by immunoassay. *J. Clin. Invest.*, 60, 43, 1977.
23. Curry, M., et al., Electroimmunoassay, radial immunoassay and radial immunodiffusion assay evaluated by quantification of human apolipoprotein B. *Clin. Chem.*, 24, 280, 1978.
24. Bury, J., et al., Immunonephelometric quantitation of the apolipoprotein C-III in human plasma. *Clin. Chim. Acta*, 145, 249, 1985.
25. Marcovina, S.M., et al., International Federation of Clinical Chemistry Standardization Project for Measurements of Apolipoproteins A-I and B. *Clin. Chem.*, 37, 1676, 1991.
26. Simo, J.M., et al., Evaluation of a fully-automated particle-enhanced turbidimetric immunoassay for the measurement of plasma lipoprotein (a). Population-based reference values in an area with low incidence of cardiovascular disease. *Clin. Biochem.*, 36, 129, 2003.
27. Noma, A., Hata, Y., Goto, Y., Quantitation of serum apolipoprotein A-I, A-II, B, C-II, C-III and E in healthy Japanese by turbidimetric immunoassay: Reference values, and age- and sex-related differences. *Clin. Chim. Acta,* 199, 147, 1991.
28. Boerma, G.J., de Bruijn, A.M., van Teunenbroek, A., Reference values for apolipoprotein A-I and apolipoprotein B in serum still depend on choice of assay techniques. *Eur. J. Clin. Chem. Clin. Biochem.*, 32, 923, 1994.
29. Otvos, J.D., Jeyarajah, E.J., Bennett, D.W. Quantification of plasma lipoproteins by proton nuclear magnetic resonance spectroscopy. *Clin. Chem.*, 37, 377, 1991.
30. Otvos, J.D., et al., Development of a proton NMR spectroscopic method for determining plasma lipoprotein concentrations and subspecies distribution from a single, rapid measurement. *Clin. Chem.*, 38, 1632, 1992.
31. Havel, R.J., Edler, H.A., Bragdon, J.H., The distribution and chemical composition of ultracentrifugally separated lipoproteins in human serum. *J. Clin. Invest.*, 34, 1345, 1955.

32. Pietzsch J, et al., Very fast ultracentrifugation of serum lipoproteins: Influence on lipoprotein separation and composition. *Biochim. Biophys. Acta,* 1254, 77, 1995.
33. Burstein, M., Scholnick, H.R., Morfin, R., Rapid method for isolation of lipoproteins from human serum by precipitation with polyanions. *J. Lipid Res.,* 11, 583, 1970.
34. Gidez, L, et al., Separation and quantitation of subclasses of human plasma high density lipoproteins by a simple precipitation procedure. *J. Lipid Res.,* 23, 1206, 1982.
35. Demacker, P.N.M., Letters to the editor: Differential determination of HDL-subfractions in clinical laboratories. *Clin. Chem.,* 35, 701, 1989.
36. Bachorik, P., Albers, J., Precipitation methods for quantification of lipoproteins, in *Methods in Enzymology, Vol. 129,* Albers, J., Segrest, J., Eds., Academic Press, Philadelphia, 1986, p. 78.
37. Warnick, G., Albers, J., A comprehensive evaluation of the heparin-manganese precipitation procedure for estimating high density lipoprotein cholesterol. *J. Lipid Res.,* 19, 65, 1978.
38. Gambert, P., et al., Direct quantitation of serum high density lipoprotein subfractions separated by gradient gel electrophoresis. *Clin. Chim. Acta,* 172, 183, 1988.
39. Rainwater, D.L., et al., Characterization of a composite gradient gel for the electrophoretic separation of lipoproteins. *J. Lipid Res.,* 38, 1261, 1997.
40. Williams, P.T., et al., Identifying the predominant peak diameter of high-density and low-density lipoproteins by electrophoresis. *J. Lipid Res.,* 31, 1131, 1990.
41. Taskinen, M.-R., Nikkila, E., High density lipoprotein subfractions in relation to lipoprotein lipase activity of tissues in man — evidence for reciprocal regulation of HDL_2 and HDL_3 levels by lipoprotein lipase. *Clin. Chem. Acta,* 112, 325, 1981.
42. Nikkila, E., et al., Regulation of lipoprotein metabolism by endothelial lipolytic enzymes, in *Treatment of Hyperlipoproteinemia,* Carlsson, J., et al., Eds., Raven Press, New York, 1984, p. 667.
43. Krauss, R., Levy, R., Fredrickson, S., Selective measurement of two lipase activities in postheparin plasma from normal subjects and patients with hyperlipoproteinemia. *J. Clin. Invest.,* 54, 1107, 1974.
44. Morikawa, W., et al., Measurement of Lp(a) with a two-step monoclonal competitive sandwich ELISA method. *Clin. Biochem.,* 28, 269, 1995.
45. Dousset, N., et al., Use of a fluorescent radiolabeled triacylglycerol as a substrate for lipoprotein lipase and hepatic triglyceride lipase. *Lipids,* 23, 605, 1988.
46. Liodakis, A., et al., Spectrofluorometric determination of lipase activity. *Biochem. Int.,* 23, 825, 1991.
47. Hendrickson, H.S., Fluorescence-based assays of lipases, phospholipases, and other lipolytic enzymes. *Anal. Biochem.,* 219, 1, 1994.
48. Duque, M., et al., New fluorogenic triacylglycerol analogs as substrates for the determination and chiral discrimination of lipase activities. *J. Lipid Res.,* 37, 868, 1996.
49. Thompson, P., et al., Postheparin plasma lipolytic activities in physically active and sedentary men after varying repeated doses of intravenous heparin. *Metabolism,* 35, 999, 1986.
50. Belfrage, P., Vaughan, M., Simple liquid-liquid partition system for isolation of labeled oleic acid from mixtures with glycerides. *J. Lipid Res.,* 10, 341, 1969.

51. Bagdade, J., Ritter, M., Subbaiah, P., Accelerated cholesteryl transfer in plasma of patients with hypercholesterolemia. *J. Clin. Invest.*, 87, 1259, 1991.
52. Barter, P., Hopkins, G., Ha, Y., The role of lipid transfer proteins in plasma lipoprotein metabolism. *Am. Heart J.*, 13, 538, 1987.
53. Tall, A., et al., Accelerated transfer of cholesteryl esters in dislipidemic plasma, role of cholesterol ester transfer protein. *J. Clin. Invest.*, 79, 1217, 1987.
54. Tato, F., et al., Relation between cholesterol ester transfer protein activities and lipoprotein cholesterol in patients with hypercholesterolemia and combined hyperlipidemia. *Atheroscler. Thromb. Vasc. Biol.*, 15, 112, 1995.
55. Inazu, A., et al., Enhanced cholesteryl ester transfer protein activities and abnormalities of high density lipoproteins in familial hypercholesterolemia. *Horm. Metab. Res.*, 24, 284, 1992.
56. Guyard-Dangermont, V., et al., Competitive enzyme-linked immunosorbent assay of the human cholesteryl ester transfer protein (CETP). *Clin. Chim. Acta,* 231, 147, 1994.
57. Ritsch, A., et al., Polyclonal antibody-based immunoradiometric assay for quantification of cholesteryl ester transfer protein. *J. Lipid Res.*, 34, 673, 1993.
58. Grandjean, P., et al., The influence of cholesterol status on blood lipid and lipoprotein enzyme changes in sedentary men after exercise. *J. Appl. Physiol.*, 89, 472, 2000.
59. Brocia, R., CETP Activity Kit, U.S. Patent Nos. 5,585,235; 5,618,683; 5,770,355; 2002.
60. National Cholesterol Education Program. Executive Summary of the Third Report of the National Cholesterol Education Program (NCEP) Expert Panel on Detection, Evaluation and Treatment of High Blood Cholesterol in Adults (Adult Treatment Panel III). *JAMA,* 285, 2486, 2001.

8

Metabolic Syndrome

Vic Ben-Ezra

CONTENTS

Introduction 147
Dyslipidemia: The Good, the Bad, and the Ugly 149
Waist Circumference: Its Association with Elevated Triglycerides, Hyperapolipoprotein B, Small Dense LDL, and Hyperinsulinemia 150
LPL Activity: A Key to Lipid Dysregulation and Insulin Resistance? 152
Leptin, Lipotoxicity, and PPARs 156
Adiponectin: A Player in Lipid Dysregulation? 158
Acylation-Stimulating Pathway (ASP): New Player in the Insulin Resistance–Dyslipidemic Relationship? 159
Summary and Conclusions 162
References 163

Introduction

In the year 2000 poor diet and physical inactivity was the second (16.6%) estimated actual cause of death in the United States totaling 400,000, second only to tobacco at 435,000 deaths (18.1%).[1] This represents an increase of one-third from the 1990 data where poor diet and inactivity accounted for an estimated 300,000 deaths, and the largest increase among all actual causes of death. The authors suggest that the 2000 data may underestimate the impact of diet and inactivity and therefore overtake deaths related to smoking.[1] These alarming figures when coupled with the NHANES III data which indicate that approximately 24% of the United States population (47 million) has the metabolic syndrome (MS),[2] present extraordinary challenges to the U.S. health care system now and in the years to come.

TABLE 8.1

National Cholesterol Education Program (NCEP): The Metabolic Syndrome

Risk Factor	Defining Level
Waist circumference	
Men	> 102 cm (approx. 40 inches)
Women	> 88 cm (approx. 35 inches)
Triglycerides	> 1.7 mmol/L (150 mg/dl)
HDL-C	
Men	< 1.03 mmol/L (40 mg/dl)
Women	< 1.29 mmol/L (50 mg/dl)
Blood pressure	> 130/80 mmHg
Fasting glucose	> 6.1 mmol/L (110 mg/dl)

The metabolic syndrome is diagnosed when three or more of these factors are present.

Dyslipidemia, often referred to as the atherogenic lipid phenotype, the atherogenic lipid profile,[3] or atherogenic dyslipidemia, often characterized by a combination of hypertriglyceridemia, low high-density lipoprotein (HDL) levels, a preponderance of small dense low-density lipoprotein (LDL) particles, and hyperapolipoproteinemia B, is closely linked to the MS and increased risk for coronary heart disease. In fact the relationship between the MS and cardiovascular disease, predominantly through lipid dysregulation, is remarkable.

NHANES III, conducted by the National Center for Health Statistics, Centers for Disease Control and Prevention, examined the relationship between NCEP-defined MS (see Table 8.1), diabetes, and the prevalence of coronary heart disease. Among participants age 50 years and older, with and without diabetes, the prevalence of the MS was 43.5%.[4] Although diabetes is surely associated with increased frequency of coronary heart disease (CHD), NHANES III data indicate that having diabetes and the MS increases the CHD risk by approximately 2.5-fold over those with diabetes alone (Figure 8.1). It should also be noted that the incidence of MS in those without diabetes is almost double that of diabetics with MS and the prevalence of the MS was approximately 60% greater than the prevalence of Type 2 diabetes in the same population.[4] These data can be interpreted to mean that there is more to the development of CHD than lipid dysregulation associated with the metabolic consequences of diabetes. Moreover, many point to insulin resistance (IR) as the main factor for abnormal lipidemia (elevated triglycerides, decreased HDL, increased apo B and small dense LDL), hyperglycemia, reduced cholesterol absorption, alterations in hepatic and lipoprotein lipase activity, and decreased plasma levels of adiponectin and increased levels of acylation-stimulating protein (ASP). The aforementioned either coexist with or contribute to dyslipidemia or elevated risk for CHD. This review will focus on those aspects of the MS, mainly IR and increased waist circumference (WC), that alter fatty acid mobilization and produce triglyceride

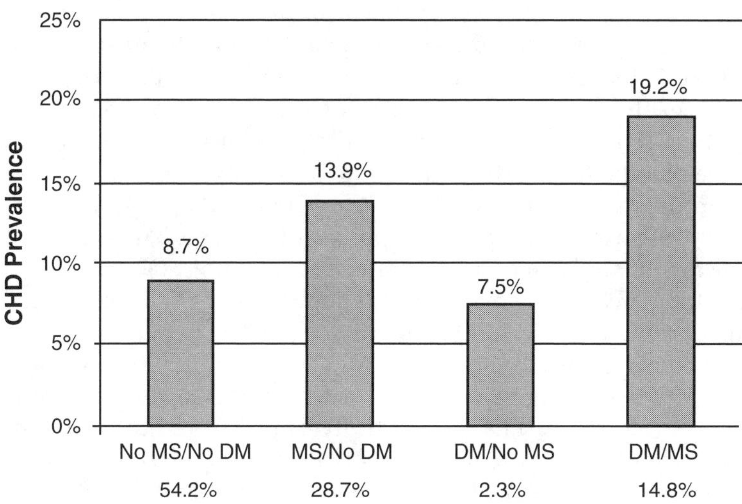

FIGURE 8.1
The relationship between CHD and MS in patients with diabetes mellitis (NHANES III).

accumulation in many non-adipose tissue sites, and how leptin, adiponectin, and ASP may play a role in this dysregulation.

Dyslipidemia: The Good, the Bad, and the Ugly

The identification of increased risk for cardiovascular disease (CVD) began with recognizing cholesterol as a primary lipid contributor of disease development. Many studies have since expanded the total cholesterol idea into examining more carefully other lipid factors such as subfractions of both HDL and LDL, HDL and LDL particle size, triglycerides, and apolipoproteins A and B. Examination of these and other factors such as insulin, and inflammatory markers like C-reactive protein (CRP) or tumor necrosis factor alpha (TNF-α) (please refer to review articles regarding details of material not covered in this monograph[5,6]), came about as a result of continued CVD development despite the reduction in total cholesterol. In fact, Sniderman et al.[7] point out that most cases of premature vascular disease found in the Framingham Study[8] had total cholesterol (TC) and LDL levels that were not very different than those individuals who did not develop premature CVD. Subsequently, both basic and prospective studies have found that CVD risk is associated with increased small dense LDL, increased triglycerides, increased apo B or apo B/apo A-1, low HDL cholesterol levels, high total cholesterol/HDL, but not as clearly or simply high levels of TC or LDL cholesterol.[8–15] In addition, in studies using LDL-lowering treatments with the outcome measures of coronary events or progression of disease, decreasing small dense LDL showed the most benefit.[16–18] Participants recruited for the AFCAPS/TexCAPS, a primary prevention study, reported at baseline with average TC and LDL-cholesterol (LDL-C) with some individuals also having low HDL-cholesterol (HDL-C) levels. Subjects were assigned lovastatin or a placebo for 1 year with the intent to compare the rate of first acute major coronary events. Baseline LDL-C, HDL-C and apo B were significant predictors of coronary events but apo B and the apo B/apo A-1 were the best on-treatment predictors of coronary events, not LDL-C.[19] Roeters van Lennep et al.[20] treated 848 patients with known coronary disease with statins and successfully reduced total cholesterol by 30%. On-treatment apo B was predictive of myocardial infarction and all-cause mortality and the apo B/apo A-1 was the strongest predictor of future cardiovascular events. On-treatment levels of TC, LDL-C and triglycerides were not associated with increased risk of cardiovascular events in these men or women with known coronary disease; however, HDL-C levels were a predictor in women. Please note that high TC or LDL-C, and or low HDL-C are not being abandoned as important risk factors to consider when examining risk for CVD. However, it is important to note that what the literature *may* be providing is additional "best practice" predictors that add, and in some cases, supplant the well-accepted measures as risk factors.

Waist Circumference: Its Association with Elevated Triglycerides, Hyperapolipoprotein B, Small Dense LDL, and Hyperinsulinemia

An enlarged waist, typically identified using NCEP ATP III guidelines of > 102 cm for men and > 88 cm for women (see Table 8.2), is linked to developing the MS and increased risk for coronary heart disease. The general hypothesis is that central fat accumulation (abdominal adiposity) results in lipid dysregulation (hypertriglyceridemia, low HDL, and increased small dense LDL levels and apo B). The evidence from a variety of population studies provides the groundwork for using a simple measure, waist circumference (WC), in conjunction with or in place of body mass index (BMI), to further or better identify individuals at risk for the MS and lipid dysregulation.[21–24] Lemieux et al.[22] suggest that using waist circumference (a correlate of increased insulin and apo B levels) and triglyceride levels (a correlate of small dense LDL) may be a more powerful tool in identifying men with an atherogenic metabolic profile. Critical cut-points for WC (≥ 90 cm) and triglycerides (≥ 2.0 mmol/L) were used to predict CAD risk factors (hyperinsulinemia, hyperapolipoprotein B, and small dense LDL). They found that using these cut-points, greater than 80% of men exhibited the atherogenic metabolic triad,

TABLE 8.2

Criteria for Metabolic Syndrome among U.S. Population ≥ 50 Years

	No Diabetes		Diabetes		
	No Metabolic Syndrome	**Metabolic Syndrome**	**No Metabolic Syndrome**	**Metabolic Syndrome**	**Total**
Percentage of population	54.2	28.7	2.3	14.8	
Criterion					
% Waist circumference (M > 102 cm; F > 88 cm)	34.4	82.0	18.5	86.0	55.0
% Triglycerides ≥ 150 mg/dl	18.0	77.8	5.1	72.1	42.8
% HDL cholesterol (M < mg/dl; F < 50 mg/dl)	16.5	70.7	2.6	69.7	39.5
Blood pressure ≥ 130/85 mmHg (%)	45.3	86.2	43.0	82.7	62.5
Fasting glucose > 110 (%)	6.2	30.9	83.0	90.2	27.2

Source: From Alexander, C.M. et al., *Diabetes*, 52, 1210, 2003. With permission.

while only 50% of men with triglyceride levels < 2.0 mmol/L but with high WC values (≥ 100 cm) had these risk factors. Validation of this model on a sample of 287 men with and without CAD found that only men with both elevated waist and triglycerides were at increased risk for CAD compared with men with low waist and triglycerides. Lemieux et al.[22] suggest that "hypertriglyceridemic waist" be used as a clinical tool to identify men at risk for CAD. Along this same line Kahn and Valdez[23] applied cut-points for elevated triglycerides (≥ 1.45 mmol/L) and enlarged WC (men ≥ 95 cm; women ≥ 88 cm) in examining 8730 adults from NHANES III with the intent to identify a state of lipid over accumulation and its metabolic consequences. Persons with enlarged waist and elevated triglycerides had higher fasting insulin, glucose, apo B, and uric acid, lower HDL cholesterol and greater prevalence of diabetes than people without enlarged waist and elevated triglycerides.

It should be noted that the NCEP cut-points for WC were determined based upon their association with BMI. Since BMI provides a more broad body view where factors like height or distribution of body fat, for example, may dilute the quality of risk factor associations, it is therefore of particular interest to discern if WC independent of BMI predicts CVD/disease risk. In addition, the NCEP WC cut-offs may in some populations or ethnic groups be too high. Okosun et al.[26] found that at the same levels of BMI (overweight: 25–29.9; obese: ≥ 30 kg/m^2) black and Hispanic men tended to have lower WC values than white men, while women across ethnic groups were similar.

Zhu et al.,[25] using NHANES III data, demonstrated that WC may be a better discriminating variable for increased risk of cardiovascular disease than BMI. However, in this study obesity-associated risk factors (HDL-C, LDL-C, glucose, blood pressure) were effectively predicted at WC of 96 cm and 85 cm for white men and women, respectively. The Canadian Heart Health Surveys data, showing waist circumference cutoffs for Caucasian men of ≥ 90 cm and women of ≥ 80 cm may be most successful for prediction of cardiovascular disease risk factors.[24]

In a series of studies[27–29] using NHANES III data, Zhu et al.[29] found that for white men, BMI in combination with WC better estimated the odds of having CVD risk factors than either measure alone, and that WC alone determined the likelihood of having CVD risks in white women. Okosun et al.[27] found that WC was strongly associated with metabolic dysregulation (hypertension, Type 2 diabetes, dyslipidemia, hypertriglyceridemia, or hyperinsulinemia) in White, Black, and Hispanic Americans independent of BMI. Lastly, Janssen et al.[28] determined that WC explains obesity-related health risk not BMI. Therefore health risks are similar across categories of BMI (normal-weight [18.5–24.9], overweight [25–29.9], class I obese [30–34.9]) if they have similar WC.

LPL Activity: A Key to Lipid Dysregulation and Insulin Resistance?

Lipoprotein lipase (LPL) has a number of roles in lipid and lipoprotein metabolism that include hydrolysis of circulating triglycerides, binding to LDL receptors and inducing receptor-mediated breakdown of very low-density lipoprotein (VLDL), and it mediates the selective uptake of cholesterol esters.[29] LPL is the major enzyme responsible for hydrolyzing triglyceride from chylomicrons and very low-density lipoprotein proteins and thereby providing fatty acids for a variety of tissues. Specifically, and most importantly, LPL can be found in adipose, heart, and skeletal muscle tissue.[30,31] For an excellent overview on LPL, see Preiss-Landl et al.[32]

LPL activity varies among tissues, adipose, heart and skeletal muscle, relative to feeding and fasting. LPL increases and decreases dramatically with feeding and fasting respectively, in adipose tissue,[33–36] while heart and skeletal LPL generally respond in the opposite direction. These changes in LPL activity promote the uptake of free fatty acids (FFAs) and thereby, storage of triglyceride in adipose tissue during feeding and diminishing triglyceride uptake by other tissues (e.g., skeletal muscle, pancreas, etc.), while the reverse condition (fasting) generally promotes sending FFAs/triglycerides to the heart and skeletal muscle for energy metabolism. Lithell et al.[36] found a 46% increase in adipose LPL and 32% decrease in skeletal muscle and heart LPL after eating in humans, while others have found 40–80% decreases in adipose, skeletal muscle, and heart tissue LPL after caloric restriction.[37,38]

Fat loss or gain has also been associated with changes in LPL. Eckel et al.[39] found a 70% decline in fasting skeletal and heart muscle LPL after a 13% body weight loss in obese women after 3 months. It should be noted that the obese women, prior to weight loss, had skeletal and heart muscle LPL that was 13% lower than normal weight controls. The implication from this study as well as those that have examined intramuscular triglyceride loss resulting from weight loss,[40,41] is that the predisposition for skeletal muscle to excessively store triglyceride is decreased, and fat storage is diminished. The effect of obesity/fat weight gain will be discussed later in association with fatty acid and/or lipid dysregulation.

As previously mentioned, LPL activity rises and falls with diet. As such, increases in insulin concurrent with plasma glucose elevation appear to upregulate skeletal muscle LPL.[37] However, if euglycemia is maintained during a hyperinsulinemic clamp, skeletal muscle LPL tends to decrease in healthy subjects. Obesity and/or insulin resistance, however, tends to cause skeletal LPL to increase in response to a euglycemic hyperinsulinemic clamp.[39,42] This rise should further exacerbate the insulin-resistant condition by increasing skeletal muscle storage of triglyceride, the result of which is linked to IR at the skeletal muscle. More recently, Goodarzi et al.[43] have found direct evidence that LPL is an IR gene using LPL haplotypes and direct quantitative measures of IR in Mexican-Americans. This data is part of the UCLA/Cedar Sinai Mexican American Coronary Artery Disease (MACAD) project that enrolls families with identified CAD. Two generations are enrolled in the study: (1) parental generation (the one with CAD and the spouse) where CAD is apparent; and (2) adult offspring and the spouses of those offspring. There were 74 families totaling 291 subjects that were both genotyped and administered the euglycemic-hyperinsulinemic clamp. The results suggest a common LPL haplotype that is protective against IR and a common haplotype that predisposes to IR in Mexican Americans. This group also found these same LPL haplotypes to protect and predispose to clinical CAD.[44]

The overexpression of muscle LPL in mice results in hyperinsulinemia and hyperglycemia. In this mouse model a mismatch occurs that appears to accelerate plasma triglyceride deposition in muscle tissue.[45] In humans it has been shown that insulin suppression of skeletal muscle LPL activity is reduced in obese women or those that have non-insulin-dependent diabetes mellitus.[46] This increased muscle LPL activity results in increased triglyceride uptake and thereby increases the potential for over-accumulation of intramuscular triglyceride. This excess triglyceride accumulation, sometimes referred to as lipotoxicity, has been closely linked to IR.[47,48]

Houmard et al.[49] reported significant increases (+ 360%) in insulin sensitivity after weight loss in morbidly obese men and women resulting from gastric bypass surgery. The improved insulin action was concurrent with significant decreases in intramuscular long-chain fatty acyl-CoAs leading the authors to conclude that, at least in part, changes in intramuscular triglyceride may be responsible for enhanced insulin action. He et al.[50] examined the effects of weight loss through caloric restriction combined with increased physical activity on muscle lipid content and droplet size in overweight and obese men and women. The intervention resulted in a decrease of 10% and 17% in weight and fat mass, respectively, along with a 16% increase in VO_{2max} and 49% increase in insulin sensitivity. The overall lipid content of the muscle did not change; however, they found that as a result of the intervention program the lipid within the muscle had dispersed into smaller and more numerous droplets. The decrease in droplet size was significantly correlated (r = –0.46) with changes in aerobic fitness. They concluded that the change in the lipid droplet size, combined with increases in oxidative enzymes, in part explains the change in insulin sensitivity. These findings may also lend some insight into the paradox of increased intramuscular triglyceride content found in endurance trained individuals who typically demonstrate excellent insulin sensitivity[51] or partly explain why intramuscular lipid is not reduced in obese subjects after diet and exercise training.[52]

Non-esterified fatty acids are believed by many to hold the key to most, if not all, IR and IR associated dyslipidemia (see Figure 8.2). The link here involves dysregulated adipocyte lipid metabolism and its effects on skeletal muscle, the liver, and the pancreatic β cells (see Figure 8.3). Data show that β-cell dysfunction is associated with elevated plasma fatty acid levels, such that increased (could lead to hyperinsulinemia) or decreased (possibly indicating a failing β cell) insulin secretion results.[53–56] However, if one looks at first-degree relatives of people with Type 2 diabetes, they typically show a poorer acute insulin response to a glucose challenge, a reduced insulin mediated glucose uptake, and significantly elevated fasting plasma FFA levels compared with those without a family history of the disease.[57,58] These people are at greater risk of developing diabetes.[57–60] Lowering the plasma FFA concentration with acipimox (i.e., drug that lowers circulating FFA) in first-degree relatives improved insulin-mediated glucose uptake as well as their

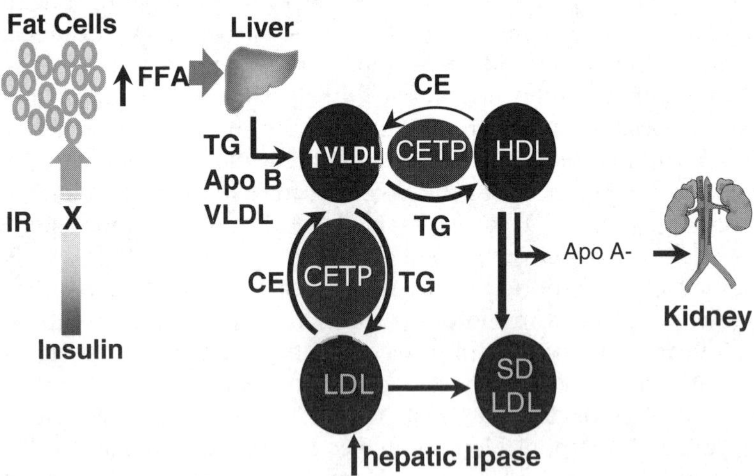

FIGURE 8.2
Mechanisms relating to insulin resistance and dyslipidemia.

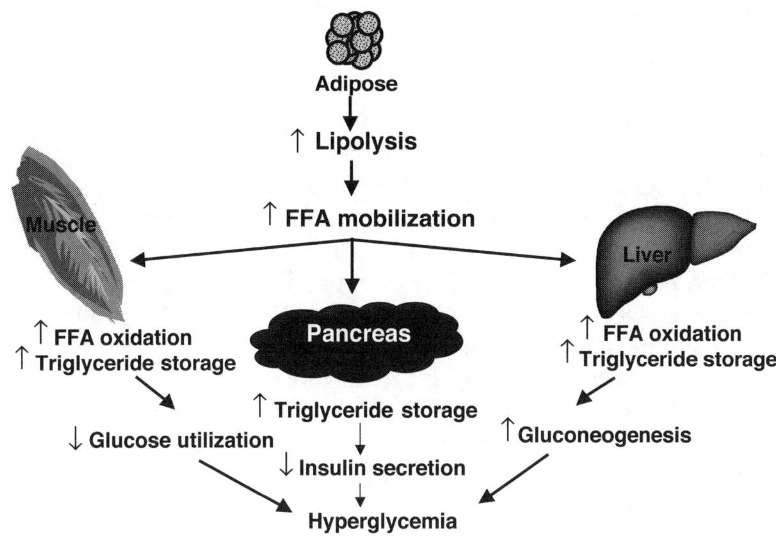

FIGURE 8.3
Increased FFA effects on other tissues.

acute insulin response[61] to a euglycemic-hyperinsulinemic clamp. A correlation ($r = -0.64$, $p < 0.006$) was found between the fall in plasma FFA and the increase in acute insulin response. These data provide further insight into the possible role that lipid dysregulation (lipotoxicity) plays in the insulin-resistance syndrome (IRS). We will also use the term insulin-resistant (IR) dyslipidemia to refer to IRS. If one examines Figure 8.3, the fat cell's oversecretion of fatty acids or underability to sequester fatty acids (discussed in the next section) appears to stimulate the liver to increase production of VLDL, triglycerides and apo B, which can lead to increased LDL, and in particular small dense LDL, while increasing the degradation of HDL and apo A-1. This mechanism is supported by data that shows increased CEPT (Guerin) and hepatic lipase activity in Type 2 diabetics.[62] The increased CEPT could promote the transfer of triglyceride to VLDL and then to LDL or from HDL directly to small dense LDL[63] which when acted upon at the liver by hepatic lipase produces small dense LDL particles.[64–66] In addition HDL, in particular HDL-2, appears to be more readily converted into HDL-3 in part by the transfer of triglyceride from VLDL to HDL (CEPT action) and its subsequent arrival at the liver where hepatic lipase hyrolyzes the triglyceride producing the more dense HDL (HDL-3).[63, 66, 67]

Leptin, Lipotoxicity, and PPARs

Leptin, a hormone primarily produced by adipocytes, appears to have significant regulatory control over food consumption, energy expenditure, fuel storage and usage, and has been implicated as the (one) link between obesity and insulin resistance.[68–70] Leptin acts by signaling the hypothalamic leptin receptors, which monitor adipose tissue mass, and produces signals that control both energy intake and energy expenditure.[68,71] Hypothalamic neurons may then be stimulated which act to stimulate sympathetic alpha-adrenergic neurons and the release of norepinephrine.[72,73] Plasma leptin levels rise with the accumulation of fat mass, and decline in response to body fat loss.[71,74] Obesity, however, appears to produce/result in hyperleptinemia and leptin resistance as evidenced by the lack of weight loss in obese individuals after exogenous leptin administration.[71,72,75] The mechanisms to explain this are not fully elucidated but may be related to alterations in the leptin receptor or the ability of leptin to cross the blood–brain barrier once hyperleptinemia develops.[76–78] Moreover, since insulin stimulates leptin production,[76–79] hyperleptinemia may be "simply" related to hyperinsulinemia. This relationship cannot explain hyperleptinemia in the face of failing pancreatic β cells, which often occurs in late stages of Type 2 diabetes. However, since leptin also mediates inhibition of insulin secretion through the β-cell leptin receptor,[81,82] this could lead to a potential role of leptin in the β cells' inability to produce and secrete insulin in sufficient quantity in Type 2 diabetes (see review by Cederberg and Enderback[83]).

Lipotoxicity (over-accumulation of tissue triglycerides) is often associated with hyperleptinemia and insulin resistance, but the association is not clear. Tissue triglyceride accumulation occurs in muscle, liver, and β cells of the pancreas, in both animal models of Type 2 diabetes, as well as Type 2 diabetic humans.[47,48,64,83] The net effect of this contributes to muscle and liver insulin resistance, a fatty liver, and pancreatic cells with impaired insulin secretion.[83–85]

Many studies have found a significant positive correlation between plasma leptin and insulin in both obese and non-obese men and women with and without diabetes.[86–88] It should also be noted that humans and animals that lack adipose tissue (lipoatrophy) are insulin-resistant, a state that is partially reversed with leptin replacement.[90–93] Leptin treatment improves insulin sensitivity,[83,84,94] possibly through decreasing the amount of intramuscular triglyceride accumulation. In this regard, leptin has been shown to protect non-adipose tissue from intracellular triglyceride accumulation by increasing the oxidation of fatty acids. This appears to be accomplished through the down-regulation of malonyl-CoA production via suppression (phosphorylation) of acetyl-CoA carboxylase thereby decreasing lipogenesis (triglyceride production) and increasing fatty acid oxidation.[70,94] The key signaling mechanism may be through AMP-kinase (AMPK). Leptin inhibits acetyl CoA carboxylase via activation of AMPK. Minokoshi et al.[95] found that leptin increases

AMPK in soleus and red gastrocnemius muscle of mice in two ways: directly by muscle incubated with leptin and indirectly through stimulation of alpha-adrenergic sympathetic nerves via leptin stimulation of hypothalamic neurons. It should be noted that increased AMPK activation is also associated with increased GLUT-4 transporter activation in contracted skeletal muscle in both non-diabetic and diabetic subjects, thus promoting glucose uptake and improving insulin sensitivity.[96–99]

AMPK stimulation in liver, muscle and adipose tissue has also been associated with glitazone treatment.[100, 101] Decreasing triglycerides in islet cells via troglitazone administration in Zucker diabetic fatty rats[85,102] prevents lipotoxicity, reduces cell apoptosis, and improves insulin sensitivity. Humans with Type 2 diabetes[103–106] or impaired glucose tolerance[107,108] also treated with troglitazone, or the newer thiazolidinediones pioglitazone and rosiglitazone, improve glycemic control and insulin sensitivity. After 12 weeks on troglitazone therapy 18 non-diabetic obese subjects, half of whom had impaired glucose tolerance, showed the following improvements: 27% increase in glucose disposal rates, 128% increase in the insulin-sensitivity index, 48% decrease in fasting insulin, and a 40% decrease in plasma insulin response to an oral glucose challenge.[108] Others have demonstrated an improved insulin secretion rate in people with IGT after troglitazone treatment.[107] Troglitazone also produced a 50% increase in insulin sensitivity in first-degree relatives of Type 2 diabetics,[109] individuals known to demonstrate insulin resistance.[59–61] Thiazolidinediones, other molecular actions are thought to work through peroxisome proliferator-activated receptors (PPARs) which regulate genes involved with adipocyte differentiation and lipid and glucose metabolism (see reviews by Olefsky,[110] Ferre,[112] and Glide and Van Bilsen[111]). The PPARs, α, β, γ, are members of a family of nuclear transcription factors that are distributed at different levels of expression in a variety of tissues. PPARα is mainly found in tissues with high rates of fatty acid oxidation such as the liver, and skeletal and cardiac muscle. It may be in part responsible for regulating muscle lipid homeostasis through regulation of genes in human skeletal muscle cells that promote fatty acid catabolism such as carnitine palmityltransferase, malonyl-CoA decarboxylase, and pyruvate dehydrogenase kinase.[113] These effects on skeletal muscle would reduce intramyocellular triglyceride accumulation and result in improved insulin sensitivity. In fact Ye et al.[114] found that activating either PPARα (with a specific chemical agonist) or (with Pioglitazone) increased whole-body insulin sensitivity and reduced muscle triglyceride and long-chain acyl-CoAs in rats fed a high-fat diet. Overall insulin sensitivity was inversely correlated with muscle long-chain acyl-CoAs (r = 0.74) and with plasma triglycerides (r = 0.77). Troglitazone[115] and rosiglitazone[106] have both been shown to decrease plasma fatty acid levels, and all three thiazolidinediones increased fatty acid uptake in skeletal muscle cells of Type 2 diabetics.[116]

PPARγ is found predominantly in adipose tissue and to a minor extent in skeletal muscle, stimulates fatty acid storage and uptake, and is involved in reducing leptin and up-regulating adiponectin expression. It is through activation of PPARγ that the glitazone family, in part, has its effects. For a pharmacological overview of the cellular and metabolic actions of thiazolidinediones please see Owens.[117]

Adiponectin: A Player in Lipid Dysregulation?

Adiponectin, a protein produced by adipocytes, is reported to be involved in glucose and fatty acid metabolism via decreased hepatic glucose production, and increased fatty acid oxidation in skeletal muscle.[118] Thus, adiponectin may be a link in the mechanisms involved with insulin resistance since it decreases triglyceride concentration in liver and skeletal muscle in obese mice.[83,84,118] Low plasma levels of adiponectin are found in individuals with insulin resistance, obesity, or coronary heart disease.[119,120] In an attempt to discriminate between obesity and IR in their relationship with adiponectin, Abbasi et al.[121] examined plasma adiponectin levels in obese and non-obese individuals, with and without insulin resistance. Fasting plasma adiponectin levels were measured in 60 non-diabetic individuals who were divided into four groups based upon their BMI (≥ 30 or < 27) and insulin sensitivity (sensitive or resistant). Insulin-resistant subjects had significantly lower adiponectin levels whether they were obese or non-obese (17.1 μg/ml vs. 16.3 μg/ml, respectively) compared with the insulin sensitive obese or non-obese (34.3 μg/ml vs. 29.8 μg/ml, respectively) subjects. Furthermore, Weyer et al.[119] found similar results when comparing Caucasians and Pima Indians over a wide range of BMI, body fat, and insulin sensitivity. Plasma adiponectin concentration was negatively correlated with percent body fat ($r = -0.43$), fasting plasma insulin ($r = -0.63$) and positively correlated with insulin sensitivity ($r = 0.59$). Faraj et al.[122] found that improved insulin sensitivity was best predicted ($r = 0.70$) by the increase in adiponectin in morbidly obese men and women who were either weight stable or reducing in weight after gastric bypass surgery. Results of these studies point to a closer association of adiponectin with insulin sensitivity than with obesity. Moreover, circulating adiponectin levels were significantly reduced in non-obese, insulin-resistant first-degree relatives of Type 2 diabetics, and negatively correlated with fasting insulin and positively correlated with insulin sensitivity.[123] It should be noted that the underlying mechanism(s) linking insulin-resistant related variables and adiponectin are as yet undefined. However, adiponectin stimulates AMPK in skeletal muscle[124] and troglitazone treatment in normal, obese, and Type 2 diabetic subjects increased plasma adiponectin concentration.[125] Both of these actions reduce triglyceride accumulation and may ameliorate insulin resistance-related lipid dysregulation. Lastly, 21 days of pioglitazone treatment resulted in a twofold increase in adiponectin while markedly decreasing endogenous glucose production via increased hepatic insulin action in Type 2 diabetics.[126] These findings provide links to the involvement of PPARγ in the insulin resistance syndrome. Insulin-resistant mouse models including lipoatrophic diabetic and obese and Type 2 diabetic mice all show a reversal of insulin resistance when adiponectin is introduced.[127]

Acylation-Stimulating Pathway (ASP): New Player in the Insulin Resistance–Dyslipidemic Relationship?

We introduced earlier in this review concepts that reveal an important metabolic "cross-talk" between adipose tissue, insulin, and the adipose tissue hormones leptin and adiponectin that may combine, in a redundant systems fashion, to regulate fuel homeostasis and lipid partitioning. Studies examining cellular signaling pathways such as the AMPK system and the PPAR network have revealed a promising mechanistic connection between adipose tissue hormones and insulin sensitivity. Insulin action is effected by a number of cytokine hormones secreted by adipose tissue (e.g., leptin, adiponectin; see above) that are involved in the regulation of energy homeostasis and lipid partitioning.[69,117,120] One such adipocyte secretagogue that has received increased attention is acylation-stimulating protein (ASP).[128] Recent review articles cover other adipocyte secretagogues (e.g., resistin, interleukin-6, TNF-α) that are not covered in this monograph.[5, 6, 83, 84, 118, 148]

ASP, which is also known as C3a-des-Arg, is another lipogenic autocrine secretion that acts similarly to insulin in function (i.e., lipogenic and inhibits hormone sensitive lipase), and therefore may provide an additional "piece" to the energy homeostasis–lipid-partitioning "puzzle" that presents as the IR-dyslipidemic state. The precursor components required to form ASP are compliment C3, adipsin, and factor B, all of which are synthesized and secreted by fully differentiated adipose cells.[128]

Similar to the function of insulin, ASP is an important biological mediator between the balance of triglyceride synthesis and degradation (lipolysis).[129] Upon binding ASP receptors, a G-coupled signal transduction pathway elicits the secondary messenger diacylglycerol (DAG) and the eventual downstream translocation of protein kinase C.[130] Currently it is believed that ASP stimulation of TG synthesis is effected through a protein kinase C-dependent mechanism that directly phosphorylates serine/threonine residues on diacylglycerol acyltransferase (DGAT),[131] the rate-limiting enzyme in TG synthesis. In addition, ASP may also influence FFA re-esterification through a phosphodiesterase 4 (PDE4)-mediated mechanism; however, the preceding upstream signaling pathway has yet to be determined.[132] Insulin, on the other hand, also effects lipid status in adipocytes primarily by TG synthesis, FFA re-esterification, and inhibition of lipolysis through stimulation of phosphatidylinositol 3-kinase in a phosphodiesterase 3 (PDE3)-dependent manner, degrading cAMP thus inhibiting hormone sensitive lipase.[132–134]

Furthermore, with the recent discovery of an ASP-specific orphan G protein-coupled receptor (C5L2) associated with a G_i subunit,[135, 136] the processes involved in ASP signaling are becoming more clear. ASP-responsive receptors are expressed in 3T3-L1 cells, human fibroblasts and human adipose tissue, and possibly in rat skeletal muscle.[137] In addition to ASP's role in TG synthesis at the adipocyte (very similar to that of insulin), glucose transport is enhanced through translocation of glucose transporters (Glut1, Glut3, and Glut4) to the adipocyte plasma membrane surface as well as in rat skeletal muscle tissue cultures.[137–139] In fact, a recent study using the rat knock-out model[139] suggests that ASP in the normophysiological state has differential effects on non-esterified fatty acids (NEFA) trapping in adipose and skeletal muscle. Essentially, in adipose tissue ASP increases LPL activity and the resultant trapping of NEFA to form TG. ASP functions in an "anti-lipotoxic" fashion at the skeletal muscle, decreasing LPL activity and thereby supporting the hydrolysis and lipolysis (i.e., oxidation) of lipid substrate.[137] In addition, ASP facilitates the "trapping" of the glycerol backbone from the glucose molecule providing an essential substrate for the esterification of fatty acids and the storage of energy for future metabolic needs. Interestingly, Weyer et al.[140] did not find an association between insulin action and ASP concentrations in an at-risk population (i.e., Pima Indians) for the development of IR and dyslipidemia. Further development of the obesity concept and the possible role that ASP "resistance" plays in fatty acid and/or lipid dysregulation will be discussed later.

The consequence of a dysregulated insulin–peripheral tissue axis (liver, skeletal muscle, and pancreatic β cell) leads to the well-defined exacerbation of lipolysis of adipose tissue TG stores. The storage and release of FFA by adipocytes is an important mechanism for energy availability. As noted earlier in this chapter, it is well known that there is differential regulation of LPL activity in adipose tissue and muscle as observed *in vivo* in the fasting and fed state with insulin-mediated LPL activity primarily affecting TG hydrolysis. Similar to LPL, several lines of evidence suggest that ASP action is also under nutritional regulation; increasing in adipose tissue and decreasing in muscle during the postprandial rise in insulin, with reciprocal changes observed during fasting.[137,141] However, ASP's main function is to trap the fatty acids (i.e., liberated during TG hydrolysis through subsequent insulin-mediated LPL activity) directly into adipocytes.[142] It is important to note here that TG clearance and fatty acid trapping occur concurrently and result from different signaling pathways (see above). Therefore, analogous to the insulin–LPL relationship with IR dyslipidemia discussed earlier, ASP has begun to receive marked attention as a possible metabolic marker of obesity-related disorders and may have considerable pathophysiological significance in the metabolic syndrome.

Abnormal function of the ASP pathway leads to a state of ineffective "fatty-acid trapping" in adipose tissue[143] comparable to that seen in insulin resistance (i.e., resulting from chronic elevated FFA concentrations). A number of disorders such as obesity, diabetes and cardiovascular diseases associated with dyslipidemia have been linked to abnormal adipose tissue metabolism and elevated FFA, as well as elevated plasma ASP concentrations.[144,145] Cianflone[144] has demonstrated that ASP levels in gynoid obese individuals are double in magnitude compared with those in an age-matched control group. Also in a recent study by the same group,[146] surgically induced weight loss showed a strong correlation between reduced plasma ASP and the change in apo B (mg/dl) ($r = 0.55$, $p = 0.009$). In the same patient group, an index of postoperative insulin sensitivity correlated well with changes in adiponectin concentrations ($r = -0.70$, $p = 0.01$). In addition, a dysfunctional ASP pathway has been demonstrated in hyper-apo B subjects.[147] Sniderman et al.[147] showed decreased binding of radiolabeled ASP in the face of elevated circulating ASP concentrations, suggesting reduced receptor number and tissue responsiveness. Recently, it has been hypothesized that a defective ASP pathway in some obese subjects, as indicated by ineffective ASP binding when exposed to elevated FFA, may be representative of an "ASP resistant" state.[148] A decreased ASP tissue responsiveness may lead to insulin resistance (i.e., secondary to elevated circulating FFA concentrations) as a result of inefficient FFA trapping and to the eventual development of the previously noted constellation of metabolic risk factors that lead to peripheral tissue lipotoxicity. It is plausible to infer that alterations in plasma ASP in Type 2 diabetics and the resultant elevations in FFA due to ineffective fatty acid trapping may encourage a hyper-apo B lipid profile. Some discrepancy exists in the literature regarding circulating plasma ASP levels in hyper-apo B patients.[147,149,150] Kildsgaard's group[149] did not find elevated plasma ASP concentrations in hyper-apo B patients while Zhang et al.[150] found elevated plasma ASP concentrations in a similar patient group. Both the Sniderman[147] and Faraj[148] reviews note that the use of the arteriovenous difference technique at the subcutaneous adipose depot of obese and or hyper-apo B patients may be a better method to determine the existence of elevated ASP. These authors report that ASP can only be detected in a capillary bed site-specific manner. Still others have measured elevated whole blood concentrations of ASP in these populations.[142,143,146] At this time it is important to note that the different methodological approaches employed throughout the literature surely contribute to some difficulties in interpreting the currently available data.

Interestingly, in Pima Indians (a group at high risk for the development of Type 2 diabetes), a recent study showed a genetic bivariate linkage with circulating ASP (↑) levels for BMI (↑) and HDL (↓), each an important risk factor for the development of the metabolic syndrome.[151] It should be noted that ASP normally enhances glucose uptake; however, paradoxically, in Pima Indians (again a population at increased risk for IR dyslipidemia) ASP levels did not correlate well with insulin action as determined by the hyperglycemic-euglycemic glucose clamp.[140] Neither radiolabeled ASP on whole plasma nor subcutaneous capillary arteriovenous difference experiments were obtained in this study so it cannot be ascertained if indeed this group was in fact ASP resistant. It is important to note, however, that obese individuals may simply have elevated ASP concentrations because of enlarged adipocytes (similar to hyperleptinemia), therefore having a greater potential to trap FFAs, thus increasing TG esterification beyond adipocyte capabilities.[148] Consequently, additional support to the heterogeneity of overweight and obesity may be phenotypically presented as either an "ASP resistant" individual with overproduction of ASP or as "ASP deficient" as noted in knock-out rat models where fasting ASP concentrations are normal yet become abnormally elevated in the postprandial state with a resultant delay in TG clearance.[152] Interestingly, obese women show a marked increase in postprandial fatty acid trapping, potentially contributing to adipocyte enlargement and quite efficient TG clearance.[153] Further studies examining circulating levels of ASP in populations at increased risk for the development of IR dyslipidemia could provide a useful insight into the potential role that ASP may play in the development of lipotoxicity-related comorbidities. The fatty-acid trapping capacity of individuals with different phenotypic presentations of obesity associated with Type 2 diabetes may be a key determinant in differentiating those individuals at greater risk for developing a hyper-apoB lipid profile.[147] Moreover, continued pursuit of basic science research using knock-out rat and mouse models may provide useful insights into the mechanisms behind ASP's regulatory contribution to IR dyslipidemia.

Summary and Conclusions

The insulin-resistance syndrome manifests itself by involving many tissues including the liver, skeletal muscle, and adipose tissue. The derangements that result affect fuel metabolism and energy homeostasis that produces increased risk for cardiovascular disease. At the center of the dysregulated metabolism, of both carbohydrate and lipid metabolism, appears to be the adipocyte where fatty acids are preferentially and "correctly" stored as triglycerides thereby not allowing triglycerides to overaccumulate in other tissues. This is intimately tied into the adipocyte's ability to secrete the hormones leptin, adiponectin, and ASP (Figure 8.4). These hormones are responsible for food intake and storage as well as influencing energy expenditure through both fat and carbohydrate metabolism. This "adipocentric" view is widely supported by both human and animal studies that present central fat deposition, and in most cases, visceral fat, as the root of dysregulated metabolism that can lead to acquiring the metabolic syndrome. So it sounds pretty simple: avoidance of the metabolic syndrome/insulin-resistance syndrome may merely, in part, lie with keeping one's waistline in check, especially as we age where the tendency is to gain weight and the incidence of the metabolic syndrome is high. Keeping an active lifestyle combined with prudent dietary considerations may in many cases avoid the onset of the metabolic syndrome, and associated lipid dysregulation and

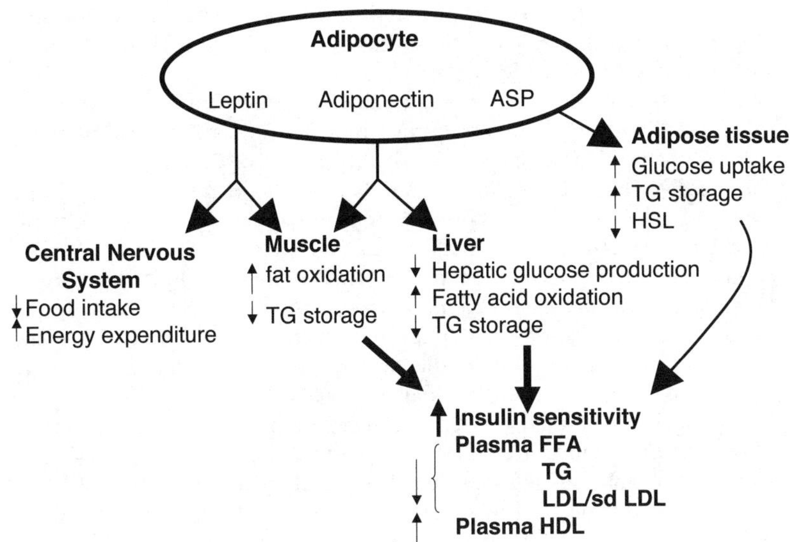

FIGURE 8.4
Adipocentric regulation of metabolism.

increased risk for cardiovascular disease. Failure to do this puts one's metabolic fate in the hands of pharmaceuticals like thiazolidinediones to correct metabolic dysregulation, or other medications, such as "statins" or niacin, which return blood lipids and lipoproteins back to the normal range.

References

1. Mokdad, A.H., et al., Actual causes of death in the United States, 2000. *JAMA*, 291(10), 1238, 2004.
2. Ford, S., Giles, W.H., and Dietz, W.H. Prevalence of the metabolic syndrome among US adults: findings from the third National Health and Nutrition Examination Survey. *JAMA*, 287(3), 356, 2002.
3. Pan, J., et al. Extended-release niacin treatment of the atherogenic lipid profile and lipoprotein (a) in diabetes. *Metabolism*, 51, 1120, 2002.
4. Alexander, C.M., Landsman, P.B., Teutsch, S.M., and Haffner, S.M. NCEP-defined metabolic syndrome, diabetes, and prevalence of coronary heart disease among NHANES III participants age 50 years and older. *Diabetes*, 52, 1210, 2003.
5. Steppan, C.M., et al. The hormone resistin links obesity to diabetes. *Nature*, 409(6818), 307, 2001.
6. Fernandez-Real, J.M. & Ricart, W. Insulin resistance and chronic cardiovascular inflammatory syndrome. *Endocrine Rev.*, 34(3), 278, 2003.
7. Sniderman, A.D., Bergeron, J., and Frohlich, J. Apolipoprotein B versus lipoprotein lipids: vital lessons from the AFCAPS/TexCAPS trial. *Can. Med. Assoc. J.*, 164, 44, 2001.

8. Kannel, W.B., Castelli, W.P., and Gordon, T. Cholesterol in the prediction of atherosclerotic disease. New perspectives based on the Framingham study. *Ann. Intern. Med.*, 90(1), 85, 1979.
9. Walldius, G., Junger, I., Holme, I., et al. High apolipoprotein B, low apolipoprotein A-I, and improvement in the prediction of fatal myocardial infarction (AMORIS study): a prospective study. *Lancet*, 358, 2026, 2001.
10. Talmud, P.J., Hawe, E., Miller, G.J., and Humphries, S.E. Non-fasting apo B and triglyceride levels as a useful predictor of coronary heart disease risk in middle-aged UK men. *Arterioscler. Thromb. Vasc. Biol.*, 22, 1918, 2002.
11. Sattar, N., Petrie, J.R., and Jaap, A.J. The atherogenic lipid phenotype and vascular endothelial dysfunction. *Atherosclerosis*, 138, 229, 1998.
12. Festa, A., et al. Low-density lipoprotein particle size is inversely related to plasminogen activator inhibitor-1 levels. The Insulin Resistance Atherosclerosis Study. *Arterioscler. Thromb. Vasc. Biol.*, 19, 605, 1999.
13. Lamarche, B., et al. Small, dense low-density lipoprotein particles as a predictor of the risk of ischemic heart disease in men. *Circulation*, 95, 69, 1997.
14. Lamarche, B., et al. Apolipoprotein A-I and B levels and the risk of ischemic heart disease during a five-year follow-up of men in the Quebec Cardiovascular Study. *Circulation*, 94, 273, 1996.
15. Stampfer, M.J., et al. A prospective study of triglyceride level, low-density lipoprotein particle diameter, and risk of myocardial infarction. *JAMA*, 276, 882, 1996.
16. Williams, K., et al. Comparison of the associations of apolipoprotein B and low-density lipoprotein cholesterol with other cardiovascular risk factors in the Insulin Resistance Atherosclerosis Study (IRAS). *Circulation*, 108, 2312, 2003.
17. Watts, G.F., et al. Independent associations between plasma lipoprotein subfraction levels and the course of coronary artery disease in the St. Thomas' Atherosclerosis Regression Study (STARS). *Metabolism*, 42, 1461, 1993.
18. Miller, B.D., et al. Predominance of dense low-density lipoprotein particles predicts angiographic benefit of therapy in the Stanford Coronary Risk Intervention Project. *Circulation*, 94, 2146, 1996.
19. Zambon, A., et al. Evidence for a new pathophysiological mechanism for coronary artery disease regression: hepatic-lipase mediated changes in LDL density. *Circulation*, 99, 1959, 1999.
20. Gotto, A.M., et al. Relation between baseline and on-treatment lipid parameters and first acute major coronary events in the Air Force/Texas Coronary Atherosclerosis Prevention Study (AFCAPS/TexCAPS). *Circulation*, 101, 477, 2000.
21. Roetters van Lennep, J.E., et al. Apolipoprotein concentrations during treatment and recurrent coronary artery disease events. *Arterioscler. Thromb. Vasc. Biol.*, 20, 2408, 2000.
22. Lemieux, I., et al. Hypertriglyceridemic waist: a marker of the atherogenic metabolic triad (hyperinsulinemia; hyperapolipoprotein B; small, dense LDL) in men. *Circulation*, 102, 179, 2000.
23. Kahn, H.S. and Valdez, R. Metabolic risk factors identified by the combination of enlarged waist and elevated triacylglycerol concentration. *Am. J. Clin. Nutr.*, 78, 928, 2003.
24. Dobbelsteyn, C.J., et al. A comparative evaluation of waist circumference, waist-to-hip ratio and body mass index as indicators of cardiovascular risk factors. The Canadian Heart Health Surveys. *Int. J. Obes.*, 25, 652, 2001.

25. Zhu, S., et al. Waist circumference and obesity-associated risk factors among whites in the third National Health and Nutrition Examination Survey: clinical action thresholds. *Am. J. Clin. Nutr.*, 76, 743, 2002.
26. Okosun, I.S., et al. Abdominal adiposity and clustering of multiple metabolic syndrome in white, black and Hispanic Americans. *Ann. Epidemiol.*, 10, 263, 2000.
27. Okosun, I.S., et al. Abdominal adiposity values associated with established body mass indexes in white, black and Hispanic Americans. A study from the Third National Health and Nutrition Examination Survey. *Int. J. Obes. Relat. Metab. Disord.*, 24, 1279, 2000.
28. Janssen, I., Katzmarzyk, P.T., and Ross, R. Waist circumference and not body mass index explains obesity-related health risk. *Am. J. Clin. Nutr.*, 79, 379, 2004.
29. Zhu, S., et al. Combination of BMI and waist circumference for identifying cardiovascular risk factors in whites. *Obes. Res.*, 12, 633, 2004.
30. Goldberg, I.J. Lipoprotein lipase and lipolysis: central roles in lipoprotein metabolism and atherogenesis. *J. Lipid Res.*, 37, 693, 1996.
31. Merkel, M., et al. Inactive lipoprotein lipase (LPL) alone increases selective cholesterol ester uptake *in vivo*, whereas in the presence of active LPL it also increases triglyceride hydrolysis and whole particle lipoprotein uptake. *J. Biol. Chem.*, 277, 7405, 2002.
32. Preiss-Landl, K., et al. Lipoprotein lipase: the regulation of tissue specific expression and its role in lipid and energy metabolism. *Curr. Opin. Lipidol.*, 13, 471, 2002.
33. Doolittle, M.H., et al. The response of lipoprotein lipase to feeding and fasting. *J. Biol. Chem.*, 265, 4570, 1990.
34. Galan, X., Llobera, M., and Ramirez, I. Lipoprotein lipase and hepatic lipase in Wistar and Sprague-Dawley rat tissues: differences in the effects of gender and fasting. *Lipids*, 29, 333, 1994.
35. Linder, C., et al. Lipoprotein lipase and uptake of chylomicron triglyceride by skeletal muscle of rats. *Am. J. Physiol.*, 37, 551, 1977.
36. Lithell, H., et al. Lipoprotein-lipase activity in human skeletal muscle and adipose tissue in the fasting and fed states. *Atherosclerosis*, 30, 89, 1978.
37. Taskinen, M.R. and Nikkila, E.A. Effect of caloric restriction on lipid metabolism in man. *Atherosclerosis*, 32, 289, 1979.
38. Taskinen, M.R. and Nikkila, E.A. Lipoprotein lipase of adipose tissue and skeletal muscle in human obesity: response to glucose and to semi-starvation. *Metabolism*, 30, 810, 1981.
39. Eckel, R.H., Yost, T.J., and Jensen, D.R. Sustained weight reduction in moderately obese women results in decreased activity of skeletal muscle lipoprotein lipase. *Eur. J. Clin. Invest.*, 25, 396, 1995.
40. Goodpaster, B.H., et. al. Intramuscular lipid content is increased in obesity and decreased by weight loss. *Metabolism*, 49, 467, 2000.
41. Greco, A., et. al. Insulin resistance in morbid obesity: reversal with intramyocellular fat depletion. *Diabetes*, 52, 144, 2002.
42. Richelsen, B., et al. Lipoprotein lipase activity in muscle tissue influenced by fatness, fat distribution, and insulin in obese females. *Eur. J. Clin. Invest.*, 23, 226, 1993.
43. Goodarzi, M.O., et al. Lipoprotein lipase is a gene for insulin resistance in Mexican Americans. *Diabetes*, 53, 214, 2004.

44. Goodarzi, M.O., et al. Determination and use of haplotypes, ethnic comparison and association of the lipoprotein lipase gene and coronary artery disease. *Genet. Med.*, 5, 322, 2003.
45. Jensen, D.R., et. al., Prevention of diet induced obesity in transgenic mice overexpressing skeletal muscle lipoprotein lipase. *Am. J. Physiol.*, 273, R683, 1997.
46. Yost, T.J., et al. Change in skeletal muscle lipoprotein lipase activity in response to insulin/glucose in non-insulin-dependent diabetes mellitus. *Metabolism*, 44, 786, 1995.
47. Goodpaster, B.H., et. al. Subcutaneous abdominal fat and thigh muscle composition predict insulin sensitivity independently of visceral fat. *Diabetes*, 46, 1579, 1997.
48. Jacob, S., et. al. Association of increased intramyocellular lipid content with insulin resistance in lean nondiabetic offspring of Type 2 diabetic subjects. *Diabetes*, 48, 1113, 1999.
49. Houmard, J.A., et al. Effect of weight loss on insulin sensitivity and intramuscular long-chain fatty acyl-coAs in morbidly obese subjects. *Diabetes*, 51, 2959, 2002.
50. He, J., Goodpaster, B.H., and Kelley, D.E. Effects of weight loss and physical activity on muscle lipid content and droplet size. *Obes. Res.*, 12, 761, 2004.
51. Goodpaster, B., et al. Skeletal muscle lipid content and insulin resistance: evidence for a paradox in endurance-trained athletes. *J. Clin. Endocrinol. Metab.*, 86, 5755, 2001.
52. Malenfant, P., et al. Elevated intramyocellular lipid concentration in obese subjects is not reduced after diet and exercise training. *Am. J. Physiol.*, 280, E632, 2001.
53. Milburn, J.L., et al. Pancreatic-cells in obesity: evidence of functional, morphologic and metabolic abnormalities by increased long-chain fatty acids. *J. Biol. Chem.*, 270, 1295, 1995.
54. Crespin, S.R., Greenough, W.B., and Steinberg, D. Stimulation of insulin secretion by long-chain free fatty acids. *J. Clin. Invest.*, 52, 1979, 1973.
55. Zhou, Y.P. and Grill, V. Long-term exposure of rat pancreatic islet to fatty acids inhibits glucose-induced insulin secretion and biosynthesis through a glucose fatty acid cycle. *J. Clin. Invest.*, 93, 870, 1994.
56. Paolisso, G., et al. Opposite effects of short- and long-term fatty acid infusion on insulin secretion in healthy subjects. *Diabetologia*, 38, 1295, 1995.
57. Warram, J., et al. Slow glucose removal rate and hyperinsulinemia precede the development of type II diabetes in the offspring of diabetic patients. *Ann. Intern. Med.*, 113, 909, 1990.
58. Pimenta, W., et al. Pancreatic-cell dysfunction as the primary genetic lesion in NIDDM. Evidence from studies in normal glucose tolerant individuals with first degree NIDDM relative. *J.A.M.A.*, 273, 1855, 1995.
59. Eriksson, J., et al. Early metabolic defects in persons at increased risk for non-insulin dependent diabetes mellitus. *N. Engl. J. Med.*, 321, 337, 1989.
60. Perseghin, G., et al. Metabolic defects in lean nondiabetic offspring of NIDDM parents: a cross-sectional study. *Diabetes*, 46, 1001, 1997.
61. Paolisso, G., et al. Lowering fatty acids potentiates acute insulin response in first-degree relatives of people with type II diabetes. *Diabetologia*, 41, 1127, 1998.
62. Baynes, C., et al. The role of insulin sensitivity and hepatic lipase in the dyslipidemia of type 2 diabetes. *Diabet. Med.*, 8, 560, 1991.

63. Guerin, M., et al. Proatherogenic role of elevated CE transfer from HDL to VLDL1 and LDL in type 2 diabetes: Impact of the degree of triglyceridemia. *Arterioscler. Thromb. Vasc. Biol.*, 21, 282, 2002.
64. Cheung, M.C., et al., Lipoprotein lipase and hepatic lipase: their relationship with HDL subspecies Lp(A-1) and Lp(A-1, A-II). *J. Lipid Res.*, 44, 1552, 2003.
65. Kuusi, T., et al. Postheparin plasma lipoprotein and hepatic lipase are determinants of hypo- and hyperalphalipoproteinemia. *J. Lipid Res.*, 30, 1117, 1989.
66. Zambon, A., et al. Common variants in the promoter of the hepatic lipase gene are associated with lower levels of hepatic lipase activity, buoyant LDL, and higher HDL-2 cholesterol. *Arterioscler. Thromb. Vasc. Biol.*, 18, 1723, 1998.
67. Deeb, S.S., et al. Hepatic lipase and dyslipidemia: interactions among genetic variants, obesity, gender, and diet. *J. Lipid Res.*, 44, 1279, 2003.
68. Zang, Y., et al. Positional cloning of the mouse obese gene and its human homologue. *Nature*, 372, 425, 1994.
69. Friedman, J.M. and Halaas, J.L. Leptin and the regulation of body weight in mammals. *Nature*, 395, 763, 1998.
70. Unger, R.H. and Orci, L. Lipotoxic diseases of nonadipose tissues in obesity. *Int. J. Obes.*, 24 (suppl 4), S28, 2000.
71. Considine, R.V., et al. Serum immunoreactive-leptin concentrations in normal-weight and obese humans. *N. Engl. J. Med.*, 334, 292, 1996.
72. Haynes, W.G., et al. Receptor-mediated regional sympathetic nerve activation by leptin. *J. Clin. Invest.*, 100, 270, 1997.
73. Seals, D.R. and Bell, C. Chronic sympathetic stimulation: consequences and cause of age-associated obesity? *Diabetes*, 53, 276, 2004.
74. Maffei, M., et al. Leptin levels in human and rodent: measurement of plasma leptin and ob RNA in obese and weight-reduced subjects. *Nat. Med.*, 1, 1155, 1995.
75. Heymsfield, S.B., et al. Recombinant leptin for weight loss in obese and lean adults: a randomized, controlled, dose-escalation trial. *J.A.M.A.*, 282, 1568, 1999.
76. Banks, W.A., et al. Leptin enters the brain by a saturable system independent of insulin. *Peptides*, 17, 305, 1996.
77. Caro, J., et al. Decreased cerebrospinal-fluid/serum leptin ratio in obesity: a possible mechanism for leptin resistance. *Lancet*, 348, 159, 1996.
78. Schwartz, M.W., et al. Cerebrospinal fluid leptin levels: relationship to plasma levels and to adiposity in humans. *Nat. Med.*, 2, 589, 1996.
79. Boden, G., et al. Effects of prolonged hyperinsulinemia on serum leptin in normal human subjects. *J. Clin. Invest.*, 100, 1107, 1997.
80. Barr, V.A., et al. Insulin stimulates both leptin secretion and production by rat white adipose tissue. *Endocrinology*, 138, 4463, 1997.
81. Seufert, J., Kieffer, T.J., and Habener, J.F. Leptin inhibits insulin gene transcription and reverses hyperinsulinemia in leptin-deficient ob/ob mice. *Proc. Natl. Acad. Sci. USA*, 96, 674, 1999.
82. Kieffer, T.J., et al. Leptin suppression of insulin secretion by the activation of ATP-sensitive K+ channels in pancreatic beta-cells. *Diabetes*, 46, 1087, 1997.
83. Cederberg, A. and Enerback, S. Insulin resistance and type 2 diabetes- an adipocentric view. *Curr. Mol. Med.*, 3, 107, 2003.
84. McGarry, J.D. Dysregulation of fatty acid metabolism in the etiology of type 2 diabetes. *Diabetes*, 51, 7, 2002.
85. Shimabukuro, M., et al. Fatty acid-induced cell apoptosis: a link between obesity and diabetes. *Proc. Natl. Acad. Sci. USA*, 95, 2498, 1998.

86. Segal, K.R., Landt, M., and Klein, S. Relationship between insulin sensitivity and plasma leptin concentration in lean and obese men. *Diabetes*, 45, 988, 1996.
87. Haffner, S.M., et al. Leptin concentrations and insulin sensitivity in normoglycemic men. *Int. J. Obes.*, 21, 393, 1997.
88. Zimmet, P.Z., et al. Is there a relationship between leptin and insulin sensitivity independent of obesity? A population-based study in the Indian Ocean nation of Mauritius. Mauritius NCD Study Group. *Int. J. Obes. Relat. Metab. Disord.*, 22, 171, 1998.
89. Milewicz, A., Miklski, E., and Bidzinska, B. Plasma insulin, cholecystokinin, galanin, neuropeptide Y and leptin levels in obese women with and without type 2 diabetes mellitus. *Int. J. Obes. Relat. Metab. Disord.*, 24 (suppl 2), S152, 2000.
90. Figlewicz, D.P., et al. Leptin reverses sucrose-conditioned place preference in food-restricted rats. *Physiol. Behav.*, 73, 229, 2001.
91. Keim, N.L., Stern, J.S. and Havel, P.J. Relation between circulating leptin concentrations and appetite during prolonged, moderate energy deficit in women. *Am. J. Clin. Nutr.*, 68, 794, 1998.
92. Rosenbaum, M., et al. Low dose leptin administration reverses effects of sustained weight-reduction on energy expenditure and circulating concentrations of thyroid hormones. *J. Clin. Endocrinol. Metab.*, 87, 2392, 2002.
93. Ebihara, K., et al. Transgenic overexpression of leptin rescues insulin resistance and diabetes in a mouse model of lipoatrophic diabetes. *Diabetes*, 50, 1440, 2001.
94. Kahn, B.B. and Flier, J.S. Obesity and insulin resistance. *J. Clin. Invest.*, 106, 473, 2000.
95. Minokoshi, Y., et al. Leptin stimulates fatty-acid oxidation by activating AMP-activated protein kinase. *Nature*, 415, 339, 2002.
96. Tomas, E., Zorzano, A., and Ruderman, N.B. Exercise and insulin signaling: a historical perspective. *J. Appl. Physiol.*, 93, 765, 2002.
97. Sakamoto, K. and Goodyear, L.J. Invited review: intracellular signaling in contracting skeletal muscle. *J. Appl. Physiol.*, 93, 369, 2002.
98. Musi, N. and Goodyear, L.J. AMP-activated protein kinase and muscle glucose uptake. *Acta Physiol. Scand.*, 178, 227, 2003.
99. Ruderman, N.B., et al. AMPK as a metabolic switch in rat muscle, liver and adipose tissue after exercise. *Acta Physiol. Scand.*, 178, 435, 2003.
100. Saha, A.K., et al. Pioglitazone treatment activates AMP-activated protein kinase in rat liver and adipose tissue *in vivo*. *Biochem. Biophys. Res. Commun.*, 314, 580, 2004.
101. Fryer, L.G., Parbu-Patel, A., and Carling, D. The anti-diabetic drugs rosiglitazone and metformin stimulate AMP-activated protein kinase through distinct signaling pathways. *J. Biol. Chem.*, 277, 25226, 2002.
102. Higa, M., et al. Troglitazone prevents mitochondrial alterations, cell destruction, and diabetes in obese prediabetic rats. *Proc. Natl. Acad. Sci. USA*, 96, 11513, 1999.
103. Raskin, P., et al. Rosiglitazone short-term monotherapy lowers fasting and postprandial glucose in patients with type II diabetes. *Diabetologia*, 43, 278, 2000.
104. Levin, K., et al. Metabolic effects of troglitazone in NIDDM patients. *Endocrinol. Metab.*, 4, 255, 1997.
105. Mudaliar, S. and Henry, R.R. New oral therapies for type 2 diabetes mellitus: the glitazones or insulin sensitizers. *Annu. Rev. Med.*, 52, 239, 2001.

106. Patel, J., Anderson, R.J., and Rappaport, E.B. Rosiglitazone monotherapy improves glycaemic control in patients with type 2 diabetes: a twelve-week, randomized, placebo-controlled study. *Diabetes Obes. Metab.*, 1, 165, 1999.
107. Cavaghan, M.K., et al. Treatment with oral antidiabetic agent troglitazone improves cell responses to glucose in subjects with impaired glucose tolerance. *J. Clin. Invest.*, 100, 530, 1997.
108. Nolan, J.J., et al. Improvement in glucose tolerance and insulin resistance in obese subjects treated with troglitazone. *N. Engl. J. Med.*, 331, 1188, 1994.
109. Levin, K., et al. Effects of troglitazone in young first-degree relatives of patients with type 2 diabetes. *Diabetes Care*, 27, 148, 2004.
110. Olefsky, J.M. Treatment of insulin resistance with peroxisome proliferator-activated receptor agonists. *J. Clin. Invest.*, 106, 467, 2000.
111. Glide, A.J. and Van Bilsen, M. Peroxisome proliferator-activated receptors (PPARS): regulators of gene expression in heart and skeletal muscle. *Acta Physiol. Scand.*, 178, 425, 2003.
112. Ferre, P. The biology of peroxisome proliferator-activated receptors: relationship with lipid metabolism and insulin sensitivity. *Diabetes*, 53 (suppl 1), 2004.
113. Muoio, D.M., et al. Peroxisome proliferator-activated receptor-α regulates fatty acid utilization in primary human skeletal muscle cells. *Diabetes*, 51, 901, 2002.
114. Ye, J-M., et al. Peroxisome proliferator-activated receptor (PPAR)-α activation lowers muscle lipids and improves insulin sensitivity in high fat-fed rats. Comparison with PPAR-γ activation. *Diabetes*, 50, 411, 2001.
115. Maggs, D.G., et al. Metabolic effects of troglitazone monotherapy in type 2 diabetes mellitus. A randomized, double-blind, placebo-controlled trial. *Ann. Intern. Med.*, 128, 176, 1998.
116. Wilmsen, H.M., et al. Thiazolidinediones upregulate impaired fatty acid uptake in skeletal muscle of type 2 diabetic subjects. *Am. J. Physiol. Endocrinol. Metab.*, 285, E354, 2003.
117. Owens, D.R. Thiazolidinediones. A pharmacological overview. *Clin. Drug Invest.*, 22, 485, 2002.
118. Havel, P.J. Update on adipocyte hormones. Regulation of energy balance and carbohydrate/lipid metabolism. *Diabetes*, 53 (suppl 1), S143, 2004.
119. Weyer, C., et al. Hypoadiponectinemia in obesity and Type 2 diabetes: close association with insulin resistance and hyperinsulinemia. *J. Clin. Endocrinol. Metab.*, 86, 1930, 2001.
120. Pischon, T., et al. Plasma adiponectin levels and risk of myocardial infarction in men. *J.A.M.A.*, 291, 1730, 2004.
121. Abbasi, F., et al. Discrimination between obesity and insulin resistance in the relationship with adiponectin. *Diabetes*, 53, 585, 2004.
122. Faraj, M., et al. Plasma acylation-stimulating protein, adiponectin, leptin, and ghrelin before and after weight loss induced by gastric bypass surgery in morbidly obese subjects. *J. Clin. Endocrinol. Metab.*, 88, 1594, 2003.
123. Pellme, F., et al., Circulating adiponectin levels are reduced in non-obese but insulin-resistant first degree relatives of type 2 diabetic patients. *Diabetes*, 52, 1182, 2003.
124. Yamauci, T., et al. Adiponectin stimulates glucose utilization and fatty-acid oxidation by activating AMP-activated protein kinase. *Nat. Med.*, 8, 1288, 2002.
125. Yu, J.G., et al. The effect of thiazolidinediones on plasma adiponectin levels in normal, obese, and type 2 diabetic subjects. *Diabetes*, 51, 2968, 2002.

126. Tonelli, J., et al. Mechanisms of early insulin-sensitizing effects of thiazolidinediones in type 2 diabetes. *Diabetes*, 53, 1621, 2004.
127. Yamauchi, T., et al. The fat-derived hormone adiponectin reverses insulin resistance associated with both lipoatrophy and obesity. *Nat. Med.*, 7, 941, 2001.
128. Cianflone, K.M., et al. Purification and characterization of acylation stimulating protein. *J. Biol. Chem.*, 264, 426, 1989.
129. Cianflone, K. Acylation stimulating protein and triacylglycerol synthesis: potential drug targets? *Curr. Pharm. Design*, 9, 1397, 2003.
130. Baldo, A., et al. Signal transduction pathway of acylation stimulating protein: involvement of protein kinase C. *J. Lipid Res.*, 36, 1415, 1995.
131. Yasruel, Z., et al. Effect of acylation stimulating protein on the triacylglycerol synthetic pathway of human adipose. *Lipids*, 26, 495, 1991.
132. Van Harmelen, V., et al. Mechanisms involved in the regulation of free fatty acid release from isolated human fat cells by acylation-stimulating protein and insulin. *J. Biol. Chem.*, 274(26), 18243, 1999.
133. Kono, T., et al. Insulin-sensitive phosphodiesterase. Its localization, hormonal, stimulation, and oxidative stabilization. *J. Biol. Chem.*, 250, 7826, 1975.
134. Solomon, S.S., et al. Effect of insulin and lipolytic hormones on cyclic AMP phosphodiesterase activity in normal and diabetic rat adipose tissue. *Endocrinology*, 96, 1366, 1975.
135. Cain, S.A. & Monk, P.N. The orphan receptor C5L2 has high affinity binding sites for complement fragments C5a and C5a des-Arg^{74}. *J. Biol. Chem.*, 277, 7165, 2002.
136. Kalant, D., et al. The chemoattractant receptor-like protein C5L2 binds C3a des-Arg^{77}/acylation-stimulating protein. *J. Biol. Chem.*, 278(13), 11123, 2003.
137. Faraj, M. and Cianflone, K.M. Differential regulation of fatty acid trapping in mouse adipose tissue and muscle by ASP. *Am. J. Physiol. Endocrinol. Metab.*, 287, E150, 2004.
138. Maslowska, M., et al. ASP stimulates glucose transport in cultured human adipocytes. *Int. J. Obes.*, 21, 261, 1997.
139. Tao, Y., et al. Acylation-stimulating protein (ASP) regulates glucose transport in rat L6 muscle cell lines. *Biochim. Biophys. Acta*, 1344(3), 221, 1997.
140. Weyer, C., et al. Insulin action and insulinemia are closely related to fasting complement C3, but not acylation stimulating protein concentration. *Diabetes Care*, 23(6), 779, 2000.
141. Faraj, M. Enhanced dietary fat clearance in postobese women. *J. Lipid Res.*, 42, 571, 2001.
142. Sniderman, A.D., et al. Of mice and men (and women) and the acylation-stimulating protein pathway. *Curr. Opin. Lipidol.*, 11, 291, 2000.
143. Murray, I., et al. Acylation-stimulating protein (ASP): structure-function determinants of cell surface binding and triacylglycerol synthetic activity. *Biochem. J.*, 342, 41, 1999.
144. Cianflone, K. The acylation stimulating protein pathway: clinical implications. *Clin. Biochem.*, 30, 301, 1997.
145. Sniderman, A.D, et al. The adipocyte, fatty acid trapping, and atherogenesis. *Arterioscler. Thromb Vas Biol.*, 18, 147, 1998.
146. Faraj, M., et al. Plasma acylation-stimulating protein, adiponectin, leptin, and ghrenlin before and after weight loss induced by gastric bypass surgery in morbidly obese subjects. *J. Clin. Endocrinol. Metab.*, 88(4), 1594, 2003.

147. Sniderman, A.D., et al. Hypertryglyceridemic hyperapoB: the unappreciated atherogenic dyslipoproteinemia in type 2 diabetes mellitus. *Ann. Intern. Med.*, 135, 447, 2001.
148. Faraj, M., et al. Diabetes, lipids, and adipocyte secretagogues. *Biochem. Cell Biol.*, 82, 170, 2004.
149. Kildsgaard, J., et al. A critical evaluation of the putative role of C3adesArg (ASP) in lipid metabolism and hyperapobetalipoproteinemia. *Mol. Immunol.*, 36, 869, 1999.
150. Zhang, X.J, et al. plasma acylation stimulating protein (ASP) as a predictor of impaired cellular biological response to ASP in patients with hyperapoB. *Eur. J. Clin. Invest.*, 28, 730, 1998.
151. Martin, L.J., et al. Bivariate linkage between acylation-stimulating protein and BMI and high-density lipoproteins. *Obes. Res.*, 12(4), 669, 2004.
152. Xia, Z., et al. Acylation stimulating protein (ASP/compliment C3adesArg) deficiency results in increased energy expenditure in mice. *J. Biol. Chem.*, 279, 4051, 2004.
153. Kalant, D., et al. Increased postprandial fatty acid trapping in subcutaneous adipose tissue in obese women. *J. Lipid Res.* 41, 1963, 2000.

9

Obesity, Lipoproteins, and Exercise

Theodore J. Angelopoulos

CONTENTS

Introduction 173
Lipoproteins, Obesity and Visceral Adiposity 174
Lifestyle Modification of Dyslipidemias 177
Conclusion 178
References 179

Introduction

Obesity refers to excess body fat and develops in response to a chronic energy surplus. The number of obese, defined as a body mass index (BMI) greater than or equal to 30 kg/m^2,[1] is on the rise. Specifically, the overall prevalence has risen in the past decade to almost one-third of the U.S. population.[2] Obesity is a serious health problem in the United States and is a major risk factor for a number of diseases. Obesity has been linked to an increase in the prevalence of chronic diseases such as cardiovascular, diabetes mellitus, cancer (certain types), arthritis, gallbladder and sleep apnea (Figure 9.1).

A common, but interesting finding is that fat location plays a relevant role in the increased health risk associated with obesity. Vague was the first to recognize the increased risk of male (android) fat patterning,[3] but many since have expanded on this finding. Waist circumference has been found to be a better predictor of cardiovascular disease (CVD) risk than BMI.

Alterations in lipoprotein profiles in obese individuals, such as increased low-density lipoprotein (LDL), are associated with increased risk for coronary heart diseases. Lipoprotein metabolism plays a central role in the etiology of coronary heart diseases. Blood lipid and lipoprotein levels may be modified with exercise and/or caloric restriction weight loss.[4–6] Some species

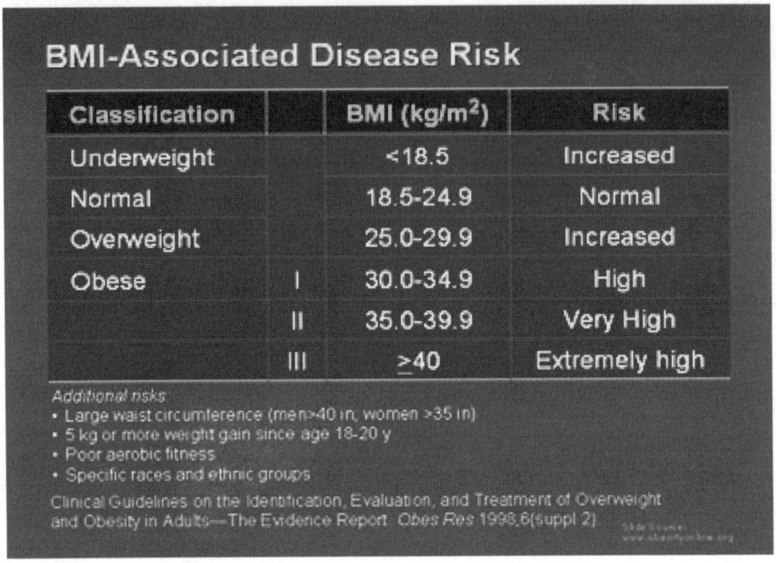

BMI-Associated Disease Risk

Classification		BMI (kg/m²)	Risk
Underweight		<18.5	Increased
Normal		18.5-24.9	Normal
Overweight		25.0-29.9	Increased
Obese	I	30.0-34.9	High
	II	35.0-39.9	Very High
	III	≥40	Extremely high

Additional risks
- Large waist circumference (men>40 in, women >35 in)
- 5 kg or more weight gain since age 18-20 y
- Poor aerobic fitness
- Specific races and ethnic groups

Clinical Guidelines on the Identification, Evaluation, and Treatment of Overweight and Obesity in Adults—The Evidence Report. *Obes Res* 1998;6(suppl 2)

FIGURE 9.1
Body mass index and risk of diseases.

of lipoproteins unfortunately are under strong genetic influence and are not altered by these lifestyle factors known to influence other lipoproteins.[7] By understanding the mechanism of exercise in the prevention of cardiovascular diseases, health professionals can better develop a plan to optimize the exercise regimen.

Lipoproteins, Obesity and Visceral Adiposity

Obesity increases the risk of developing CVD. At a BMI (in kg/m^2) of greater than 30, there are substantial increases in both men and women in reference to LDL count and significant decreases in high-density lipoprotein (HDL),[8–10] as compared to a BMI of 25. LDL particle size is a good predictor for coronary heart disease (CHD) risk. Indeed, Schaefer et al.[11] found that CHD patients have smaller LDL particles than control subjects. Increases in triglycerol (TG) and remnant-like particles, decreases in HDL cholesterol, and alterations in LDL particle size are common in obese and diabetic subjects.[12,13]

Obesity commonly exists as a state of insulin resistance (IR), and a possible early stage in the development of Type 2 diabetes (referred to here on out as simply "diabetes"). The link between the two is so strong that the term "diabesity" has even been proposed.[12] A BMI of over 35 has been shown to

Lipids and Lipoproteins & Resting BP in Insulin-Sensitive and Insulin-Resistant Obese Subjects†

	Insulin Sensitive (n = 17)	Insulin Resistant (n = 26)
Total cholesterol (mmol/L)	5.14 ± 0.80	4.84 ± 0.91
Triglycerides (mmol/L)	1.50 ± 0.85	2.02 ± 0.87*
LDL cholesterol (mmol/L)	3.28 ± 0.72	3.00 ± 0.85
HDL cholesterol (mmol/L)	1.16 ± 0.47	0.91 ± 0.31*
TC/HDL cholesterol	5.0 ± 1.8	5.7 ± 1.8
Systolic BP (mm Hg)	137.2 ± 14.5	139.7 ± 14.8
Diastolic BP (mm Hg)	72.5 ± 11.1	75.6 ± 8.2

†Postmenopausal women.
Data are mean ± SD.
*P = 0.01.

Brochu M et al. *J Clin Endocrinol Metab.* 2001;86:1020-1025.

FIGURE 9.2
Lipids and lipoproteins and resting BP in insulin-sensitive and insulin-reistant obese subjects.

increase the risk of diabetes to 93 times that of a BMI of less than 20.[13] Highlighting the relationship between obesity and the subsequent development of diabetes is a study on a group of morbidly obese individuals who underwent bariatric surgery. After 2 years only 0.2% of the surgery group had progressed to diabetes (weight loss of 28 kg) compared with 6% who did not undergo the surgery.[14]

Due to this close link it should be obvious that similar population trends exist for diabetes as were already outlined for obesity. Accordingly, in 1995 there were an estimated 135 million Type 2 diabetics worldwide,[15] with 12.1 million estimated to reside in the United States in 2002.[16] Nationally this represents an increase of 9% (1 million from 2000), and 17% from 1997. The same estimates project the number to rise to 17.4 million by 2020, a rise of 24% in regard to percentage of population. At the national level the combined direct and indirect costs of diabetes for 2002 were estimated at $132 billion.

Pioneering work by Reaven identified several metabolic abnormalities (i.e., dyslipidemias) that commonly coexist with insulin resistance and the increased risk associated with them.[17] Despite the problems associated with using the Homeostasis Model Assessment of IR (HOMA) to evaluate IR in highly insulin-resistant individuals, a solid relationship still exists between the level of HOMA and clustering of CVD risk factors.[18] However, the relationship between IR and increased CV risk does not seem to rely solely upon the presence of obesity. Rather, IR has often been shown to be associated independently with an increased risk of CHD.[19,20] IR has been shown to be positively associated with plasma viscosity. It is possible that this may explain the link between the metabolic syndrome and vascular complications that accompany it.[21] Once diabetes develops, hyperglycemia *per se* is an obvious candidate for the increased risk associated with diabetes due to structural changes in lipoproteins,[22] and the formation of advanced glycation end products that stimulate vascular injury.[23] What should be made clear is that hyperglycemia is unlikely to be related to the increased risk associated with non-diabetic IR states due to the fact that it is typically a late development in the etiology of diabetes, as will be explained later. Also downplaying the role of hyperglycemia is the observation that there is a poor correlation between the duration of diabetes and macrovascular disease.[22]

The effects of diabetes on plasma lipid composition, often referred to as "diabetic dyslipidemia," are highly related to the clustering of metabolic abnormalities associated by Reaven. They are suspected to contribute to a significant amount of the elevated CVD risk associated with IR states. It has more recently been said that increased levels of small dense LDL particles is the true hallmark of diabetic dyslipidemia. Due to a decreased ability to bind receptors, they have been shown to confer an increased atherosclerotic risk.[24,25] Furthermore, the presence of small dense LDL particles is associated with high triglycerides and low HDL-cholesterol (HDL-C) levels.[26] It is probable that these abnormalities contribute to the elevated risk of IR, independent of diabetic status, due to the fact that diabetic dyslipidemia does not immediately correct itself with normalization of glycemia, and are also observed in a prediabetic state.[26] It is possible that the role of such plasma lipid abnormalities has been overestimated as common risk factors, and accounts for only 25–30% of the observed increased CVD risk.[27] Of particular importance, however, is the observation that plasma total cholesterol levels are often within normal range in obese individuals with excess visceral adiposity.

Alterations in lipoproteins are also associated with aging and gender. Schaefer and colleagues[11] had reported an increase in fasting TG concentrations with age. There is an 80% increase between the age of 20 and approximately 50 years. LDL concentrations increased by 30% in the same age bracket. Noted reasons on these alterations are delayed chylomicron remnant clearance in the elderly compared with younger populations. These include a decline in the fractional catabolic rate of LDL, perhaps caused by a decline in the number of LDL receptors, an age-associated increase in visceral adiposity.[28] This also may increase the rate of cholesterol synthesis. A noted increase of dietary fat intake in older populations and inactivity are also to be blamed. Very low-density lipoprotein apolipoprotein (apo) B-100 secretion being elevated in the elderly coupled with delayed clearance also accounts for the increases in TG and LDL.

In the very elderly population, those people aged 80 and above, both TG and LDL are significantly lower compared with middle-aged individuals,[11] most probably due to the reduction in BMI and decreased apo B-100 production in these subjects.[29,30]

Gender differences exist with lipoproteins, and it is now accepted that women have significantly higher concentrations of HDL cholesterol and apo

A-I than men. The ratio of HDL_3/HDL_2 is gender dependent.[31] The hormones presumably reflect the gender differences in HDL levels: androgens increase the activity of the enzyme HL and estrogens cause a decrease.[32] Even premenopausal women a have higher apo A-I secretion than men.[33] In addition, girls tend to be more susceptible to LDL decreases from weight loss compared with boys. This was concluded in a study of obese children who lost weight after intervention of diet and exercise.[34]

Lifestyle Modification of Dyslipidemias

Regular exercise has been recommended as an important strategy for the prevention and treatment of obesity. Much information has been accumulated regarding the beneficial effects of exercise. It is generally accepted that exercise training positively affects many of the components of the plasma lipoprotein-lipid profile that partly determines the person's CVD risk.[35–45] Intervention trials involving aerobic exercise training showed favorable decreases in TG[38,39,46,47] and LDL[48–51] only when combined with weight loss, even with Type 2 diabetic patients.[52] Exercise alone in most cases does not reduce plasma LDL-C.[53] Interestingly, Kokkinos et al.[54] observed that LDL-C and TG levels were positively associated with BMI but inversely correlated with the distance run per week, the frequency of exercise per week and the durations of the exercise per session. Durstine et al.[51] argued that exercise training does not always alter total cholesterol and LDL-C unless a reduction in dietary fat intake is brought about and body weight loss is a part of the exercise training program, or both. Halle et al.[55] concluded that increases in physical activity in hypocholesterolemic men lowered TG and small LDL concentrations, while Williams and colleagues[56] reported that distance per week and reduced body fat mass correlated significantly with decreases in small LDL levels. Woolf-May et al.[50] reported a decrease in LDL with short walking of 5–10 min per bout, but performing more than one bout of walking per day. Finally, LDL oxidation is important in assessing cardiovascular risk. Decreased LDL oxidation reduces the risk of arteriosclerosis, and a decreased LDL was observed following a 10-month exercise program.[59]

Generally, the beneficial effects of regular exercise on blood lipids are observed even after training at low training volumes. To observe clinically significant gains, energy expenditures of 1200 to 2200 kcal/week must be attained.[57,58] As such, there is likely a dose–response relationship between training volume and blood lipid changes.

Endurance exercise training induces significant reductions in TG. Studies reporting decreases in TG with exercise often show exercise-induced weight loss and a reduction in TG that is related to baseline values. The higher the baseline concentration, the greater the exercise-induced reductions.[53,54,60,61]

Beneficial changes in TG may also occur independent of changes in body mass.[62]

A comprehensive review of the effects of exercise on HDL-C has been undertaken by Durstine and Haskell.[63] The majority of studies report favorable increases in HDL,[64–69] and a dose–response relationship. Thresholds established from cross-sectional and longitudinal exercise training studies indicate that 15–20 miles/week of brisk walking or jogging, which elicit between 1200 and 2200 kcal of energy expenditure per week, increases HDL-C by 2–8 mg/dl.[51]

Exercise training volume (kilocalories expended during the exercise training program) is important for favorable changes in HDL concentration. It appears that reduction in body weight and fat mass may also be important for changes in HDL concentration in overweight individuals. Thompson et al.[53] found no significant changes in HDL concentration in overweight men after prolonged exercise training without weight loss. The same result was observed by Nicklas and colleagues.[70] It appears that the effectiveness of endurance training, without concomitant weight loss, is blunted in obese people. Finally, previous studies have shown that exercise training has little effect on HDL levels in subjects with initially low HDL cholesterol.[71,72]

In summary, sufficient exercise appears to induce favorable changes in lipids and lipoproteins in the obese state. Some of the beneficial effects of exercise, however, may be blunted in obese people if exercise is not combined with caloric restriction that induces weight loss. Van Gaal and colleagues[73] had shown that even 5–10% weight loss, when combined with exercise, significantly decreases TG levels and increases LDL particle size. A meta-analysis published by Dattilo et al.[74] showed that for every kilogram decreased in body weight during a weight loss process, HDL increases by 0.009 mmol/L and plasma total cholesterol, LDL and TG decrease by 0.05, 0.02 and 0.015 mmol/L, respectively.

Conclusion

Obesity is accompanied by changes in lipid–lipoprotein profiles that increase one's risk for CVD. Lifestyle modifications have shown some beneficial changes in lipids and lipoproteins of obese individuals. The impact of lifestyle modifications may be optimum when sufficient exercise is combined with caloric restriction that induces weight loss. The level of individual response may be influenced by training volume, amount of weight loss, and genetics.

References

1. Clinical Guidelines on the identification, evaluation, and treatment of overweight and obesity in adults — The Evidence Report. National Institutes of Health. *Obes. Res.* 6 Suppl 2:51S–209S, 1998.
2. Flegal KM, Carroll MD, Ogden CL, Johnson CL. Prevalence and trends in obesity among US adults, 1999–2000. *JAMA* 288:1723–1727, 2002.
3. Vague J. The degree of masculine differentiation of obesities: a factor determining predisposition to diabetes, atherosclerosis, gout, and uric calculous disease. 1956. *Obes Res* 4:204–212, 1996.
4. Sasaki J, Shindo M, Tanaka H, et al. A long-term aerobic exercise program decreases the obesity index and increases the high density lipoprotein cholesterol concentration in obese children. *Int J Obes* 11:339–345, 1987.
5. Pacy PJ, Webster J, Garrow JS. Exercise and obesity. *Sports Med* 3:89–113, 1986.
6. Sopko G, Jacobs DR Jr, Jeffery R, et al. Effects on blood lipids and body weight in high risk men of a practical exercise program. *Atherosclerosis* 49:219–229, 1983.
7. Thompson P, Tsongalis G, Seip RL, et al. Apoprotein E genotype and changes in serum lipids and maximal oxygen uptake with exercise training. *Metabolism* 53:193–202, 2004.
8. Howard BV, Ruotolo G, Robbins DC. Obesity and dyslipidemia. *Endocrinol Metab Clin North Am* 32:855–867, 2003.
9. Schaefer E. Lipoproteins, nutrition, and heart disease. *Am J Clin Nutr* 75:191–212, 2002.
10. Troxler RG, Schwertner HA. Cholesterol, stress, lifestyle, and coronary heart disease. *Aviat Space Environ Med* 56:660–665, 1985.
11. Schaefer E, Lichtenstein A, Lamon-Fava S, et al. Lipoproteins, nutrition, aging, and atherosclerosis. *Am J Clin Nutr* 61Suppl:726S–40S, 1995.
12. Brown SA, Upchurch S, Anding R, et al. Promoting weight loss in type II diabetes. *Diabetes Care* 19:613–624, 1996.
13. Siegel R, Cupples A, Schaefer E, et al. Lipoproteins, apolipoproteins, and low density lipoprotein size among diabetics in the Framingham Offspring Study. *Metabolism* 45:1267–1272, 1996.
14. Astrup A, Finer N. Redefining type 2 diabetes: 'diabesity' or 'obesity dependent diabetes mellitus'? *Obes Rev* 1:57–59, 2000.
15. Han TS, Richmond P, Avenell A, Lean ME. Waist circumference reduction and cardiovascular benefits during weight loss in women. *Int J Obes Relat Metab Disord* 21:127–134, 1997.
16. Sjostrom CD, Lissner L, Wedel H, Sjostrom L. Reduction in incidence of diabetes, hypertension and lipid disturbances after intentional weight loss induced by bariatric surgery: the SOS Intervention Study. *Obes Res* 7:477–484, 1999.
17. King H, Aubert RE, Herman WH. Global burden of diabetes, 1995–2025: prevalence, numerical estimates, and projections. *Diabetes Care* 21:1414–1431, 1998.
18. Hogan P, Dall T, Nikolov P. Economic costs of diabetes in the US in 2002. *Diabetes Care* 26:917–932, 2003.
19. Reaven GM. Banting lecture 1988. Role of insulin resistance in human disease. *Diabetes* 37:1595–1607, 1988.

20. Ohnishi H, Saitoh S, Ura N, Takagi S, Obara F, Akasaka H, et al. Relationship between insulin resistance and accumulation of coronary risk factors. *Diabetes Obes Metab* 4:388–393, 2002.
21. Bressler P, Bailey SR, Matsuda M, DeFronzo RA. Insulin resistance and coronary artery disease. *Diabetologia* 39:1345–1350, 1996.
22. Reaven GM. Insulin resistance and compensatory hyperinsulinemia: role in hypertension, dyslipidemia, and coronary heart disease. *Am Heart J* 121:1283–1288, 1991.
23. Caimi G, Sinagra D, Scarpitta AM, Lo PR. Plasma viscosity and insulin resistance in metabolic syndrome. *Int J Obes Relat Metab Disord* 25:1856–1857, 2001.
24. Kreisberg RA. Diabetic dyslipidemia. *Am J Cardiol* 82:67U–73U, 1998.
25. Hayden JM, Reaven PD. Cardiovascular disease in diabetes mellitus type 2: a potential role for novel cardiovascular risk factors. *Curr Opin Lipidol* 11:519–528, 2000.
26. Goldberg IJ. Clinical review 124: Diabetic dyslipidemia: causes and consequences. *J Clin Endocrinol Metab* 86:965–971, 2001.
27. Krauss RM. Heterogeneity of plasma low-density lipoproteins and atherosclerosis risk. *Curr Opin Lipidol* 5:339–349, 1994.
28. Miller N. Why does plasma low density lipoprotein concentration in adults increase, with age? *Lancet* 1:263–267, 1984.
29. Pouliot MC, Després JP, Nadeau A, et al. Visceral obesity in men: associations with glucose tolerance, plasma insulin, and lipoprotein levels. *Diabetes* 41:826–834, 1992.
30. Tchernof A, Lamrarche B, Prud'homme, et al. The dense LDL phenotype: association with plasma lipoprotein levels, visceral obesity and hyperinsulinemia in men. *Diabetes Care* 19:629–637, 1996.
31. Eisenberg S. High density lipoprotein metabolism. *J Lipid Res* 25:1017–1058, 1984.
32. Packard C, Sheperd J. Intravascular metabolism of high-density lipoproteins, in Betteridge D, Illingworth D, Sheperd J (Eds), *Lipoproteins in Health and Disease*, Vol. 1. New York: Oxford University Press, pp 17–30, 1999.
33. Schaefer E, Zech L, Jenkins L. Human apolipoprotein A-I and A-II metabolism. *J Lipid Res* 36:1155–1167, 1982.
34. Sothern MS, Despinasse B, Brown R, et al. Lipid profiles of obese children and adolescents before and after significant weight loss: differences according to sex. *South Med J* 93:278–282, 2000.
35. Williams PT, Stefanick ML, Vranizan KM, et al. The effects of weight loss by exercise or by dieting on plasma high-density lipoprotein (HDL) levels in men with low, intermediate, and normal-to-high HDL at baseline. *Metabolism* 43:917–924, 1994.
36. Despres JP, Lamarche B. Low-intensity endurance exercise training, plasma lipoproteins and the risk of coronary heart disease. *J Intern Med* 236:7–22, 1994.
37. Bain SC, Jones AF. Brisk walking and high density lipoprotein cholesterol. *BMJ* 300:195–196, 1990.
38. Krauss RM. Exercise, lipoproteins, and coronary artery disease. *Circulation* 79:1143–1145, 1989.
39. Weintraub MS, Rosen Y, Otto R, et al. Physical exercise conditioning in the absence of weight loss reduces fasting and postprandial triglyceride-rich lipoprotein levels. *Circulation* 79:1007–1014, 1989.

40. Butler RM, Goldberg L. Exercise and prevention of coronary heart disease. *Prim Care* 16:99–114, 1989.
41. Raz I, Rosenblit H, Kark JD. Effect of moderate exercise on serum lipids in young men with low high density lipoprotein cholesterol. *Arteriosclerosis* 8:245–251, 1988.
42. Hagan RD, Upton SJ, Wong L, et al. The effects of aerobic conditioning and/or caloric restriction in overweight men and women. *Med Sci Sports Exerc* 18:87–94, 1986.
43. Haskell WL. The influence of exercise training on plasma lipids and lipoproteins in health and disease. *Acta Med Scand Suppl* 711:25–37, 1986.
44. Haskell WL. The influence of exercise on the concentrations of triglyceride and cholesterol in human plasma. *Exerc Sport Sci Rev* 12:205–244, 1984.
45. Blair SN, Cooper KH, Gibbons LW, et al. Changes in coronary heart disease risk factors associated with increased treadmill time in 753 men. *Am J Epidemiol* 118:352–359, 1983.
46. Nieman DC, Brock DW, Butterworth D, et al. Reducing diet and/or exercise training decreases the lipid and lipoprotein risk factors of moderately obese women. *J Am Coll Nutr* 21:344–350, 2002.
47. Katzel LI, Bleecker ER, Rogus EM, et al. Sequential effects of aerobic exercise training and weight loss on risk factors for coronary disease in healthy, obese middle-aged and older men. *Metabolism* 46:1441–1447, 1997.
48. Lakka HM, Tremblay A, Despres JP, et al. Effects of long-term negative energy balance with exercise on plasma lipid and lipoprotein levels in identical twins. *Atherosclerosis* 172:127–133, 2004.
49. Okura T, Nakata Y, Tanaka K. Effects of exercise intensity on physical fitness and risk factors for coronary heart disease. *Obes Res* 11:1131–1139, 2003.
50. Woolf-May K, Kearney E, Owen A, et al. The efficacy of accumulated short bouts versus single bouts of brisk walking in improving aerobic fitness and blood lipid profiles. *Health Educ Res* 14:803–815, 1999.
51. Durstine JL, Grandjean PW, Cox CA, et al. Lipids, lipoproteins, and exercise. *J Cardiopulm Rehabil* 22:385–398, 2002.
52. Lehmann R, Vokac A, Niedermann K, et al. Loss of abdominal fat and improvement of the cardiovascular risk profile by regular moderate exercise training in patients with NIDDM. *Diabetologia* 38:1313–1319, 1995.
53. Thompson PD, Yurgalevitch SM, Flynn MM, et al. Effect of prolonged exercise training without weight loss on high-density lipoprotein metabolism in overweight men. *Metabolism* 46:217–223, 1997.
54. Kokkinos P, Holland J, Narayan P. Miles run per week and high-density lipoprotein cholesterol levels in healthy, middle aged men. *Arch Intern Med* 155:415–420, 1998.
55. Halle M, Berg A, Konig D. Differences in the concentration and composition of low-density lipoprotein subfraction particles between sedentary and trained hypocholesterolemic men. *Metabolism* 46:186–191, 1997.
56. Williams PT, Krauss RM, Vranizan KM, et al. Changes in lipoprotein subfractions during diet-induced and exercise-induced weight loss in moderately overweight men. *Circulation* 81:1293–1304, 1990.
57. Durstine JL, Thompson PD. Exercise in the treatment of lipid disorders. *Cardiol Clin* 19:471–488, 2001.
58. Durstine JL, Grandjean PW, Davis P. The effects of exercise training on serum lipids and lipoproteins: a quantitative analysis. *Sports Med* 31:1033–1062, 2001.

59. Vasankari TJ, Kujala UM, Vasankari TM, et al. Reduced oxidized LDL levels after a 10-month exercise program. *Med Sci Sports Exerc* 30:1496–1501, 1998.
60. Grandjean PW, Crouse S, O'Brien B. The effects of menopausal status and exercise training on serum lipids and the activities of intravascular enzymes related to lipid transport. *Metabolism* 47:377–383, 1998.
61. Kokkinos P, Narayan P, Colleran J. Effects of moderate intensity exercise on serum lipids in African-American men with severe systemic hypertension. *Am J Cardiol* 81:415–420, 1998.
62. Lamarche B, Després JP, Pouliot MC, et al. Is body fat a determinant factor in the improvement of carbohydrate and lipid metabolism following aerobic exercise training in obese women. *Metabolism* 41:826–834, 1992.
63. Durstine JL, Haskell WL. Effects of exercise training on plasma lipids and lipoproteins. *Exerc Sport Sci Rev* 22:477–521, 1994.
64. Stefanick ML, Mackey S, Sheehan M, et al. Effects of diet and exercise in men and postmenopausal women with low levels of HDL cholesterol and high levels of LDL cholesterol. *N Engl J Med* 339:12–20, 1998.
65. Williams PT, Krauss RM, Vranizan KM, et al. Effects of exercise-induced weight loss on low density lipoprotein subfractions in healthy men. *Arteriosclerosis* 9:623–632, 1989.
66. Williams PT, Krauss RM, Stefanick ML, et al. Effects of low-fat diet, calorie restriction, and running on lipoprotein subfraction concentrations in moderately overweight men. *Metabolism* 43:655–663, 1994.
67. Williams PT, Krauss RM, Vranizan KM, et al. Effects of weight-loss by exercise and by diet on apolipoproteins A-I and A-II and the particle-size distribution of high-density lipoproteins in men. *Metabolism* 41:441–449, 1992.
68. Hardman AHA, Jones P, Norgan N. Brisk walking and plasma high density lipoprotein cholesterol concentration in previously sedentary women. *BMJ* 229:1204–1225, 1989.
69. Whitehurst M, Menendez E. Endurance training in older women. *Physician Sports Med* 19:95–104, 1991.
70. Nicklas BJ, Katzel LI, Busby-Whitehead J, et al. Increases in high-density lipoprotein cholesterol with endurance exercise training are blunted in obese compared with lean men. *Metabolism* 46:556–561, 1997.
71. Zmuda JM, Yurgalevitch SM, Flynn MM, et al. Exercise training has little effect on HDL levels and metabolism in men with initially low HDL cholesterol. *Atherosclerosis* 137:215–221, 1998.
72. Lokey EA, Tran ZV. Effects of exercise training on serum lipid and lipoprotein concentrations in women: a meta-analysis. *Int J Sports Med* 10:424–429, 1989.
73. Van Gaal LF, Wauters MA, De Leeuw IH. The beneficial effects of modest weight loss on cardiovascular risk factors. *Int J Obes Relat Metab Disord* 21 Suppl 1:S5–S9, 1997.
74. Dattilo A, Kris-Etherton PM. Effects of weight reduction on blood lipids and lipoproteins: a meta-analysis. *Am J Clin Nutr* 56:320–328, 1992.

10

Pharmacological Treatments of Lipid Abnormalities

Sachin M. Navare and Paul D. Thompson

CONTENTS

Introduction 183
Targets for Therapy 184
Goals for Therapy 185
Therapeutic Lifestyle Changes 186
Pharmacotherapy 187
Statins 189
Bile Acid Binding Resins 194
Nicotinic Acid 197
Fibrates 199
Cholesterol Absorption Inhibitors 200
Other Therapies 202
Selection of Drug 204
Monitoring 204
Summary 205
References 205

Introduction

Cholesterol is an essential component of mammalian cell membranes and also serves as a source of steroid hormones and bile acids. Although vital for cellular growth and metabolism, its deposition into the arterial wall produces atherosclerosis.[1] Cholesterol is transported primarily as cholesteryl ester, which is water insoluble, and therefore must be transported in the water world of the bloodstream in specialized particles called lipoproteins. At least three major classes of lipoproteins are involved in transport of cholesterol. Very low-density lipoprotein (VLDL) is a triglyceride-rich particle that transports triglycerides (TGs) and cholesterol from the liver. Low-density lipoprotein (LDL) is a cholesterol-rich particle produced by the delipidation of VLDL. LDL transports cholesterol to various tissues including the arterial wall and returns cholesterol to the liver via the LDL receptor. HDL also has a major role in returning cholesterol to the liver as part of the general process known as "reverse cholesterol transport." There is overwhelming evidence that elevation in LDL-cholesterol (LDL-C) leads to the development of atherosclerosis. There is also strong evidence that elevations in TG and subnormal levels of HDL increase atherosclerotic risk. Atherosclerosis is the single most common cause of mortality in the United States accounting for almost 1.5 million deaths each year.[2] Nearly half of these deaths result from coronary artery disease (CAD). Thus treatment of the lipoprotein disorders forms the cornerstone for CAD risk reduction.

Targets for Therapy

The National Cholesterol Education Program (NCEP) Adult Treatment Panel (ATP) first published guidelines for the detection, evaluation and treatment of hyperlipidemia in 1988. The latest reiteration of these guidelines (NCEP ATP III), published in 2001, provides a simple, evidence-based, approach to management of dyslipidemia and forms the basis of the current review.[3]

ATP III identifies LDL-C as the major atherogenic lipoprotein. Extensive evidence obtained from animal, genetic, and epidemiological studies as well as clinical trials shows a strong direct relationship between levels of LDL-C and CAD events in populations with and without established CAD.[4–7] This relationship is linear and is observed over a broad range of LDL-C levels.[8] Moreover, interventions which reduce LDL-C levels reduce both short- and long-term CAD morbidity and mortality.[9] Recent clinical trials have shown that a 1% reduction in LDL reduces CAD risk by 2%. Angiographic studies have also demonstrated favorable effects on coronary lesions with LDL reduction.[10] Thus, ATP III uses LDL-C as the primary target for cholesterol-lowering therapy.

ATP III also recognizes the risk inherent in elevated VLDL levels.[11–13] Consequently, in patients at LDL goal, but whose TGs are > 200 mg/dl, non-HDL cholesterol, calculated as total cholesterol minus the HDL-C, becomes a secondary target of therapy.

HDL-C is not a distinct target of therapy in ATP III, although the risk associated with low HDL levels is recognized. Epidemiological studies have shown that CAD risk correlates inversely with HDL-C levels.[14] A 1% decrease in HDL-C is associated with a 2–3% increase in risk of CAD while a high HDL-C is considered a negative risk factor. Low HDL is associated with other atherogenic risk factors such as glucose intolerance and high TGs. Also, present strategies to increase HDL-C alter other risk factors, making it impossible to prove that increasing HDL-C alone reduces CAD events. Nevertheless, despite the absence of conclusive evidence of its value, ATP III encourages interventions that raise HDL.

Goals for Therapy

The fundamental principle of the ATP III guidelines is that the intensity of intervention is directly related to the degree of CAD risk. Therefore, the first step is to determine the 10-year CAD risk using non-LDL traditional risk factors (Table 10.1) and risk estimates provided by the Framingham Heart Study (Figure 10.1).

LDL-C treatment goals are categorized into three levels of risk (Table 10.2). Patients with the highest risk include those with existing CAD and those whose risk is equivalent to that of patients with CAD ("CAD risk equivalents"). This latter group includes diabetics, patients with non-CAD atherosclerotic disease, and those with a 10-year calculated risk > 20% since this is the approximate risk of a recurrent myocardial infarction or sudden death in patients with diagnosed CAD. The LDL-C goal for these patients is < 100 mg/dl, although an update released on July 13, 2004 suggests that a goal < 70 mg/dl is an appropriate therapeutic strategy for these high-risk patients.[15] Patients with intermediate risk are those with multiple (≥ 2) risk factors. ATP III designates a LDL-C goal of < 130 mg/dl for this category. This group is further categorized into two subgroups, one whose 10-year CAD risk is 10–20% and one whose risk is < 10%. Patients with 0–1 risk factors have the lowest risk and a LDL-C goal of < 160 mg/dl.

TABLE 10.1

Major CHD Risk Factors

Positive risk factors
1. Cigarette smoking
2. Hypertension (BP ≥ 140/90 mmHg or on antihypertensive medication)
3. Low HDL cholesterol (< 40 mg/dl)
4. Family history of premature CHD (CHD in male first degree relative < 55 years; CHD in female first degree relative < 65 years)
5. Age (men ≥ 45 years; women ≥ 55 years)
Negative risk factors
1. High HDL-C > 60 mg/dl

Men

Estimate of 10-Year Risk for Men

(Framingham Point Scores)

Age	Points
20-34	-9
35-39	-4
40-44	0
45-49	3
50-54	6
55-59	8
60-64	10
65-69	11
70-74	12
75-79	13

Total Cholesterol	Points				
	Age 20-39	Age 40-49	Age 50-59	Age 60-69	Age 70-79
<160	0	0	0	0	0
160-199	4	3	2	1	0
200-239	7	5	3	1	0
240-279	9	6	4	2	1
≥280	11	8	5	3	1

	Points				
	Age 20-39	Age 40-49	Age 50-59	Age 60-69	Age 70-79
Nonsmoker	0	0	0	0	0
Smoker	8	5	3	1	1

HDL (mg/dL)	Points
≥60	-1
50-59	0
40-49	1
<40	2

Systolic BP (mmHg)	If Untreated	If Treated
<120	0	0
120-129	0	1
130-139	1	2
140-159	1	2
≥160	2	3

Point Total	10-Year Risk %
<0	< 1
0	1
1	1
2	1
3	1
4	1
5	2
6	2
7	3
8	4
9	5
10	6
11	8
12	10
13	12
14	16
15	20
16	25
≥17	≥ 30

10-Year risk ____%

Women

Estimate of 10-Year Risk for Women

(Framingham Point Scores)

Age	Points
20-34	-7
35-39	-3
40-44	0
45-49	3
50-54	6
55-59	8
60-64	10
65-69	12
70-74	14
75-79	16

Total Cholesterol	Points				
	Age 20-39	Age 40-49	Age 50-59	Age 60-69	Age 70-79
<160	0	0	0	0	0
160-199	4	3	2	1	1
200-239	8	6	4	2	1
240-279	11	8	5	3	2
≥280	13	10	7	4	2

	Points				
	Age 20-39	Age 40-49	Age 50-59	Age 60-69	Age 70-79
Nonsmoker	0	0	0	0	0
Smoker	9	7	4	2	1

HDL (mg/dL)	Points
≥60	-1
50-59	0
40-49	1
<40	2

Systolic BP (mmHg)	If Untreated	If Treated
<120	0	0
120-129	1	3
130-139	2	4
140-159	3	5
≥160	4	6

Point Total	10-Year Risk %
< 9	< 1
9	1
10	1
11	1
12	1
13	2
14	2
15	3
16	4
17	5
18	6
19	8
20	11
21	14
22	17
23	22
24	27
≥25	≥ 30

10-Year risk ____%

FIGURE 10.1
Score sheet for 10-year CAD risk for men and women using the Framingham risk scores.

Therapeutic Lifestyle Changes

ATP III offers two major modalities for lowering LDL-C: therapeutic lifestyle changes (TLC) and drug therapy. TLC offers a variety of non-pharmacologic approaches to lower elevated cholesterol level. ATP III considers TLC as the most cost-effective means of reducing the risk of CAD. The major components of TLC are:

TABLE 10.2

Classification of CHD Risk and LDL Goals

Risk Category	Criteria	LDL-C Goal (mg/dl)	Non-HDL-C Goal (mg/dl)	LDL Level to Initiate TLC (mg/dl)	LDL Level to Initiate Drug Therapy (mg/dl)
High	1. Existing CHD 2. CHD equivalents 3. ≥ 2 risk factors (10-year risk)	< 100	< 130	≥ 100	> 100
Intermediate	≥ 2 risk factors	< 130	< 160		
	10-year risk 10–20%	< 130	< 160	≥ 130	≥ 130
	10-year risk < 10%	< 130	< 160	≥ 130	≥ 160
Low	0–1 risk factors	< 160	< 190	≥ 160	≥ 190

1. Reduction in dietary saturated fat intake to < 7% of total calories and cholesterol intake to < 200 mg/day. This may reduce LDL-C by 6–10%.
2. The use of viscous (formerly called "soluble") fiber and plant stanol/sterols. A viscous fiber intake of 5–10 g reduces LDL-C by 5% while 2–3 g of stanols/sterols daily reduce LDL-C by 6–15%.
3. Weight reduction.
4. Increased regular physical activity.

The last two modalities are mainly recommended for treatment of metabolic syndrome but may reduce LDL-C in some patients.

Pharmacotherapy

The initial step in managing serum lipids and CAD risk is to determine if the lipid levels are abnormal and what element requires treatment. This will ultimately determine the treatment approach. Screening can be based on a non-fasting sample, but if the TGs are elevated, a fasting sample must be obtained. The severity of lipid abnormalities can be classified as in Table 10.3.

The next step is to exclude secondary causes of hyperlipidemia because treatment of the secondary cause often cures the lipid abnormality (Table 10.4). Hypothyroidism, diabetes, and the nephrotic syndrome should be excluded by thyroid-stimulating hormone, glucose, hemoglobin A1c, and urinary protein measurements, respectively. The patient's medication list should also be reviewed since many drugs can produce secondary hyperlipidemia.

TABLE 10.3

Classification of Severity of Lipoprotein Abnormalities

Total Cholesterol (mg/dl)	
Desirable	< 200
Borderline high	200–239
High	≥ 240
Triglycerides (mg/dl)	
Normal	< 150
Borderline high	150–199
High	200–499
Very high	≥ 500
LDL-C (mg/dl)	
Optimal	< 100
Above optimal	100–129
Borderline high	130–159
High	160–189
Very high	≥ 190
HDL-C (mg/dl)	
Low	< 40
High	> 60

TABLE 10.4

Secondary Causes of Lipoprotein Abnormalities

1. Diabetes mellitus
2. Hypothyroidism
3. Nephrotic syndrome
4. Drugs
    a. Alcohol ingestion
    b. HIV-protease inhibitors
    c. Beta blockers
    d. Thiazide diuretics
    e. Cyclosporine
    f. Glucocorticoids
    g. Oral estrogens
    h. Isotretinoin
    i. Sertaline hydrochloride

The final step is to identify the goals of therapy and to select an appropriate pharmacological agent if dietary modification, weight loss, and physical activity fail to correct the problem. Unfortunately, hygienic interventions fail

TABLE 10.5

Summary of Effects of Various Medications on Lipoprotein Concentrations

Drug Class	LDL	HDL	TG
Statins	↓↓↓↓	↑↑	↓↓↓
Sequestrants	↓↓ to ↓↓↓	↑	↑↓
Ezetimibe	↓↓	↑	↓
Fibrates	↓ to ↓↓	↑↑↑	↓↓↓↓
Nicotinic acid	↓ to ↓↓	↑↑↑↑	↓↓↓

in most patients with severe lipid abnormalities and pharmacologic therapy is required.

Lipoprotein disorders are usually chronic conditions requiring lifelong therapy. Hence, safety, tolerability and cost effectiveness are as important as efficacy, in selecting drug therapy. Currently five classes of medications are available for treating lipid disorders. Each class affects the major lipoproteins differently (Table 10.5).

The initial drug choice should be tailored to the lipoprotein abnormality. Statins are the drugs of choice for patients with a predominantly LDL abnormality, whereas either a fibrate or niacin could be initial therapy for a patient with elevated TGs. These medicines can be used as monotherapy or in combination. Use of drugs in combination increases the efficacy of the therapy and allows use of lower doses of each medication. This strategy may reduce the side effects of individual therapy, but in some instances, such as the combination of statins with the fibric acid derivative, gemfibrozil, combined therapy can increase the risk of side effects.

Statins

Introduction

Since the introduction of lovastatin in 1987, statins have revolutionized the treatment of lipoprotein disorders. They are the most powerful drugs for reducing LDL-C and have consistently been shown to reduce the risk of all atherosclerotic clinical events.[16–21]

Pharmacology

As of June 2004, six statins are FDA approved. Cerivastatin, a seventh drug approved in 1997, was voluntarily withdrawn from the market in 2001 by its manufacturer due to a high rate of fatal rhabdomyolysis. The statins owe their activity to a moiety, resembling hydroxymethyl-glutaric acid, which

TABLE 10.6

Pharmacology of Statins

Drug	Form	Solubility	Half-Life (h)	Bioavailability (%)	Elimination
Atorvastatin	Active	Lipophilic	13–30	14	98% hepatic
Fluvastatin	Active	Hydrophilic	0.5–3	24	Hepatic
Lovastatin	Prodrug	Lipophilic	2–4	30	10% renal; 83% hepatic
Pravastatin	Active	Hydrophilic	2–3	17	20% renal; 70% hepatic
Rosuvastatin	Active	Hydrophilic	19	20	10% renal; 90% hepatic
Simvastatin	Prodrug	Lipophilic	1–3	< 5	13% renal; 60% hepatic

may be present in open (acid, active) form or closed (lactone, inactive) form. Of the six statins, only lovastatin and simvastatin are inactive lactones (prodrugs), which are converted to hydroxy acids (active forms) in the liver. Lovastatin and pravastatin are fungal derivatives, simvastatin is semi-synthetic while the remainder are purely synthetic compounds. The predominant route of elimination is through the bile after hepatic transformation. In addition, the kidneys also eliminate all statins, although the percentage varies greatly among the different statins (Table 10.6).

Mechanism of Action

All statins are competitive inhibitors of the enzyme 3-hydroxy-3-methylglutaryl CoA (HMG CoA) reductase.[22] HMG CoA reductase catalyses the conversion of HMG to mevalonate, the rate-limiting step in cholesterol synthesis. This decreases hepatic cholesterol content and produces an up-regulation of LDL receptors on the hepatic cell surface.[23] The LDL receptors facilitate the uptake of apolipoprotein (apo)-B containing lipoproteins, predominantly LDL-C, by the liver. However, intermediate-density lipoprotein (IDL) and VLDL remnants are also removed via the LDL receptor and this may account for some of the triglyceride-lowering effects of the statins.[24,25] Statins also reduce the hepatic production of VLDL by an effect on apo-B secretion.[26]

Lipid-Lowering Effects

Effects on LDL

Statins reduce LDL-C by 18–63%. There is considerable variation among the different statins in their effect on LDL-C (Table 10.7). The reduction in LDL-C with statins is dose-dependent, but the relationship between dose and degree of LDL reduction is log-linear. In general, each doubling of the statin dose decreases LDL-C by an additional 6%.[27]

TABLE 10.7

Summary of Lipid-Lowering Effects of Statins

Drug	Starting Dose (mg)	Maximum FDA Approved Dose (mg)	Equivalent Dose (mg) (LDL ↓ by 30–35%)	LDL Reduction (%)	HDL Increase (%)	TG Reduction (%)
Atorvastatin	10	80	10	37–57	5–13	17–53
Fluvastatin	20	80	80	18–31	3–11	12–25
Lovastatin	20	80	40	24–40	2–10	6–27
Pravastatin	20	80	40	24–34	2–12	15–24
Rosuvastatin	5–10	40	5	45–63	8–14	10–35
Simvastatin	20	80	20	35–46	8–16	12–34

Effects on HDL

Statin therapy increases HDL-C by 5–10%, with greater increases seen in patients with low HDL and high TGs. Rosuvastatin increases HDL-C up to 10%, an effect greater than the other statins. In general, HDL-C increases with higher doses of the statin, but with atorvastatin increasing the dose lessens the increase in HDL-C.[28,29]

Effects on TG

All statins lower TG concentrations by 7–30%. The effect of statins on TGs is related to the baseline TG level. In a pooled analysis involving 2689 subjects, statins did not reduce TGs in patients with TGs < 150 mg/dl, but in patients with baseline TGs > 250 mg/dl, statins produced significant dose-dependent TG reductions of 22–45%.[30] The magnitude of the TG reduction in hypertriglyceridemic subjects with different statins is directly proportional to the statin's effect on LDL.

Administration

All statins can be given in once-daily dosing. High-dose fluvastatin and lovastatin are slightly more effective when given in divided doses. Statins are generally administered at night because of their short half-lives and the fact that cholesterol synthesis is greater at night. Atorvastatin and rosuvastatin are the exceptions and can be administered at any time of the day, or even every other day, because of their long half-lives. Food increases the bioavailability of lovastatin, reduces the absorption of pravastatin and has no effect on the absorption of other statins. Therefore, lovastatin should be given with food, pravastatin on an empty stomach, whereas other statins can be given at any time.

Drug Interactions

Various drugs can reduce statin clearance and produce higher statin blood levels via effects on the cytochrome P450 (CP450) system or on the newly discovered statin glucuronidation pathway.[31,32] Interaction of the statins with other drugs, therefore, varies with the metabolic pathways of both the statin and the concomitant medication. Much has been made about the susceptibility of various statins to drug interaction, but caution should be used with all statins when combined with agents known to affect the CP450 system. The CY3A4 isoenzyme of the CP450 system is responsible for metabolism of atorvastatin, lovastatin and simvastatin, while the CY2C9 isoenzyme is responsible for metabolism of fluvastatin. Pravastatin is metabolized predominantly by sulfonation, independent of the CP450 system. Drugs, which inhibit CY3A4 (such as macrolide antibiotics, azole antifungal agents, antidepressants, and protease inhibitors), inhibit glucuronidation (such as gemfibrozil) or decrease statin excretion from skeletal muscle (such as cyclosporine) (Table 10.8), increase serum levels of statins and predispose to statin-induced myopathy.[33] Individual statins may have special situations either increasing their safety or risk. For example in the ALERT trial, which randomized 2102 renal transplant recipients on cyclosporine to either fluvastatin or placebo, the incidence of serious adverse events, such as ≥ 3-fold increase in alanine aminotransferase or ≥ 5-fold increase in creatinine kinase concentrations and non-fatal rhabdomyolysis, did not differ significantly between groups.[34] In contrast, rosuvastatin maximal concentrations and area under the curve are increased 11- and 7-fold when this agent is administered with cyclosporine, suggesting that this agent should be avoided in transplant patients.[35]

TABLE 10.8

Risk Factors for Statin-Induced Myopathy

1. Advanced age
2. Hypothyroidism
3. Small body habitus and frailty
4. Multi-system disease (renal insufficiency, DM)
5. Multiple medications
6. Perioperative periods
7. Combination with the following medications
    a. Fibrates (especially gemfibrozil)
    b. Cyclosporine
    c. Azole antifungals (ketoconazole, itraconazole)
    d. Macrolide antibiotics (erythromycin, clarithromycin)
    e. HIV protease inhibitors
    f. Nefazodone
    g. Verapamil
    h. Amiodarone
    i. Grapefruit juice (>1 quart/day)
    j. Alcohol abuse

Side Effects

A variety of adverse effects have been attributed to the statins. Major side effects include hepatotoxicity and myopathy, which are rare. Common side effects are myalgia and constipation.

Hepatotoxicity is feared by the public, but is extremely rare, occurring in < 1% of patients at high doses.[36] Asymptomatic elevation of transaminase levels occurs in 0.5–2.0% of patients, is dose dependent, and generally reverses with either dose reduction or continued administration.[37,38] Progression to permanent liver damage almost never occurs with statins, but patients with elevated transaminase levels should be monitored, and the statin should be discontinued if the levels rise > 3 times the upper limit of normal.

Statins can produce a variety of muscle complaints.[33,39] These have been variously defined by differing authorities, but include:

1. Myositis and rhabdomyolysis (generally defined as CK > 10 × upper limits of normal [ULN] plus muscle symptoms)
2. Increased CK < 10 ULN with or without symptoms
3. Myalgia with normal CK values
4. Muscle weakness
5. Muscle cramps

The management of statin myopathy has been discussed in detail elsewhere.[33] In general, physicians should use the lowest dose of statin necessary to reach the therapeutic goal and warn patients to discontinue the drug and seek medical care if they develop important muscle pain, weakness or dark urine. The incidence of asymptomatic small elevations in CK is not known, since this information is rarely reported in clinical trials. Different approaches have been recommended to monitoring muscle enzymes and symptoms during statin therapy. We suggest that statins be stopped if the CK level is greater than 10 times the upper limits of normal (ULN). CK levels should be monitored at least monthly if the CK is 5–10 times ULN and the patient is asymptomatic. CK elevations < 5 times ULN can be treated with benign neglect in asymptomatic patients. Myalgias are common with a reported incidence of 5%. Interestingly, the incidence of myalgia in clinical trial is similar between placebo and drug therapy groups,[38] but most clinicians are convinced that these medications can induce myalgia. Reducing the statin dose may relieve the symptoms, as may switching to another statin. Rare patients may experience severe myositis characterized by muscle pain, weakness associated with CK > 10 times ULN. Failure to discontinue statin therapy in this setting can lead to rhabdomyolysis, renal failure and even death. Fatal rhabdomyolysis is extremely rare (less than 1 death/million prescriptions).[39] The incidence rate is similar for all statins except for cerivastatin (16–80 times higher than other statins).[39] Risk factors for statin myopathy have been presented (Table 10.8).

Clinical Trials

Multiple large trials have proven the efficacy of statins in both the primary and secondary prevention of CAD.[16–20,40] They reduce the risk of myocardial infarction, cardiac mortality, revascularization procedures and peripheral vascular disease. They also reduce the risk of stroke and overall mortality in patients with established CAD. The findings of major statin trials are summarized in Table 10.9.

Bile Acid-Binding Resins

Introduction

These agents, once a mainstay of lipid-lowering therapy, are predominantly used as adjuncts to other drugs in patients requiring additional LDL-C reductions and as single agents in children and patients seeking to avoid long-term statin use.

Pharmacology and Mechanism of Action

The resins currently available in the United States are cholestyramine, colestipol and colesevelam. They are not absorbed into the systemic circulation. These agents bind bile acids in the gut thus interrupting their enterohepatic circulation. Depleting the hepatic bile-acid pool increases hepatic cholesterol 7-alpha-hydroxylase activity, the rate-limiting step in bile synthesis. The increased diversion of cholesterol to bile acid synthesis depletes hepatic cholesterol, producing up-regulation of hepatic LDL receptors and increased clearance of LDL-C from the blood.[41] However, HMG CoA reductase and phosphatidic acid phosphatase activity are also up-regulated, increasing cholesterol and TG synthesis, respectively, because bile acids suppress activity of these enzymes.[42]

Administration

Cholestyramine and colestipol are generally administered as powders mixed in water or fruit juice. A packet or scoopful contains 4 g of cholestyramine or 5 g of colestipol.[3] The usual dose is 2–6 packets daily. Micronized colestipol is also available as 1 g tablets. Colesevelam is available as 625 mg tablets and administered in up to six tablets daily. Approximately 5 g of colestipol

TABLE 10.9
Summary of Clinical Trials of Statins

Trial	Agent	Patients	Duration (years)	Baseline Lipids	LDL	HDL	TG	Coronary Events	Revascularization	Cardiac Mortality	Total Mortality	Stroke
WOSCOPS	Pravastatin 40 mg	6596	4.9	LDL 192 TG 164 HDL 44	↓26%	↑5%	↓12%	↓31%	↓37%	↓28%	↓22%	↓11% (NS)
AFCAPS/ TexCAPS	Lovastatin 20–40 mg	6605	5.2	LDL 150 TG 158 HDL 36	↓25%	↑6%	↓13%	↓25%	↓33%	NS	NS	NS
HPS	Simvastatin 40 mg	20,536	5	LDL 188 TG 135 HDL 46	↓29%	↑3%	↓14%	↓27%	↓24%	↓18%	↓12%	↓25%
4S	Simvastatin 10/40 mg	4444	5.4	LDL 188 TG 135 HDL 46	↓35%	↑8%	↓10%	↓34%	↓37%	↓42%	↓30%	↓27%
CARE	Pravastatin 40 mg	4159	5	LDL 139 TG 135 HDL 39	↓28%	↑5%	↓14%	↓25%	↓27%	↓24%	↓9%	↓31%
LIPID	Pravastatin 40 mg	9014	6.1	LDL 150 TG 138 HDL 36	↓25%	↑5%	↓11%	↓29%	↓24%	↓24%	↓23%	↓19%

NS, not significant; ↓, reduction; ↑, elevation; LDL, low-density lipoprotein; HDL, high-density lipoprotein; TG, triglycerides.

are equivalent to 4 g of cholestyramine in their LDL-lowering effect.[27] Colesevelam is 4–6 times more potent as a bile-acid sequestrant than the other two agents.[43] The powdered resins are impalatable for many patients and their physical bulk makes them inconvenient. Colesevelam is more easily administered and better tolerated than other sequestrants.

Lipid-Lowering Effects

Given alone, resins lower LDL-C 10–24% depending on the dose, and produce an additive effect when combined with a statin.[3,44] The statin inhibition of HMG CoA increases the efficacy of the resin. In a trial comparing LDL lowering with atorvastatin and colesevelam, the LDL-C reduction with atorvastatin 80 mg was not significantly different from the combination of colesevelam 3.8 g and atorvastatin 10 mg.[45] Resins increase HDL-C approximately 3–5%. Resins often increase TG levels by up-regulating activity of phosphatidic acid phosphatase and are not indicated in patients with hypertriglyceridemia.[46]

Drug Interactions

Resins non-specifically bind coadministered drugs such as warfarin, digitalis, thyroxine, non-steroidal anti-inflammatory agents, oral hypoglycemic agents, statins and gemfibrozil. These interactions can be avoided by administering the other drugs either 1 h before or 4 h after the administration of the resin. Colesevelam apparently does not interfere with the absorption of these drugs and need not be administered separately.[47]

Side Effects

Up to 39% of patients experience constipation, bloating, epigastric fullness, flatulence and nausea, giving these drugs a high rate of discontinuation.[48,49] Administration of viscous fiber or prune juice may help avoid constipation. Colesevelam is less likely to cause GI side effects and is better tolerated.[50]

Clinical Trials

The Lipid Research Clinics Coronary Primary Prevention Trial (LRC-CPPT) involved 3806 men with hypercholesterolemia but without known coronary disease.[48,49] Cholestyramine treatment reduced mean LDL-C by 12% compared with placebo and decreased non-fatal myocardial infarction and cardiac death by 19%, new-onset angina by 20% and new positive exercise tests by 25%, but did not alter total mortality. In the Familial Atherosclerosis Treatment Study (FATS) coronary atherosclerosis regression trial, intensive lipid lowering with colestipol in combination with either lovastatin or niacin reduced the frequency of progression of coronary lesions, increased the frequency of regression, and reduced the incidence of cardiovascular events by 70%.[51]

Nicotinic Acid

Introduction

Niacin or nicotinic acid is a water-soluble compound that functions as a B-vitamin at low doses and as a lipid-lowering agent at high doses. A related compound nicotinamide lacks any lipid-lowering effect and functions only as a vitamin.[3]

Pharmacology

Niacin is available in two forms: immediate release or crystalline (nicotinic acid), and sustained release or extended release (Niaspan) forms. The crystalline form has to be administered several times in a day and has a high incidence of flushing. Sustained release formulations cause less flushing than immediate release preparations, but have a higher incidence of hepatotoxicity.[52]

Mechanism of Action

Niacin has multiple potential actions, but its major effect is to inhibit lipolysis in peripheral tissues thereby reducing the availability of free fatty acids for hepatic TG synthesis. Reduced substrate for hepatic triglyceride synthesis ultimately reduces hepatic secretion of apo-B and VLDL.[53]

The mechanism by which niacin increases HDL is less clear. It appears to decrease the hepatic uptake of apo AI, thereby reducing HDL catabolism.

Lipid-Lowering Effects

Niacin increases HDL-C 15–40%, an effect greater than any other currently available lipid-lowering drug.[3,52,54] The reduction in TGs is more modest, in the range of 20–35%, with up to 50% reductions seen in patients with hypertriglyceridemia. The effect on LDL-C is variable (5–25% reduction). The effect on HDL-C and TG concentrations is log-linear, with significant changes seen at low doses whereas high doses are required to produce clinically important effects on LDL-C.[55]

Administration

Niacin produces flushing, which can be reduced by slowly increasing the dose. Crystalline niacin is usually started at doses of 100 mg four times daily and increased by 100 or 250 mg per dose weekly to 1 g four times a day. Long-release preparations are started at 500 mg at bedtime and increased by not more than 500 mg weekly to 1.5–2.0 g/day. The most important niacin dose is the bedtime dose since niacin inhibits lipolysis, which is greater overnight and during other periods of fasting.

Side Effects

The most common side effect is prostaglandin-mediated cutaneous vasodilatation causing flushing and pruritus.[27] Most patients develop tachyphylaxis and tolerance to flushing after prolonged use. Flushing can be reduced by taking the drug with food, or by using aspirin 325 mg or ibuprofen 200 mg 30 min before or with the dose. Niacin can also worsen glucose tolerance, activate gout and peptic ulcers, and produce conjunctivitis, nasal stuffiness, acanthosis nigricans, ichthyosis and rarely, retinal edema.[3]

A serious side effect is hepatotoxicity, including jaundice and fulminant hepatitis.[52–54] The onset of hepatotoxicity is unpredictable, requiring regular monitoring of serum transaminase levels at 4–6-month intervals throughout therapy. Niacin should be discontinued if transaminase levels are persistently elevated. Hepatotoxicity should also be suspected if there is a dramatic reduction in lipoprotein levels.[56] The risk of hepatotoxicity is higher with higher doses and with the use of sustained release formulations.[3]

Clinical Trials

The Coronary Drug Project (CDP) was a large secondary prevention trial, which compared five lipid-lowering drugs including nicotinic acid in 8341 patients with known CAD.[57] Treatment with nicotinic acid reduced major coronary events by 25% and on long-term follow-up (15 years) resulted in an 11% decrease in total mortality.[58] In the Stockholm study, 555 patients with myocardial infarction were randomized to either placebo or the combination of nicotinic acid and clofibrate. Lipid-lowering therapy lowered serum cholesterol by 13% and TGs by 19% and reduced CAD mortality by 36% and total mortality by 28%.[59]

Fibrates

Introduction

Fibric acid derivatives or fibrates are effective for lowering TGs and increasing HDL-C. Three fibrates are currently approved in the United States: clofibrate, gemfibrozil and fenofibrate, although clofibrate is difficult to obtain. Two more fibrates are available in Europe: bezafibrate and ciprofibrate.

Pharmacology

Absorption of gemfibrozil is approximately 44% higher when given 0.5 h before meals, whereas fenofibrate absorption is 35% higher when given with meals.[60] Both gemfibrozil and fenofibrate should be used cautiously in patients with renal insufficiency since they are partially renally cleared.

Mechanism of Action

Fibrates activate the nuclear transcription factor, peroxisome proliferator-activated receptor (PPAR)-alpha producing[61–63]:

1. Activation of lipoprotein lipase (LPL) and decreased expression of the LPL inhibitor, apo C-III. Increased LPL activity helps clear triglyceride-rich particles.
2. Increased oxidation of fatty acids in the liver and muscle, reducing the synthesis of VLDL-TGs.
3. Increased synthesis of apo A-I and A-II, which increases HDL-C.

Lipid-Lowering Effects

Fibrates reduce TGs by 30–35% in normal subjects and up to 55% in severely hypertriglyceridemic patients, and increase HDL-C by 10–15%. These changes are greater in patients with very high TGs and low HDL-C.[60] The effects on LDL are variable. Fibrates may decrease LDL-C by 10–20% in normotriglyceridemic patients, but can increase LDL in hypertriglyceridemic subjects by facilitating the transformation of VLDL to LDL via increased LPL activity and VLDL delipidation.[64,65]

Indications

Fibrates are useful for managing elevated TG levels, for increasing HDL-C especially in hypertriglyceridemic subjects, and in combination with resins or ezetimibe for statin intolerant patients with elevated LDL-C levels.

Side Effects

The most common side effects of gemfibrozil are upper gastrointestinal disturbances such as dyspepsia. Both gemfibrozil and fenofibrate can increase liver function tests (LFTs), which in our experience seems most common in patients with steatohepatitis. Treatment should be continued unless the patient is symptomatic or the LFTs are > 3 times ULN. Fibrates increase the biliary secretion of cholesterol, increasing the likelihood of gallstone disease.[66] Fibrates have also been associated with myositis and rhabdomyolysis in patients receiving concomitant therapy with statins especially with concomitant azotemia.[66] Fenofibrate may be safer than gemfibrozil in combination with statins because it dose not affect the glucuronidation clearance pathway and is not metabolized by the CYP3A4 system.[67,68]

Fibrates have been implicated in increased carcinogenesis in animal studies, and there was increased mortality from cancer in the WHO clofibrate trial.[69] However, other human trials have failed to show increased incidence of cancer with fibrates.

Clinical Trials

Several primary and secondary prevention trials have examined the role of fibrates in CAD[69–72] (Table 10.10). In the WHO clofibrate trial, clofibrate reduced coronary events. Total mortality was increased, mainly due to the diseases of gastrointestinal and biliary tracts, reducing the enthusiasm for the use of fibrates. However, subsequent primary and secondary prevention trials with gemfibrozil reduced CAD and did not increase total mortality. Not all trials, however, have shown a reduction in CAD events. The BIP secondary prevention trial failed to show any reduction in coronary ischemic events and revascularization with bezafibrate[70] and in the Coronary Drug Project, clofibrate did not reduce recurrent coronary events.[57]

Cholesterol Absorption Inhibitors

Introduction

Ezetimibe belongs to a new class of lipid-lowering drugs, which selectively inhibit intestinal absorption of cholesterol and phytosterols.[73]

TABLE 10.10

Summary of Clinical Trials of Fibrates

Trial	Agent	Type	Patients	Duration (years)	TC	HDL	TG	Mortality	Coronary Events	MI	Stroke
WHO	Clofibrate	Primary prevention	15,745	5.3	↓11%	NA	↓24%	↑43%	↓20%	25%	NA
HHS	Gemfibrozil	Primary prevention	4081	5	↓14%	↑8%	↓34%	ND	↓34%	↓37%	ND
BIP	Bezafibrate	Secondary prevention	3090	6.2	↓6.5%	↑18%	↓21%	ND	ND	13%	ND
VA-HIT	Gemfibrozil	Secondary prevention	2531	5	↓4%	↑6%	↓31%	ND	↓22%	↓23%	↓29%

NA, not available; ND, no difference; ↓, reduction; ↑, elevation; HDL, high-density lipoprotein; TG, triglycerides.

Pharmacology

Ezetimibe's absorption is not affected by food, it can be given daily or even every other day because of its half-life of 24 h, and it does not interact with other medications.[60]

Mechanism of Action

Ezetimibe interacts with the Nieman Pick Like Protein 1 in the intestine to inhibit absorption of dietary and biliary cholesterol by up to 54%.[74] Reduced delivery of cholesterol to the liver depletes hepatic stores, up-regulates hepatic LDL-receptor activity thereby increasing LDL-C clearance.

Lipid-Lowering Effects

Ezetimibe alone reduces LDL-C by approximately 18%, produces small (5%) non-significant reductions in TGs and small (3.5%) but significant increases in HDL-C.[75,76] Statin administration increases intestinal cholesterol absorption. Ezetimibe reduces intestinal cholesterol absorption, making ezetimibe very effective in combination with statins. For example, ezetimibe 10 mg plus atorvastatin 10 mg reduces LDL-C 53%, similar to the 54% reduction achieved with the 80 mg or maximum dose of atorvastatin.[77] Similar data are available with other statins.[78–80]

Indications

Ezetimibe is useful, therefore, either as single therapy in patients intolerant of statins or in combination with other lipid-lowering agents for reducing TC, LDL-C and apo-B in patients with primary hypercholesterolemia.

Other Therapies

Fish Oils

Oils derived from fatty fish (salmon, mackerel, tuna, sardines and herring) are rich in such n-3 (omega) fatty acids as eicosapentanoic acid (EPA) and docosahexanoic acid (DHA), which can be used to reduce TG levels.[81] Plant sources of omega-3 fatty acids, including flaxseed, canola oil, soybean oil and nuts, are not as effective as fish oils in reducing TGs.[82]

Mechanism of Action

The mechanism by which omega-3 fatty acid (FA) reduces TGs is not known, but is thought to involve both decreased production and increased catabolism of TG-rich lipoproteins.

Lipid-Lowering Effects

High omega-3 FA intakes are required to reduce TG levels. An intake of 3 g per day is associated with a 30% TG reduction and 9 g/day reduces TGs by as much as 50%.[83] Reduction in TG levels may be accompanied by increases in LDL-C levels. Commercial fish oil capsules are approximately 30% EPA by weight. Postmyocardial infarction patients treated with 1 g of EPA daily, which is approximately equal to three fish oil capsules, experienced a 30% reduction in cardiovascular events and a 45% reduction in sudden death.[84] Fish oils also reduce platelet aggregation and may reduce blood pressure.[81]

Side Effects

The doses of fish oil required to reduce TGs can produce nausea, abdominal bloating, flatulence and diarrhea. Patients may note a fishy odor and an after-taste. Platelet inhibition may lead to nosebleeds and easy bruiseability.[81] Also, since each 1 g capsule contains 9 g of fat, patients often gain weight.

Indications

Fish oils are used to treat hypertriglyceridemia. They can be added to statins in patients in whom the addition of fibrates or niacin to a statin is contraindicated or not tolerated. The ATP-III panel recommends consumption of fish oils as an optional treatment modality due to the lack of strong data supporting its use.

Clinical Trials

A fish diet was superior to high-fiber and low-fat diets for reducing cardiovascular events in patients with known CAD in the Diet and Reinfarction trial.[85] In the GISSI prevention study, recent myocardial infarction patients treated with 1 g of EPA from fish oils daily experienced a significantly lower incidence of cardiovascular events, due to a 30% reduction in cardiovascular deaths, including a 45% reduction in sudden deaths.[84]

Selection of Drug

Statins are usually the drugs of first choice for LDL-C lowering therapy. They are the most effective LDL-C lowering agents currently available, easy to administer and safe. The different statins produce different degrees of LDL-C reduction and are metabolized by different routes. Therefore, the initial choice of statin depends on the magnitude of LDL-C reduction required to reach the LDL goal and the presence of associated medical disorders or concomitant drug therapy, since the later may influence statin metabolism.

For patients requiring large reductions in LDL-C levels, rosuvastatin or atorvastatin may be the statins of first choice, whereas in patients requiring only modest reductions in LDL-C, pravastatin or simvastatin may achieve the therapeutic goals. Pravastatin and fluvastatin may be the preferred drugs for patients receiving concomitant therapy with drugs that inhibit the CYP3A4 enzymes, such as macrolide antibiotics and HIV-protease inhibitors. Similarly, in post-transplant patients receiving cyclosporine, pravastatin or fluvastatin may be preferred drugs.

Ezetimibe and bile-acid sequestrants are the next most effective LDL-C lowering drugs. They can be used as a monotherapy, when only mild reductions in LDL-C are required, especially in young patients. However, their major use is in addition to a statin to maximize LDL-C reduction. In general, doubling the dose of a statin produces only an additional 6% LDL-C reduction, whereas adding either ezetimibe or a bile-acid sequestrant to a starting dose of a statin can produce reductions in LDL-C similar to those achieved by the maximal statin dose. This may be beneficial in patients who are unable to tolerate higher doses of a statin and to reduce the risk of statin side effects. Adding ezetimibe or a resin to the maximal dose of a statin produces further reduction in LDL-C. Ezetimibe is better tolerated by patients than resins.

Nicotinic acid and fibrates are not primary LDL-C reducing agents and hence are usually not the first line of therapy for LDL elevations. However, these agents may be used if additional LDL-C lowering is required after maximal doses of statins and absorption inhibitors or if other agents are not tolerated. Nicotinic acid and fibrates may be used as initial agents in patients whose primary lipoprotein abnormality is elevated TGs and/or low HDL.

Monitoring

Baseline liver function tests (LFTs) and measurement of creatine kinase, fasting blood sugar and thyroid-stimulating hormone levels are recommended before therapy. The maximal response to statins occurs within 3 weeks of drug initiation whereas other medications may require 6–8 weeks. Follow-up lipid levels should be obtained as soon as any effect will be detectable to provide the patient with appropriate feedback. LFTs with statin therapy should be obtained after 12 weeks of treatment since LFTs often increase transiently in the first 12 weeks of therapy. LFTs can then be measured annually thereafter during statin therapy. We recommend monitoring LFTs during niacin therapy every 4 months. Statin-treated patients should be warned of the risk for myopathy and told to stop the drug and report promptly for a creatine kinase determination if symptoms appear. Once treatment goals are achieved, follow-up visits should be scheduled every 6–12 months.

Summary

Most patients with important vascular disease or increased risk of vascular disease will require lipid-lowering therapy to reduce their risk of recurrent or primary CAD events. Available lipid-lowering medications are extremely effective in reducing LDL-C and TGs and in increasing HDL-C. These agents can be used individually or in combination therapy, and most agents have been documented to reduce CAD events.

References

1. Steinberg D. The cholesterol controversy is over. Why did it take so long? *Circulation*, 80, 1070, 1989.
2. American Heart Association. Heart Disease and Stroke Statistics — 2004 Update. American Heart Association, Dallas, 2003.
3. Third report of the National Cholesterol Education Program (NCEP) Expert Panel on detection, evaluation, and treatment of high blood cholesterol in adults (Adult Treatment Panel III). *Circulation*, 106, 3143, 2002.
4. Wilson P.W. et al. Prediction of coronary heart disease using risk factor categories. *Circulation*, 97, 1837, 1998.
5. Kannel W.B. et al. Overall and coronary heart disease mortality rates in relation to major risk factors in 325,348 men screened for the MRFIT. Multiple Risk Factor Intervention Trial. *Am Heart J*, 112, 825, 1986.
6. Lipid Research Clinics Program. The Lipid Research Clinics Coronary Primary Prevention Trial results. I: Reduction in the incidence of coronary heart disease. *JAMA*, 251, 351, 1984.
7. Lipid Research Clinics Program. The Lipid Research Clinics Coronary Primary Prevention Trial Results. II: The relationship of reduction in incidence of coronary heart disease to cholesterol lowering. *JAMA*, 251, 365, 1984.

8. Stamler J., Wentworth D., Neaton J.D. Is relationship between serum cholesterol and risk of premature death from coronary heart disease continuous and graded? Findings in 356,222 primary screenees of the Multiple Risk Factor Intervention Trial (MRFIT). *JAMA*, 256, 2823, 1986.
9. Grundy S.M. Cholesterol-lowering trials: a historical perspective. In: Grundy SM, editor. *Cholesterol Lowering Therapy: Evaluation of Clinical Trial Evidence.* Marcel Dekker, New York, 2000, pp 1–329.
10. Rossouw J.E. Lipid-lowering interventions in angiographic trials. *Am J Cardiol*, 76, 86C, 1995.
11. Austin M.A., Hokanson J.E., Edwards K.L. Hypertriglyceridemia as a cardiovascular risk factor. *Am J Cardiol*, 81, 7B, 1998.
12. Assmann G. et al. The emergence of triglycerides as a significant independent risk factor in coronary artery disease. *Eur Heart,* Suppl M, M8, 1998.
13. Havel R.J. Remnant lipoproteins as therapeutic targets. *Curr Opin Lipidol*, 11, 615, 2000.
14. Gordon D.J. et al. High-density lipoprotein cholesterol and cardiovascular disease. Four prospective American studies. *Circulation*, 79, 8, 1989.
15. Grundy S.M. et al. National Heart, Lung, and Blood Institute; American College of Cardiology Foundation; American Heart Association. Implications of recent clinical trials for the National Cholesterol Education Program Adult Treatment Panel III guidelines. *Circulation*, 110, 227, 2004.
16. Downs J.R. et al. Primary prevention of acute coronary events with lovastatin in men and women with average cholesterol levels: results of AFCAPS/TexCAPS. Air Force/Texas Coronary Atherosclerosis Prevention Study. *JAMA*, 279, 1615, 1998.
17. Long-Term Intervention with Pravastatin in Ischemic Disease (LIPID) Study Group. Prevention of cardiovascular events and death with pravastatin in patients with coronary heart disease and a broad range of initial cholesterol levels. *N Engl J Med*, 339, 1349, 1998.
18. Shepherd J. et al. Prevention of coronary heart disease with pravastatin in men with hypercholesterolemia. West of Scotland Coronary Prevention Study Group. *N Engl J Med*, 333, 1301, 1995.
19. Scandinavian Simvastatin Survival Study Group. Randomized trial of cholesterol lowering in 444 patients with coronary heart disease: the Scandinavian Simvastatin Survival Study (4S). *Lancet*, 344, 1383, 1994.
20. Sacks F.M. et al. The effect of pravastatin on coronary events after myocardial infarction in patients with average cholesterol levels. Cholesterol and Recurrent Events Trial investigators. *N Engl J Med*, 335, 1001, 1996.
21. LaRosa J.C., He J., Vupputuri S. Effect of statins on risk of coronary disease: a meta-analysis of randomized controlled trials. *JAMA*, 282, 2340, 1999.
22. Endo A. The discovery and development of HMG-CoA reductase inhibitors. *J Lipid Res*, 33, 1569, 1992.
23. Bilheimer D.W. et al. Mevinolin and colestipol stimulate receptor-mediated clearance of low-density lipoprotein from plasma in familial hypercholesterolemia heterozygotes. *Proc Natl Acad Sci USA*, 80, 4124, 1983.
24. Broyles F.E. et al. Effect of fluvastatin on intermediate density lipoprotein (remnants) and other lipoprotein levels in hypercholesterolemia. *Am J Cardiol*, 76, 129A, 1995.

25. Bakker-Arkema R.G. et al. Efficacy and safety of a new HMG-CoA reductase inhibitor, atorvastatin, in patients with hypertriglyceridemia. *JAMA*, 275, 128, 1996.
26. Arad Y., Ramakrishnan R., Ginsberg H.N. Lovastatin therapy reduces low-density lipoprotein apoB levels in subjects with combined hyperlipidemia by reducing the production of apoB-containing lipoproteins: implications for the pathophysiology of apoB production. *J Lipid Res*, 31, 567, 1990.
27. Knopp R.H. Drug treatment of lipid disorders. *N Engl J Med*, 341, 498, 1999.
28. Jones P. et al. Comparative dose efficacy study of atorvastatin versus simvastatin, pravastatin, lovastatin, and fluvastatin in patients with hypercholesterolemia (the CURVES study). *Am J Cardiol*, 81, 582, 1998.
29. Jones P.H. et al. STELLAR Study Group. Comparison of the efficacy and safety of rosuvastatin versus atorvastatin, simvastatin, and pravastatin across doses. *Am J Cardiol*, 92, 152, 2003.
30. Stein E.A., Lane M., Laskarzewski P. Comparison of statins in hypertriglyceridemia. *Am J Cardiol*, 81, 66B, 1998.
31. Prueksaritanont T. et al. Glucuronidation of statins in animals and humans: a novel mechanism of statin lactonization. *Drug Metab Dispos*, 30, 505, 2002.
32. Prueksaritanont T. et al. Mechanistic studies on metabolic interactions between gemfibrozil and statins. *J Pharmacol Exp Ther*, 301, 1042, 2002
33. Thompson P.D., Clarkson P., Karas R.H. Statin-associated myopathy. *JAMA*, 289, 1681, 2003.
34. Holdaas H. et al. Assessment of Lescol in Renal Transplantation (ALERT) Study Investigators. Effect of fluvastatin on cardiac outcomes in renal transplant recipients: a multicentre, randomised, placebo-controlled trial. *Lancet*, 361, 2024, 2003.
35. Product Information: Crestor(R), rosuvastatin calcium. AstraZeneca Pharmaceuticals LP, Wilmington, DE (PI revised 8/2003) reviewed 9/2003.
36. Pedersen T.R., Tobert J.A. Benefits and risks of HMG-CoA reductase inhibitors in the prevention of coronary heart disease: a reappraisal. *Drug Saf*, 14, 11, 1996.
37. Hsu I., Spinler S.A., Johnson N.E. Comparative evaluation of the safety and efficacy of HMG-CoA reductase inhibitor monotherapy in the treatment of primary hypercholesterolemia. *Ann Pharmacother*, 29, 743, 1995.
38. Bradford R.H. et al. Expanded Clinical Evaluation of Lovastatin (EXCEL) study results. I. Efficacy in modifying plasma lipoproteins and adverse event profile in 8245 patients with moderate hypercholesterolemia. *Arch Intern Med*, 151, 43, 1991.
39. Pasternak R.C. et al. ACC/AHA/NHLBI Advisory on the Use and Safety of Statins. *Circulation*, 106, 1024, 2002.
40. Heart Protection Study Collaborative Group. MRC/BHF Heart Protection Study of cholesterol lowering with simvastatin in 20536 high-risk individuals: a randomized placebo-controlled trial. *Lancet*, 3607, 2002.
41. Shepherd J. et al. Cholestyramine promotes receptor-mediated low-density-lipoprotein catabolism. *N Engl J Med*, 302, 1219, 1980.
42. Shepherd J. Mechanism of action of bile acid sequestrants and other lipid-lowering drugs. *Cardiology*, 76 Suppl 1, 65; discussion 71, 1989.
43. Davidson M.H. et al. Colesevelam hydrochloride (cholestagel): a new, potent bile acid sequestrant associated with a low incidence of gastrointestinal side effects. *Arch Intern Med*, 159, 1893, 1999.

44. The Pravastatin Multicenter Study Group II. Comparative efficacy and safety of pravastatin and cholestyramine alone and combined in patients with hypercholesterolemia. *Arch Intern Med*, 153, 1321, 1993.
45. Hunninghake D. et al. Coadministration of colesevelam hydrochloride with atorvastatin lowers LDL cholesterol additively. *Atherosclerosis*, 158, 407, 2001.
46. Crouse JR 3rd. Hypertriglyceridemia: a contraindication to the use of bile acid binding resins. *Am J Med*, 83, 243, 1987.
47. Donovan J.M. et al. Drug interactions with colesevelam hydrochloride, a novel, potent lipid-lowering agent. *Cardiovasc Drugs Ther*, 14, 681, 2000.
48. The Lipid Research Clinics Coronary Primary Prevention Trial results. I. Reduction in incidence of coronary heart disease. *JAMA*, 251, 351, 1984.
49. The Lipid Research Clinics Coronary Primary Prevention Trial results. II. The relationship of reduction in incidence of coronary heart disease to cholesterol lowering. *JAMA*, 251, 365, 1984.
50. Davidson M.H. et al. Colesevelam hydrochloride (cholestagel): a new, potent bile acid sequestrant associated with a low incidence of gastrointestinal side effects. *Arch Intern Med*, 159, 1893, 1999.
51. Brown G. et al. Regression of coronary artery disease as a result of intensive lipid-lowering therapy in men with high levels of apolipoprotein B. *N Engl J Med*, 323, 1289, 1990.
52. McKenney J.M. et al. A comparison of the efficacy and toxic effects of sustained- vs. immediate-release niacin in hypercholesterolemic patients. *JAMA*, 271, 672, 1994.
53. Kamanna V.S., Kashyap M.L. Mechanism of action of niacin on lipoprotein metabolism. *Curr Atheroscler Rep*, 2, 36, 2000.
54. Knopp R.H. et al. Contrasting effects of unmodified and time-release forms of niacin on lipoproteins in hyperlipidaemic subjects: clues to mechanism of action of niacin. *Metabolism*, 34, 642, 1985.
55. Illingworth D.R. et al. Comparative effects of lovastatin and niacin in primary hypercholesterolemia: a prospective trial. *Arch Intern Med*, 154, 1586, 1994.
56. Tato F., Vega G.L., Grundy S.M. Effects of crystalline nicotinic acid-induced hepatic dysfunction on serum low-density lipoprotein cholesterol and lecithin cholesteryl acyl transferase. *Am J Cardiol*, 81, 805, 1998.
57. Coronary Drug Project Research Group. Clofibrate and niacin in coronary heart disease. *JAMA*, 231, 360, 1975.
58. Canner P.L. et al. Fifteen year mortality in Coronary Drug Project patients: long-term benefit with niacin. *J Am Coll Cardiol*, 8, 1245, 1986.
59. Carlson L.A., Rosenhamer G. Reduction of mortality in the Stockholm Ischemic Heart Disease Secondary Prevention Study by combined treatment with clofibrate and nicotinic acid. *Acta Med Scand*, 223, 405, 1988.
60. *Physicians Desk Reference*. Medical Economics Company, Montvale, NJ, 2004.
61. Schoonjans K., Staels B., Auwerx J. Role of the peroxisome proliferator-activated receptor (PPAR) in mediating the effects of fibrates and fatty acids on gene expression. *J Lipid Res*, 37, 907, 1996.
62. Fruchart J.C., Brewer H.B. Jr, Leitersdorf E. Consensus for the use of fibrates in the treatment of dyslipoproteinemia and coronary heart disease. Fibrate Consensus Group. *Am J Cardiol*, 81, 912, 1998.
63. Vu-Dac N. et al. Fibrates increase human apolipoprotein A-II expression through activation of the peroxisome proliferator-activated receptor. *J Clin Invest*, 96, 741, 1995.

64. Leaf D.A. et al. The hypolipidaemic effects of gemfibrozil in type V hyperlipidaemia. A double blind, crossover study. *JAMA*, 262, 3154, 1989.
65. Pauciullo P. et al. Serum lipoproteins, apolipoproteins and very low density lipoprotein subfractions during 6-month fibrate treatment in primary hypertriglyceridemia. *Intern Med*, 228, 425, 1990.
66. Palmer R.H. Effects of fibric acid derivatives on biliary lipid composition. *Am J Med*, 83, 37, 1987.
67. Prueksaritanont T. et al. Mechanistic studies on metabolic interactions between gemfibrozil and statins. *J Pharmacol Exp Ther*, 301, 1042, 2002.
68. Prueksaritanont T. et al. Effects of fibrates on metabolism of statins in human hepatocytes. *Drug Metab Dispos*, 30, 1280, 2002.
69. Report from the Committee of Principal Investigators: WHO cooperative trial on primary prevention of ischemic heart disease with clofibrate to lower serum cholesterol: final mortality follow-up. *Lancet*, 324, 600, 1984.
70. Secondary prevention by raising HDL cholesterol and reducing triglycerides in patients with coronary artery disease: the Bezafibrate Infarction Prevention (BIP) study. *Circulation*, 102, 21, 2000.
71. Frick M.H. et al. Helsinki Heart Study: primary-prevention trial with gemfibrozil in middle-aged men with dyslipidemia. Safety of treatment, changes in risk factors, and incidence of coronary heart disease. *N Engl J Med*, 317, 1237, 1987.
72. Rubins H.B. et al. Gemfibrozil for the secondary prevention of coronary heart disease in men with low levels of high-density lipoprotein cholesterol. Veterans Affairs High-Density Lipoprotein Cholesterol Intervention Trial Study Group. *N Engl J Med*, 341, 410, 1999.
73. Sudhop T. et al. Inhibition of intestinal cholesterol absorption by ezetimibe in humans. *Circulation*, 106, 1943, 2002.
74. Altmann S.W. et al. Niemann-Pick C1 Like 1 protein is critical for intestinal cholesterol absorption. *Science*, 303, 1201, 2004.
75. Dujovne C.A. et al. Efficacy and safety of a potent new selective cholesterol absorption inhibitor, ezetimibe, in patients with primary hypercholesterolemia. *Am J Cardiol*, 90, 1092, 2002.
76. Knopp R.H., et al. Effects of ezetimibe, a new cholesterol absorption inhibitor, on plasma lipids in patients with primary hypercholesterolemia. *Eur Heart J*, 24, 729, 2003.
77. Ballantyne C.M. et al. Effect of ezetimibe coadministered with atorvastatin in 628 patients with primary hypercholesterolemia: a prospective, randomized, double blind trial. *Circulation*, 107, 2409, 2003.
78. Melani L. et al. Efficacy and safety of ezetimibe coadministered with pravastatin in patients with primary hypercholesterolemia: a prospective, randomized, double-blind trial. *Eur Heart J*, 24, 717, 2003.
79. Melani L. et al. Efficacy and safety of ezetimibe coadministered with pravastatin in patients with primary hypercholesterolemia: a prospective, randomized, double-blind trial. *Eur Heart J*, 24, 717, 2003.
80. Kerzner B. et al. Efficacy and safety of ezetimibe coadministered with lovastatin in primary hypercholesterolemia. *Am J Cardiol*, 91, 418, 2003.
81. Stone N.J. Fish consumption, fish oil, lipids, and coronary heart disease. *Circulation*, 94, 2337, 1996.

82. Kestin M. et al. N-3 Fatty acids of marine origin lower systolic blood pressure and triglycerides but raise LDL cholesterol compared with n-3 and n-6 fatty acids from plants. *Am J Clin Nutr*, 51, 1028, 1990.
83. Rambjor G.S. et al. Eicosapentaenoic acid is primarily responsible for hypotriglyceridemic effect of fish oil in humans. *Lipids*, 31 Suppl, S45, 1996.
84. Gruppo Italiano per lo Studio della Sopravvivenza nell'Infarto miocardico. Dietary supplementation with n-3 polyunsaturated fatty acids and vitamin E after myocardial infarction: results of the GISSI-Prevenzione trial. *Lancet*, 354, 447, 1999.
85. Burr M.L. et al. Effects of changes in fat, fish, and fibre intakes on death and myocardial reinfarction: diet and reinfarction trial (DART). *Lancet*, 2, 757, 1989.

11

New Insights on the Role of Lipids and Lipoproteins in Cardiovascular Disease: The Modulating Effects of Nutrition

Kirsten F. Hilpert, Amy E. Griel, Tricia Psota, Sarah Gebauer, Yumei Coa, and Penny M. Kris-Etherton

CONTENTS

Introduction 212
The Effect of Nutrients on Lipids and Lipoproteins 213
  Total Fat 213
  Saturated Fatty Acids 217
  Trans Fatty Acids 218
  Monounsaturated Fatty Acids 219
  Polyunsaturated Fatty Acids 220
    n-6 PUFA 220
    n-3 PUFA 221
  Dietary Cholesterol 222
  Dietary Fiber 222
    Epidemiologic Evidence of Fiber and Heart Disease 222
    The Role of Dietary Fiber in Lipid Management 224
  Glycemic Index/Glycemic Load 225
  Conclusion 227
Effects of Dietary Patterns on Lipids and Lipoproteins 228
  NCEP Recommendations 228
  Portfolio Diet 230
  Lifestyle Heart Program 231
  Mediterranean Diet 232
  Dietary Approaches to Stop Hypertension (DASH) Diet 233
Effects of Weight Loss Diets on Lipids and Lipoproteins 233
  Low-Fat Diets 234
  Moderate-Fat Diets with MUFA 234
  High-Protein Diets 235

Emerging Lipid and Lipoprotein CVD Risk Factors Affected by Diet 236
Diet Effects on LDL Particle Size 236
The Effects of a Changing Macronutrient Profile on LDL Particle Size 237
Effects of High-Fat, Moderate-Fat Diets 237
Effects of High-Protein, Low-Carbohydrate Diets 237
Other Dietary Interventions – Type of Fat, Dietary Fiber, and Multiple Dietary Strategies 239
HDL Particle Size 240
Postprandial TG 242
Lipoprotein (a) 244
Science-Based Dietary Guidelines for Health 246
Summary 246
References 248

Introduction

The first lipoprotein particle identified was high-density lipoprotein (HDL) that was isolated from horse serum in 1929.[1] Since the discovery of plasma lipoproteins (reviewed in Ref. 2), remarkable progress has been made in understanding their role in the development and progression of cardiovascular disease (CVD). The progress was catalyzed by the development of a method for the quantitative measurement of different serum lipoproteins isolated by ultracentrifugation.[3] Historically, a panel of plasma lipid and lipoprotein abnormalities has been a primary intervention target for reducing risk of CVD.[4] With respect to plasma lipids and lipoproteins, an elevated total and LDL cholesterol (LDL-C) have a long-standing history of being the major risk factors for CVD. Low HDL cholesterol (HDL-C) and elevated triglyceride (TG) levels have been identified more recently as important risk factors for CVD. In addition, other lipoprotein constituents (e.g., apolipoproteins A and B) have been shown to have important biological functions related to CVD. During the past 10 years, it has become abundantly clear that each lipoprotein fraction is remarkably heterogeneous with respect to both composition and biological function.[5]

Numerous epidemiologic studies have shown beneficial effects of single nutrients as well as dietary patterns on morbidity and mortality related to CVD. Over the past several decades, a major scientific effort has been devoted to identifying the mechanisms by which diet impacts overall CVD risk via modification of lipids and lipoproteins. Research has demonstrated that nutrition can modulate both lipoprotein composition and function in ways that span the spectrum from anti-atherogenic to pro-atherogenic. Dietary factors that affect lipids and lipoproteins include saturated fatty acids (SFA), monounsaturated fatty acids (MUFA), polyunsaturated fatty acids (PUFA), *trans* fatty acids (TFA), dietary cholesterol, dietary sterols and stanols, and soluble fiber. Weight status including gaining or losing weight markedly affects plasma lipids and lipoproteins. Modifications of lipids and lipoproteins by these dietary factors can substantially reduce risk of CVD. Other dietary and lifestyle interventions, such as dietary patterns that include fruits, vegetables, whole grains, low-fat dairy products, fish and nuts, along with physical activity, also can significantly reduce risk of CVD that can be explained mechanistically, in large part, by changes in lipids and lipoproteins.

The focus of this chapter is to review the current understanding of the effects that diet has on lipids and lipoproteins with emphasis on a discussion of the maximal effects that can be expected given ideal adherence to a dietary intervention that is low in SFA, TFA, dietary cholesterol and high in plant sterols/stanols and soluble fiber. In addition, observational evidence of the association between diet and CVD morbidity and mortality is discussed to provide a rationale for the numerous clinical studies that have evaluated the effects of diet on lipids and lipoproteins, important risk factors for CVD.

The Effect of Nutrients on Lipids and Lipoproteins

It is well established that elevated levels of total cholesterol (TC), LDL-C, and TG increase CVD risk, while a high level of HDL-C reduces CVD risk. These lipid risk factors are the focal point for cholesterol-lowering treatment guidelines developed by the third Adult Treatment Panel of the National Cholesterol Education Program.[6] The well-known effects of nutrients on TC, LDL-C, HDL-C, and TG are reviewed in Table 11.1. The total fat content of the diet is comprised of a mixture of individual fatty acids. Dietary sources of fat are described in Table 11.2. Furthermore, different food sources of fat differ substantially in their fatty acid profiles (Figure 11.1). This section reviews studies demonstrating the effects of total fat, SFA, *trans* fatty acids, MUFA, PUFA, dietary cholesterol, fiber, and the glycemic index/glycemic load on lipids and lipoproteins.

Total Fat

Numerous studies have been conducted that have compared the plasma lipid and lipoprotein responses to different blood cholesterol-lowering diets that vary in the amount of total fat and carbohydrate. Low-fat/high-carbohydrate diets (18–30% of kilocalories [kcal] total fat) have been compared with higher fat diets (30–40% of kcal) that provide similar amounts of SFA (4–12% of kcal) and dietary cholesterol (< 100–410 mg/day). Consistently, a low-fat, high-carbohydrate diet compared with a higher fat diet (both

TABLE 11.1

Expected Lipid Response of Selected Dietary Components

Dietary Component	NHLBI Evidence Statement[6]	Expected Lipid Response			
		LDL-C	TC	HDL-C	TG
Total fat	Unsaturated fat does not raise LDL-C when substituted for CHO; it is not necessary to restrict total fat intake for LDL-C reduction, provided SFA are reduced	↔	↔	↑	↓[a]
Saturated fat	There is a dose response relationship between SFA and LDL-C; diets high in SFA raise LDL-C and reducing dietary SFA lowers LDL-C	↑↑↑	↑↑↑	↑	↓[a]
Trans fat	*Trans* fatty acids raise LDL-C and intake should be kept as low as possible	↑↑↑	↑↑↑	↔[a] or ↓[b]	↔
Cholesterol	Higher intakes of dietary cholesterol raise LDL-C	↑	↑	↑	↔
n-6 PUFA	Linoleic acid, a PUFA, reduces LDL-C levels when substituted for SFA in the diet; PUFAs also can cause small reductions in HDL-C when compared with MUFA; controlled clinical trials indicate that substitution of PUFA for SFA reduces risk for CHD	↓↓	↓↓	↔ or ↓	↓[a]
n-3 PUFA	The mechanisms whereby they might reduce coronary events are unknown and may be multiple; prospective and clinical evidence suggest that higher intakes of n-3 fatty acids reduce risk for CHD events and mortality	↔ or ↑[c]	↔	↑	↓↓↓
MUFA	MUFA lowers LDL-C relative to SFA; mUFA does not lower HDL-C nor raise TG; to lower LDL-C, energy derived from SFA can be reduced if weight loss is desirable or replaced with either CHO or MUFA when weight loss is not a goal	↔ or ↓[d]	↔	↑	↓a

(continued)

TABLE 11.1 (CONTINUED)

Expected Lipid Response of Selected Dietary Components

Dietary Component	NHLBI Evidence Statement[6]	Expected Lipid Response LDL-C	TC	HDL-C	TG
Carbohydrate	When CHO is substituted for SFA, LDL-C decreases; however, very high intakes of CHO (>60% total kcal) can reduce HDL-C and raise TG; viscous fiber may attenuate this response	↓[d]	↓[d]	↔ or ↓	↔ or ↑
Viscous fiber	Use dietary sources of viscous fiber (5–10 g/day) to reduce LDL-C	↓	↓	↑	↔ or ↓
Plant stanols/ sterols	Use 2–3 g/day to enhance LDL-C lowering	↓↓↓	↓↓	↔	↔
Soy protein	Soy protein can cause small reductions in LDL-C, especially when it replaces animal food products	↓	↓	↔	↔ or ↓
Weight reduction (– 10 lb)	Weight reduction of even a few pounds will reduce LDL-C regardless of the nutrient composition of the diet, but weight reduction achieved through a calorie-controlled low-SFA and cholesterol diet will enhance and sustain LDL-C lowering	↓↓	↓↓	↑	↓↓[e]

↑, increase; ↓, decrease; ↔, no change.

[a] When substituted for dietary carbohydrate.

[b] Compared with saturated fatty acids.

[c] Increases LDL size.

[d] When substituted for saturated fatty acids.

[e] TG may rebound after maintenance of weight loss, when consuming a high-carbohydrate, low-fat, low-fiber diet.

relatively low in SFA and cholesterol) decreases LDL-C levels similarly.[7–19] Low-fat diets, however, decrease HDL-C and since HDL-C is proportionately decreased as LDL-C, the ratio of LDL-C to HDL-C does not change.[20] On a moderate-fat diet, however, when unsaturated fat replaces SFA, LDL-C decreases proportionately more than HDL-C thereby decreasing the LDL:HDL-C ratio.[21] Low-fat, high-carbohydrate diets increase fasting TGs versus moderate-fat diets, both of which are low in saturated fat. Viscous fiber may attenuate the hypertriglyceridemic response to dietary carbohydrate.[6] Within the range of total fat evaluated in the controlled feeding studies conducted to date, there is a linear dose-response relationship between total fat content of the diet and the changes in HDL-C and TG.[22]

In some individuals, low-fat, high-carbohydrate diets, compared with higher fat diets, induce atherogenic dyslipidemia,[6] which is characterized by

TABLE 11.2

Sources of Fatty Acids in the Diet

Type (Chemical Structure[a])	Dietary Source
Saturated Fat	
Butyric (4:0)	Butterfat
Lauric (12:0)	Coconut oil, palm kernel oil
Myristic (14:0)	Butterfat, coconut oil
Palmitic (16:0)	Palm oil, animal fat
Stearic (18:0)	Cocoa butter, animal fat
Unsaturated Fat	
Monounsaturated	
Oleic (18:1)	Olive oil, canola oil, peanuts, avocado, sunflower oil
Elaidic or *trans* fat (18:1)	Hydrogenated vegetable oil and ruminant fat
Polyunsaturated	
n-6 fatty acids	
Linoleic (18:2)	Vegetable oils (e.g., soybean, corn, safflower)
Arachidonic (20:4)	Lard, meat
n-3 fatty acids	
α-Linolenic (18:3)	Soybean oil, canola oil, walnuts, flaxseed
EPA (20:5)	Fish oils, algae
DHA (22:6)	Fish oils, algae

EPA, eicosapentanoic acid; DHA, docosahexanoic acid.

[a] Carbon chain length:double bond.

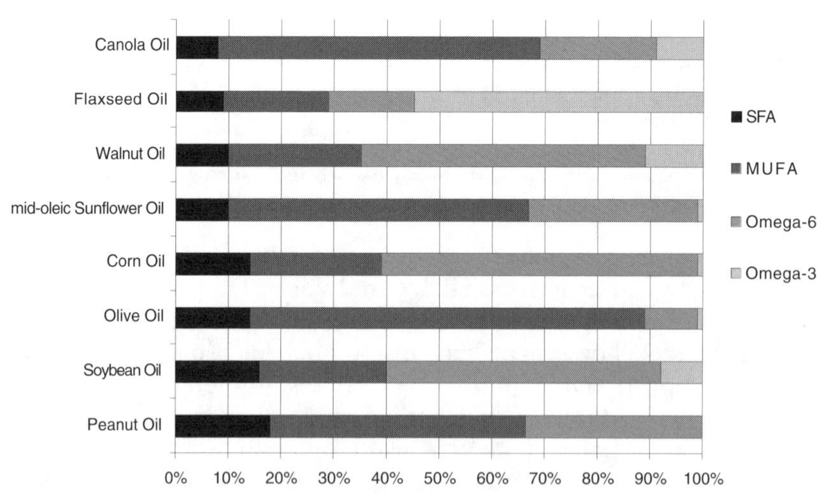

FIGURE 11.1
Fatty acid composition of common oils. Source: USDA Nutrient Database, release 15.

small dense LDL particles, high TG and low HDL-C levels. In sedentary, overweight or obese populations, in particular, low-fat, high-carbohydrate diets increase the prevalence of this phenotype. This phenotype is associated with increased risk of coronary heart disease (CHD).[23]

Saturated Fatty Acids

The Seven Countries Study was a classic epidemiologic study that reported a strong positive correlation between SFA intake and CHD mortality rates, as well as a significant association between total SFA intake and TC.[24] Subsequent epidemiologic studies also have found correlations with classes of SFA and TC levels and incidence of CHD.[25,26] In a more recent analysis of the study, strong positive associations were reported between 25-year death rates from CHD and average intake of the four major saturated fatty acids: lauric, myristic, palmitic, and stearic acid ($r > 0.8$).[27] Specifically, intakes of lauric acid (12:0) and myristic acid (14:0) were most strongly associated with TC ($r = 0.84$, $r = 0.81$, respectively).

Clinical trials confirm the associations between SFA and TC observed in epidemiologic studies. The early studies by Keys et al.[28] and Hegsted et al.[29] in the 1960s evaluated the effect of individual fatty acids on TC in humans using regression analysis on data from many clinical studies. Predictive equations estimate that SFA raises TC compared with carbohydrates and MUFA (which both have neutral effects), while PUFA lowers TC. Clinical studies also have demonstrated the LDL-C raising effect of SFA.[30,31] For every 1% increase in energy from SFA, LDL-C levels will increase approximately 0.033–0.045 mmol/L.[21,32,33] In addition to raising TC and LDL-C, SFA also has been shown to increase HDL-C levels. It is estimated that for every 1% increase in SFA, HDL-C will increase by 0.011–0.013 mmol/L.[21,32,33]

In the Dietary Effects on Lipoproteins and Thrombogenic Activity (DELTA) Study, an average American diet (AAD) (34% kcal total fat, 15% kcal SFA) was compared with a Step I diet (28.6% kcal total fat, 9% kcal SFA), and a low-SFA diet (25.3% kcal total fat, 6.1% kcal SFA).[34] TC was reduced 5% and 9% on the Step I and low-SFA diets, respectively, compared with the AAD (both $p < 0.01$). LDL-C and HDL-C were reduced similarly by 7% and 11%, respectively, on both the Step I and low-SFA diets versus the AAD (both $p < 0.01$).

In addition to equations that incorporate classes of fatty acids, equations have been generated to predict how alterations in individual dietary fatty acids affect TC, LDL-C, and HDL-C. Recent regression analyses have demonstrated that stearic acid (18:0) has no affect on TC, LDL-C, and HDL-C,[35] while myristic acid (14:0) is more hypercholesterolemic than lauric acid (12:0) and palmitic acid (16:0).[36] A recent meta-analysis of 60 controlled trials determined the effects of different SFA relative to carbohydrate (CHO) on the TC/HDL-C ratio.[37] Although lauric acid was found to increase LDL-C the most, it decreased the ratio of TC/HDL-C due to a greater increase in

HDL-C levels relative to TC. Myristic and palmitic acids had little effect on the ratio due to similar increases in both TC and HDL-C. Stearic acid reduced the ratio due to slight increases in HDL-C.

Trans Fatty Acids

Elaidic acid (t-18:1) is the predominant *trans* fatty acid found in some hydrogenated fats which are used in commercially prepared baked products, fried foods, and margarine. In the Seven Countries Study, the average intake of elaidic acid was positively associated with TC ($r = 0.70$, $p < 0.01$) and 25-year mortality rates from CHD ($r = 0.78$, $p < 0.001$).[27] This association has been confirmed by other epidemiologic studies as well.[38,39] Using follow-up data from the Nurses' Health Study, Hu et al.[26] found that compared with equivalent energy from CHO, the relative risk (RR) for a 2% increment in energy from *trans* fatty acids was 1.93 ($p < 0.001$). The RR for *trans* fatty acids was higher than that for 5% of energy from SFA, and 5% from total fat (RR = 1.17, $p = 0.10$, and RR = 1.02, $p = 0.55$, respectively). Studies have shown that *trans* fatty acids increase CHD risk by various lipid-mediated mechanisms including raising LDL-C, lowering HDL-C, and raising TG.[40] In addition, LDL particle size is decreased,[41] and lipoprotein (a) is increased[42–44] by *trans* fatty acids (reviewed in a later section).

A recent clinical trial conducted by Judd et al.[45] evaluated the effects of replacing carbohydrates with *trans* fatty acids on LDL-C. Subjects were fed diets providing approximately 15% of energy from protein, 39% from total fat, and 46% from CHO. TC was increased by 5.8% and LDL-C was increased by 10% when *trans* fatty acids replaced 8% of the energy provided by CHO. When 8% of the energy provided by CHO was replaced with a combination of 4% *trans* fatty acids and 4% stearic acid, TC was increased by 5.6% and LDL-C was increased by 8.7%. In a review of the *trans* fat studies that have been conducted, a linear dose-dependent relationship was reported between *trans* fatty acid intake and the LDL:HDL ratio from intakes of 0.5–10% of total calories.[46] The magnitude of this effect is greater for *trans* fatty acids than for SFA.

Several clinical trials have reported an HDL-C-lowering effect of *trans* fat when compared with saturated fat. In a study conducted by Mensink et al.,[47] subjects were placed on three diets that were identical in nutrient composition except that 10% of total calories were either from oleic acid, *trans* isomers of oleic acid, or SFA. The mean HDL-C level was the same on the SFA and oleic acid diets, but was 0.17 mmol/L lower on the *trans* fatty acid diet ($p < 0.0001$). Likewise, a high *trans* fat diet (9.2% kcal *trans* fat, 12.9% kcal SFA) produced a greater reduction in HDL-C by 0.36 mmol/L compared with a high SFA diet (0% kcal *trans* fat, 22.9% kcal SFA).[48] These studies and others[49] indicate that *trans* fatty acids are unfavorable due to their HDL-C-lowering effect in addition to their LDL-C raising effect.

Lichtenstein et al.[50] conducted a clinical trial evaluating the effects of different types of hydrogenated fats on lipids and lipoproteins. The experimental diets provided 30% energy from total fat and were identical except for fat source. Two-thirds of the fat was provided by soybean oil (< 0.5 g *trans* fat per 100 g of fat), semi-liquid margarine (< 0.5 g per 100 g), soft margarine (7.4 g per 100 g), shortening (9.9 g 100 g), stick margarine (20.1 g per 100 g), or butter (1.25 g per 100 g). The soybean-oil diet compared with the butter diet resulted in reductions of TC, LDL-C, and HDL-C of 10%, 12%, and 3%, respectively. The semi-liquid margarine diet compared with the butter diet resulted in reductions of 10%, 11%, and 4%, respectively. The stick margarine diet resulted in reductions of 3%, 5%, and 6%, respectively. Although all of the vegetable fat diets resulted in decreases in TC, LDL-C, and HDL-C compared with the butter diet, stick margarine (containing the highest amount of *trans* fatty acid) decreased LDL-C the least and decreased HDL-C the most compared with the other vegetable fats. This resulted in a 4% increase in the TC:HDL-C ratio, whereas the other vegetable fats slightly decreased the ratio. The soybean oil and semi-liquid margarine diets, which contained the lowest amount of *trans* fat, had the most beneficial effects on blood lipoproteins. The soybean oil caused the greatest reduction in TC and LDL-C and the smallest reduction in HDL-C, resulting in the greatest decrease in the TC:HDL-C ratio of 6%. The semi-liquid margarine diet resulted in a 5% reduction in the TC:HDL-C ratio. This study demonstrates that increases in *trans* fat result in a dose–response increase in LDL-C. The study also indicates that at levels higher than typically consumed in the diet, which is approximately 2.6% kcal, *trans* fatty acids decrease HDL-C.

The effects of *trans* fatty acids on TC, LDL-C, and HDL-C have been compared with other fatty acids via the development of blood cholesterol predictive equations. Results indicate that *trans* fatty acids increase TC and LDL-C less than SFA, but lower HDL-C more than SFA.[36]

Monounsaturated Fatty Acids

Unsaturated fat (both MUFA and PUFA) as well as carbohydrate can be used to replace saturated and *trans* fatty acid calories, which are both targets for reduction in cholesterol-lowering diets. Oleic acid, the primary MUFA in the diet, has been shown to have a neutral effect on TC. Epidemiologic studies have found inverse associations between MUFA intake and risk of CHD and ischemic heart disease (IHD) after adjusting for SFA and dietary cholesterol.[26,51,52] Furthermore, the Seven Countries Study showed that rates of coronary artery disease (CAD) were low despite moderately high total fat intakes when SFA was replaced with MUFA.[24] Mortality rate from CHD is lower in Mediterranean populations and they consume a diet that differs in many ways from a Western diet, including widespread use of olive oil, a major source of oleic acid, as their principal source of fat.

Grundy and Mattson[14,30] have demonstrated that replacing SFA with MUFA lowers LDL-C levels without lowering HDL-C. Kris-Etherton et al.[53] demonstrated that replacing SFA with MUFA (37% kcal total fat, 22% kcal MUFA, 47% kcal CHO) versus CHO (30% kcal total fat, 15% kcal MUFA and 54% kcal CHO) resulted in comparable decreases in LDL-C (6.3% and 7.0%, respectively). The blood cholesterol-lowering diet high in CHO and low in fat decreased HDL-C by 7.7% and increased TG by 6.9%, whereas the diet high in MUFA only decreased HDL-C by 4.1% and decreased TG by 4.6%.[54] Furthermore, a meta-analysis conducted by Garg et al.[55] found that diets high in MUFA vs. high in carbohydrate reduce fasting TG levels by 19%, decrease VLDL-C by 22%, and moderately increase HDL-C without negatively affecting LDL-C.

Polyunsaturated Fatty Acids

Epidemiologic studies from within-population and cross-population studies provide mixed results regarding whether PUFA (n-3 and n-6) is inversely associated with CVD mortality. Many studies have shown an association between dietary PUFA and reduced CVD mortality after adjusting for SFA;[56] however other studies, such as the Seven Countries Study, reported no significant association between PUFA intake and CVD.[24,27]

n-6 PUFA

Specific associations with linoleic acid (LA), the predominant n-6 fatty acid, and coronary disease risk also have been inconsistent. A cross-population study in healthy men found an inverse association between n-6 levels in adipose tissue and mortality rate from CAD.[57] In contrast, a recent study in an Israeli population consuming PUFA as 10% of total energy did not find an association between LA intake and acute myocardial infarction (AMI).[58] However, there was a positive association between arachidonic acid, the long chain derivative of LA, with AMI ($p = 0.004$). After multivariate adjustment, however, there was no indication of an adverse association between LA and AMI.

Some of the earliest clinical trials evaluated the effects of diets high in PUFA, ranging from 13% to 21% of energy, on TC and CHD events.[59–62] Three of these studies reported a 13–15% decrease in TC, which was accompanied by a 25–43% decrease in CHD events.[59–61] Predictive equations have demonstrated that a 1% increase in PUFA results in a reduction of TC by 0.024 mmol/L.[28,29] The TC-lowering effect is approximately half of the cholesterol-raising effect of SFA.[28,29] More recent predictive equations developed for individual fatty acids demonstrate that LA is the strongest TC and LDL-C-lowering fatty acid.

Some studies have shown that LA raises HDL-C when compared with stearic acid (18:0).[53] A study by Mattson and Grundy,[30] however, reported an HDL-C-lowering effect (-5 ± 1.7 mg/dl, $p < 0.02$) of PUFA at very high levels (28% of kcal) in normotriglyceridemic individuals. Other studies have reported no significant change in HDL-C with a high PUFA intake.[63]

n-3 PUFA

The cardioprotective effects of marine-derived long-chain n-3 fatty acids, eicosapentanoic acid (EPA) and docosahexanoic acid (DHA), are well established.[64] An inverse association between n-3 fatty acids and CAD has been found in numerous epidemiologic studies. In the Seven Countries Study, a non-significant negative correlation ($r = -0.28$) was observed between fish consumption and CAD mortality despite large differences in fish consumption among the cohorts. An inverse correlation also was found in the 25-year follow-up of the study with n-3 fatty acid intake and 25-year CAD mortality rates ($r = -0.36$).[27] In the Zutphen Study,[65] an increase in fish consumption from 0 to 45 g/day was associated with a progressive decrease in the risk of CAD after 20 years ($p < 0.05$). Epidemiologic studies also have found an association between α-linolenic acid (ALA), specifically, and CHD risk. In the Health Professionals Follow-Up Study, a 1% increase in ALA intake was associated with a 40% lower risk of CHD.[66]

In the GISSI Prevention Study,[67] the largest prospective clinical trial to test the efficacy of n-3 fatty acids for secondary prevention of CHD, subjects were randomized to the EPA + DHA supplement group (850 mg/day of omega-3 fatty acid ethyl esters), with and without 300 mg/day of vitamin E. Individuals in the supplement group compared with the control group experienced a 15% reduction in the primary endpoint of death, nonfatal myocardial infarct, and nonfatal stroke ($p < 0.02$). In addition, all-cause mortality and sudden death were reduced by 20% ($p = 0.01$) and 45% ($p < 0.001$), respectively, compared with the control group, with Vitamin E providing no benefit.

The mechanisms proposed by which n-3 fatty acids protect against CHD include increased stabilization of atherosclerotic plaques, decreased production of adhesion molecules, chemoattractants, eicosanoids, cytokines, and increased endothelial relaxation and vascular compliance.[68] In addition, n-3 fatty acids are known to influence the lipid profile. Overall, studies have observed slight increases in LDL-C (5–10%) and HDL-C (1–3%) and substantial decreases in TG levels (25–20%) with marine-based n-3 fatty acid supplementation (< 7 g n-3 fatty acids/day).[64]

The primary effect of marine sources of n-3 fatty acids on the lipid profile is due to their TG-lowering effects. In a review of 44 intervention studies by Harris,[69] supplementation of 0.5–25 g of n-3 fatty acids from fish oils for an average of 6 weeks elicited a substantial decrease in TG levels (10–20%), while LDL-C and HDL-C concentrations did not change. In addition, a study of longer duration (16 weeks) found that a low dose of n-3 PUFA from fish oil (1 g/day) decreased fasting TG levels by 21%.[70] Consumption of 3–4 g/day of EPA and DHA results in a 25% decrease in TG in normolipemic (TG less than 2 mmol/L) and 34% decrease in TG in hypertriglyceridemic patients (TG greater than 2 mmol/L).[64] The characteristic TG-lowering effect appears specific to marine sources of n-3 fatty acids and is generally not observed with plant sources of n-3 fatty acids. However, a TG-lowering effect was found at very high levels (38 g) of ALA intake.[64]

In addition, marine-derived n-3 fatty acids have been shown to increase HDL-C levels 5–15% in recent supplementation trials.[71–75] Likewise, slightly elevated LDL-C levels have been a consistent finding in the n-3 fatty acid supplementation trials.[76–79] In a review, LDL-C was increased by 4.5% in normolipemic patients and 10.8% in the hypertriglyceridemic patients consuming 3–4 g/day of EPA and DHA.[64] Several studies suggest that the elevation of LDL-C probably relates to an increase in LDL particle size.[77,79]

Dietary Cholesterol

Some epidemiologic studies have shown positive associations between cholesterol intake and CHD risk, including the Seven Countries Study, the Honolulu Heart Program, and the Western Electric Study,[27,80,81] while others have not.[66,82] Numerous studies have demonstrated that there is a positive linear relationship between dietary cholesterol intake and both TC and LDL-C. Based on a meta-analysis of 27 controlled feeding studies, each increase of 100 mg of dietary cholesterol results in an increase in TC by about 0.5 to 1 mmol/L, 80% of which is due to increases in LDL-C.[22] In addition, dietary cholesterol also has a modest HDL-C-raising effect,[83,84] especially in individuals who are hyper-responders.[85,86]

Dietary Fiber

Epidemiologic Evidence of Fiber and Heart Disease

Several large epidemiologic studies have reported a strong inverse correlation between dietary fiber (refined or whole grain) and CHD. The Health Professionals Follow-up Study tracked 43,757 U.S. male health professionals, aged 40–75 years who were initially free of diagnosed CHD and diabetes, for 6 years.[87] The age-adjusted relative risk for total myocardial infarction was 0.59 among men with the highest quartile of total dietary fiber intake (median 28 g/day) compared with men with the lowest quartile (median 12.4 g/day). The relative risk for fatal myocardial infarction in the highest quartile was 0.45 compared with the lowest quartile of fiber intake. In the Nurses' Health Study, Wolk et al.[88] reported that an increase of 10 g/day dietary fiber was associated with a 20% reduction in CHD risk. In the Alpha-Tocopherol, Beta-Carotene Cancer Prevention Study, Pietinen et al.[89] followed 21,930 male Finnish smokers for 6 years and reported a significant reduction in both coronary morbidity and mortality associated with increased intake of dietary fiber. A recent meta-analysis of ten prospective cohort studies (91,058 men and 245,186 women) found that each 10 g/day increment of total dietary fiber was associated with a 14% reduction in risk of all coronary events and 27% reduction in coronary mortality.[90] In all four of these studies, a stronger association was observed between cereal fiber and CHD risk than between vegetable or fruit fiber. Using data from the NHANES I Epidemiologic Follow-up Study (n = 9,776), Bazzano et al.[91] found that water-soluble dietary fiber intake reduced CHD events 15% and CVD events 10% when comparing participants with the highest intake (5.9 g/day) to those with the lowest intake (0.9 g/day). However, not every study shows this relationship. Liu et al.[92] studied 39,876 female health professionals in the Women's Health Study over 6 years and found a non-significant inverse association between dietary fiber and risk for CVD and myocardial infarction after multiple adjustments for smoking, CVD risk factors, and dietary variables.

The importance of whole grains as a source of fiber has been demonstrated in several studies.[93,94] A study using the Iowa Women's Health Study database matched women on total grain fiber intake, but differed in the proportion of fiber consumed from whole vs. refined grain.[95] Interestingly, after adjusting for multiple confounding factors, women who consumed a higher amount of whole grains (4.7 g whole grain/2000 kcal and 1.9 g refined grain/2000 kcal) had a 17% lower mortality rate (RR = 0.83, 95% CI, 0.73–0.94) than women who consumed a greater proportion of refined grains (4.5 g/2000 kcal and 1.3 g whole grain/2000 kcal). Death due to CHD was also significantly different between groups after adjustment for age and energy intake; however, this difference lost significance when multiple confounding factors (i.e., education, hypertension, diabetes, BMI, etc.) were entered into the model. Furthermore, a prospective cohort study in 3588 men and women aged 65 years or older reported that dark breads (wheat, rye, pumpernickel) were associated with a lower risk of CVD (hazard ratio 0.76, 95% CI, 0.64–0.09) compared with cereal fiber from other sources.[96] A recent meta-analysis of 12 population-based cohort studies found that whole-grain foods significantly reduced the risk of CHD by approximately 26% after adjustment for multiple CHD risk factors.[97] The inverse association of whole grains was stronger than for cereal fiber, fruits, or vegetables, suggesting that three servings of whole grains per day may be important to cardiovascular health.

Overall, epidemiologic studies lend convincing support to the hypothesis that individuals with a higher intake of dietary fiber, especially from whole grains,[93,94,98–102] have a lower risk of CVD than those who consume a diet poor in fiber. The new recommendations from the National Academy of Science for fiber intake are 38 and 25 g/day for young men and women, respectively, based on an intake of 14 g of fiber per 1000 kcal.[22] In addition, several studies suggest that the cardioprotective benefit of regular whole grain consumption may be conferred via favorable effects on risk factors associated with CVD, including hypertension,[103–105] Type 2 diabetes,[104,106–108] and other metabolic risk factors.[106,107] Therefore, consistent with the Dietary Guidelines 2005 Report, the public should consume three servings of whole grains per day to decrease risk of chronic disease.

The Role of Dietary Fiber in Lipid Management

Numerous studies have demonstrated that diets rich in soluble fiber are more effective in lowering blood cholesterol levels than are diets rich in insoluble fiber.[109–115] The key soluble fibers are β-glucan (found in oats, barley, and yeast), psyllium (found in husks of blonde psyllium seed), and pectin (found in fruit). Several properties of soluble fiber, including viscosity, bile acid-binding capacity, and potential cholesterol synthesis-inhibiting capacity after fermentation in the colon,[116,117] contribute to its cholesterol-lowering effect.[118]

A meta-analysis of eight studies reported that 10 g/day of psyllium reduced TC and LDL-C by 4% and 7%, respectively.[119] Another meta-analysis of 67 controlled dietary studies performed by Brown et al.[120] found that for each gram of soluble fiber from oats, psyllium, pectin, or guar gum, TC concentrations decreased by 0.037, 0.028, 0.070, and 0.026 mmol/L (1.42, 1.10, 2.69, and 1.13 mg/dl), respectively. LDL-C decreased by 0.032, 0.029, 0.055, and 0.033 mmol/L (1.23, 1.11, 1.96, and 1.20 mg/dl), respectively, demonstrating that the cholesterol-lowering effects of these soluble fibers are comparable. Furthermore, two servings of oats (2.6 g soluble fiber) has been shown to elicit a 2–3% cholesterol-lowering effect beyond what is achieved by a blood cholesterol-lowering diet alone.[121] Beneficial effects of fiber intake also have been observed in healthy populations. In a study of normolipidemic and normotensive subjects (n = 53,), increased dietary fiber intake (30.5 g/day total fiber and 4.11 g/day soluble fiber) over 3 months significantly reduced LDL-C by 12.8%, while TG and HDL-C did not change.[122] Interest in barley as another source of β-glucan is on the rise.[123–126] The addition of 3 or 6 g/day β-glucan from barley to a Step I diet has been shown to further lower TC (4% and 9%, respectively) and LDL-C (13.8% and 17.4%, respectively) concentrations in mildly hypercholesterolemic men and women.[123] Overall, these studies achieve modest reductions in TC of 2–18%. This is important because a reduction in TC of just 1% could reduce CVD mortality by 2%.[127]

In addition to lowering blood cholesterol levels, a high-fiber intake prevents or attenuates the hypertriglyceridemic response to a high-carbohydrate diet.[128] The traditional adoption of a high-carbohydrate, low-fat diet can produce an unfavorable lipid profile by decreasing HDL-C and increasing TG.[129] The mechanism has not been confirmed with some studies concluding that the hypertriglyceridemic response is the result of reduced VLDL-TG clearance,[130] while others attribute it to increased VLDL-TG secretion because of increased hepatic fatty acid availability resulting from increased influx of fatty acids and decreased hepatic fatty acid oxidation.[131,132] Elevated levels of blood TG are considered an independent risk factor for CHD;[133,134] a 1 mmol/L increase in fasting blood TG is associated with a 76% and 31% increase in CVD risk in women and men, respectively.[135] Several studies note that increasing dietary fiber diminishes the adverse effects of a low-fat, high-CHO diet on HDL-C and TG concentrations.[109,120,123,136]

An extensive review of 14 studies by Anderson[128] found that high-CHO (60% kcal CHO), low-fiber (6 g/1000 kcal) diets elicited higher fasting serum TG levels by a mean of 53% (95% CI, 34–71%), compared with low-CHO (< 45% kcal CHO), low-fiber diets. The opposite was true for high-CHO, high-fiber (29 g/1000 kcal) diets, which modestly lowered TG by 10% (95% CI, –2% to –17%) compared with low-CHO (42% kcal CHO), low-fiber (7.5 g/1000 kcal) diets. Even modest increases in dietary fiber from 10 to 22 g/1000 calories has been associated with a 10% reduction in fasting serum TG levels in Type 2 diabetic patients consuming a moderate-CHO diet (55% kcal CHO).[137] Garg et al.[138] conducted an innovative study comparing the TG response of two diets matched for fiber content (25 g/day), but varied in levels of carbohydrate in hypertriglyceridemic diabetic individuals (n = 8). The high-CHO diet (60% kcal CHO) resulted in a 27.5% ($p < 0.002$) increase in plasma TG compared with the low-CHO diet (35% kcal CHO).

Emerging evidence suggests that increases in blood TG levels may contribute to increased concentrations of small, dense LDL particles, which are atherogenic.[139] A recent study of 36 overweight men aged 50–75 years found that consumption of two large servings of oats daily (about 14 g/day dietary fiber) substantially decreased small, dense LDL-C (– 17.3%) and LDL particle number (– 5.0%) compared with the wheat control (+ 60.4% and + 14.2%, respectively).[140] More importantly, although carbohydrate intake increased and total and saturated fat intakes decrease, HDL-C and TG levels remained stable in subjects who consumed the high-fiber oat cereals. Other emerging data suggest that dietary fiber is inversely associated with C-reactive protein, a marker of inflammation.[141,142]

The association between increased dietary fiber consumption and improved lipid profiles indicates a causal relationship between fiber, blood lipids, and heart disease. Further research is needed to define the optimal ratio of fiber to carbohydrate in the diet. However, when instituting a low-fat, high-carbohydrate diet, care should be taken to simultaneously increase fiber-dense foods with carbohydrate content.

Glycemic Index/Glycemic Load

The traditional approach of classifying carbohydrates is based on their chemical structure (starch, sugars, fiber). Over the past two decades, an alternative approach, which characterizes dietary CHO on the basis of their effects on postprandial glycemia has been intensely debated. The glycemic index (GI), defined as the area under the 2-h glycemic curve after consumption of a food containing 50 g CHO, divided by the area under the curve for a standard food (white bread or glucose) also containing 50 g CHO,[143,144] may be superior to the traditional schema in elucidating the effects of CHO-rich foods on glucose and lipid metabolism. In theory,[145] lowering the postprandial rise in glucose and insulin improves insulin sensitivity and reduces hepatic TG synthesis and secretion. This results in reduced fasting TG concentrations and reciprocal increased HDL-C levels.

Excessive postprandial hyperglycemia has been linked to all-cause and CVD mortality,[146–148] increased carotid intima media thickness,[149,150] and impaired endothelial function.[151,152] As a consequence of hyperglycemia, hyperinsulemia has been implicated in the development of dyslipidemia (i.e., high TG and low HDL-C).[153,154] Therefore, controlling postprandial hyperglycemia via CHO intake may alleviate dyslipidemia associated with excessive insulin.

Scores for high-GI, moderate-GI, and low-GI foods are > 70, 56–69, and < 55, respectively, using glucose as the standard.[155] Several large-scale epidemiologic studies have demonstrated that the average GI and glycemic load (the product of the GI of a specific food multiplied by its CHO content) of the diet are significant independent predictors of risk of Type 2 diabetes[156–158] and CVD.[157] Furthermore, studies show that total carbohydrate intake or sugar intake is not associated with increased risk. More importantly, high-GI diets are associated with lower HDL-C concentrations in both healthy[159–161] and diabetic populations.[162] In the studies of healthy populations, reductions in GI range from 16% to 22% when comparing the highest and lowest quintiles of intake.[159–161] This corresponds with significant increases in HDL-C of 9–20%. Similar results have been observed in individuals with diabetes.[162] The effect of GI on blood TG was evaluated in the Nurses' Health Study.[159] When comparing the two extreme quintiles of glycemic load (117 vs. 180), TG levels were 144% higher in women with a BMI > 25 and 40% higher in women of normal weight (BMI ≤ 25).

Clinical studies generally show that when the amount of carbohydrate is held constant, foods with a higher GI increase fasting blood TG. In 10 of 11 studies reviewed by Miller,[163] a reduction in GI of greater than 12 points lowered TG levels by an average of 9%. Individual variations in lipid response to low-GI diets has been observed.[164] Thirty subjects were treated with a high-GI diet (GI = 84) for 1 month, a low-GI diet (GI = 73) for 1 month, and finally a high-GI diet. Individuals diagnosed with type IIa hypercholesterolemia showed little lipid response, whereas subjects with a variety of types of hypercholesterolemia (IIb and IV), characterized by hypertriglyceridemia, experienced significant reductions in TG (about 20%), LDL-C (7–10%), and TC (7–9%).[164] These results need to be confirmed, however, since the diets also differed in fiber, fat, and energy content. In a partially controlled feeding study, 15 patients with Type 2 diabetes consumed a low-GI diet (GI = 60) for 6 weeks and a high-GI diet (GI = 87) for 6 weeks.[165] The study investigators provided the starchy food portion of the diet. The diets were similar in macronutrient profile (23% kcal fat, 57% kcal CHO). Serum TG increased almost 10% on the high-GI diet and decreased 15% on the low GI-diet, however due to the low sample size, this difference was not statistically different. In a metabolic ward study, 12 overweight (30–35 BMI) men consumed two diets *ad libitum* for 6 days in a crossover fashion. The diets represented an American Heart Association (AHA) phase 1 diet (30% kcal total fat, 10% kcal SFA, and 55% kcal CHO) and a low-fat, low-GI diet (32% kcal total fat, 14% kcal SFA, and 37% kcal CHO).[166] The AHA diet induced a 28% increase in TG levels and a reciprocal 10% reduction in HDL-C, resulting in a significant increase in TC:HDL-C. The opposite was true for the low-GI diet; plasma TG fell 35% and LDL particle size increased by 1.6%. Although difficult to interpret due to differences in the diets, this study highlights the rapid effects of these diets on lipid metabolism and suggests that a low-GI, high-protein diet may be beneficial compared with a traditional low-fat diet.

Low GI-diets also may protect against HDL-C lowering of traditional high-CHO diets. Luscombe et al.[167] conducted a partially controlled feeding study in which 21 diabetic individuals consumed three diets: a high-GI diet (GI = 63), a low-GI diet (GI = 43), and a high-MUFA, high-GI diet (GI = 59) in a crossover design. Over each 4-week period, 45% of energy was provided as key CHO foods, and subjects were instructed on menus for implementing the intervention diets. This resulted in similar intakes of energy, fiber, and macronutrients across treatments. The low-GI diet and high-MUFA diet had comparable effects on the lipid profile, whereas the low-GI diet elicited higher HDL-C levels (6%) compared with the high-GI diet. TG levels were 18% lower; however, this was not statistically different. In contrast, individuals with impaired glucose tolerance experienced a significant reduction in HDL-C and no change in TG levels, when they consumed a low-GI diet for 4 months vs. a high-GI diet.[168]

Studies have also evaluated the impact of GI in the context of weight loss diets. A study by Heilbronn et al.[169] in 55 overweight men and women found that both high-GI and low-GI diets reduced TG to a similar extent with concurrent weight loss (~ 5%). HDL-C did not change in either diet; however, LDL-C levels were reduced more (8%) in subjects on the low-GI diet. A study comparable in design also reported similar LDL-C-lowering results with no changes in TG levels in 20 individuals with Type 2 diabetes.[170] Other studies utilizing low-GI diets as a means to lose weight also report no changes in TG or HDL-C.[171,172]

The GI can be easily manipulated by food choice selection and offers promise for treating dyslipidemia. Incorporating low-GI foods into a low-fat, high-CHO diet may prevent CHO-induced hypertriglyceridemia. The GI effects on HDL-C are inconclusive and further research is needed. It must also be noted that results from many studies demonstrate considerable heterogeneity in the lipid response to a low-GI diet.[145] Although controversial, the GI concept has been shown to be useful in the dietary management of diabetes, hyperglycemia, and hyperlipidemia.[173,174]

Conclusion

Diet plays an important role in modifying CVD risk, partly due to the effects of nutrients on lipids and lipoproteins. Saturated fatty acids, *trans* fatty acids, dietary cholesterol, and simple carbohydrates adversely affect lipids and lipoproteins, while unsaturated fatty acids and complex carbohydrates rich in fiber beneficially affect lipids and lipoproteins. It is important to modify diet appropriately to modify plasma lipids and lipoproteins in a way that minimizes coronary disease risk.

Effects of Dietary Patterns on Lipids and Lipoproteins

Several dietary patterns have been studied extensively and found to have specific effects on lipids and lipoproteins, which are reviewed in Table 11.3. The traditional dietary plans recommended by the National Cholesterol Education Program (NCEP) to treat hypercholesterolemia are the Step I and Step II diets.[175] Step I diet guidelines include limiting total and saturated fat and dietary cholesterol, while the Step II diet recommends further reductions in saturated fat and dietary cholesterol (Table 11.3). Currently, the NCEP recommends the Therapeutic Lifestyle Changes (TLC) diet, which incorporates several dietary manipulations to maximally lower LDL-C.[6] Other dietary patterns for managing lipids and lipoproteins include vegetarian diets, very low-fat diets, and Mediterranean-style diets. Many clinical studies have evaluated the effects of these diets on blood lipids and lipoproteins. Typically, these diets lower TC and LDL-C levels, while the effects on TG and HDL-C levels vary on the basis of diet composition and lifestyle program. The availability of several different dietary patterns for the management of dyslipidemia provides many options for patients and clinicians. This aids in optimizing diet adherence, resulting in maximal lipid lowering in response to diet.

NCEP Recommendations

Numerous free-living and controlled clinical trials have assessed the effects of Step I and Step II diets on the lipid profile across populations of varying ages, including individuals with CAD,[176] normal blood lipids,[177] hypercholesterolemia,[178] and combined hypercholesterolemia and hypertriglyceridemia.[179] The results of these studies consistently show beneficial effects on TC and LDL-C levels, while the effects on HDL-C and TG levels are specific to each intervention. When Yu-Poth et al.[180] examined 37 dietary intervention studies in a meta-analysis assessing NCEP guidelines in free-living subjects, a Step I diet decreased TC, LDL-C, and TG levels by 10%, 12%, and 8%, respectively, while a Step II diet resulted in decreases of 13%, 16%, and 8%, respectively, and a 7% decrease in HDL-C levels. Although Step I and Step II diets decreased HDL-C levels, the TC:HDL-C ratio also decreased 10%, which reduces overall CVD risk. When following a Step I or Step II diet, a

TABLE 11.3

Lipid Response of Selected Dietary Patterns

Diet	Description	Expected Lipid Response			
		TC	**LDL-C**	**HDL-C**	**TG**
Step I[175]	Total fat < 30%, SFA 8–10%, cholesterol < 300 mg/day	↓	↓	↓	↑, ↓ or ↔
Step II[175]	Total fat < 30%, SFA < 7%, cholesterol < 200 mg/day	↓↓	↓↓	↓	↑, ↓ or ↔
Therapeutic Lifestyle Changes[6]	Total fat 25–35%, SFA < 7%, cholesterol < 200 mg/day For further LDL-C lowering: Add plant stanol/sterols (2 g/day) Add viscous fiber (10–25 g/day) Add moderate physical activity to expend 200 kcal/day	↓↓↓	↓↓↓	↓ or ↔	↔
Portfolio[182–184]	Low-fat vegetarian diet containing a dietary portfolio that included a plant sterol ester-enriched margarine, oats, barley, and psyllium, soy milk and soy meat analogs, fruits and vegetables, and whole almonds; eggplant and okra were also used as additional sources of viscous fiber	↓↓↓↓	↓↓↓↓	↔	↔
Lifestyle Heart[185]	Low-fat, plant-based diet that uses fruits, vegetables, whole grains, beans, and soy products in their natural forms, moderate quantities of egg whites and nonfat dairy or soy products and only small amounts of sugar and white flour; moderate aerobic exercise, stress management training, smoking cessation, and group psychosocial support were also included	↓↓	↓↓	´	´
Indo-Mediterranean Diet[190]	Rich in whole grains (at least 400–500 g of whole grains), fruits, vegetables, walnuts and almonds, legumes, rice, maize, wheat, and 3–4 servings/day of mustard seed or soybean oil	↓	↓	↑	↓
DASH[136]	Rich in fruits and vegetables (9 servings/day) and low-fat dairy products (2–3 servings/day), with increased fish, nuts, legumes and is low in saturated and total fat and sodium	↓	↓	↓	↔

↑, increase; ↓, decrease; ↔, no change.

1-kg decrease in body weight decreased TG by 0.011 mmol/L ($r = 0.35$, $p < 0.01$) and increased HDL-C by 0.011 mmol/L ($r = -0.38$, $p < 0.02$). Therefore, TG levels decrease[180] or remain unchanged[177–179] when following a Step I or Step II diet for weight loss. However, TG levels would be expected to increase if there is no weight loss.[176]

The TLC diet incorporates several dietary manipulations such as plant stanols/sterols and viscous fiber and emphasizes weight loss and physical activity to maximally lower LDL-C.[6] The expected combined effect of the TLC diet is a 20–30% decrease in LDL-C levels. The approximate contribution of each lifestyle change to a reduction in LDL-C is: 8–10% by limiting SFA intake to < 7% of calories, 3–5% by limiting dietary cholesterol to < 200 mg, up to 5% with the addition of 5–10 g/day of viscous fiber, about 5–8% for a weight loss of approximately 10 pounds, and 6–15% with the consumption of 2 g/day plant stanol/sterol esters.[6]

In hypercholesterolemic individuals, consuming a TLC diet (15% kcal protein, 58% kcal CHO, and 30% kcal total fat: 7% kcal SFA, 10% kcal MUFA, and 10% kcal PUFA, and 75 mg cholesterol per 1000 kcal) compared with a Western diet (15% kcal protein, 47% kcal CHO, 38% kcal fat: 16% kcal SFA, 16% kcal MUFA, and 6% kcal PUFA, and 180 mg cholesterol per 1000 kcal) significantly lowers TC, LDL-C, and HDL-C levels by 9%, 11%, and 7% (all $ps < 0.001$), respectively; however VLDL-C levels remain unchanged and TG levels increase 7% ($p = 0.265$). Consistent with the effects on LDL-C and HDL-C, apolipoprotein (apo) B and apo A-I levels were ~ 6% lower after consumption of the TLC diet compared with the Western diet ($p < 0.001$).[178]

The influence of gender on lipid response to the TLC diet (26% kcal total fat, 4% kcal SFA, and 45 mg cholesterol/1000 kcal) vs. an average American diet (AAD: 35% kcal total fat, 14% kcal SFA, and 147 mg cholesterol/1000 kcal) was evaluated in moderately hypercholesterolemic adults.[181] Following the TLC diet, TC, LDL-C, and apo B levels were significantly decreased when compared with an AAD (respectively, men: 19%, 21%, and 18%; women: 12%, 15%, and 9%; $p < 0.05$ for both groups); however, the reductions in TC and apo B were greater in men than women ($p < 0.05$). Fasting TG levels were not affected by the TLC diet in men, but were increased 14% in women ($p < 0.05$). Yet, postprandial TG levels measured after a standard fat load were greater in men than women ($p < 0.05$). LDL particle size decreased 11% in men and 21% in women ($p < 0.05$). These data indicate that middle-aged men may have a more favorable lipoprotein response to a low-fat, low-cholesterol diet than postmenopausal women.[181]

Portfolio Diet

The Portfolio diet is designed to maximally lower LDL-C levels by employing a variety of dietary interventions, each of which has hypocholesterolemic properties. The Portfolio diet is a vegetarian diet rich in soy protein, almonds, plant sterols and viscous fibers primarily from oats, barley, and psyllium.[182]

When the effects of the Portfolio diet (22.4% kcal protein: 96.8% as vegetable protein, 50.6% kcal CHO, 27.0% kcal total fat, 4.3% kcal SFA, 11.8% kcal MUFA, 9.9% kcal PUFA, 10 mg cholesterol/1000 kcal, and 30.7 g fiber/1000 kcal) were evaluated in hypercholesterolemic adults, TC levels decreased by 22.4% and LDL-C levels by 29.0%, respectively ($p < 0.001$); while HDL-C and TG levels decreased non-significantly.[182,183] Consistent with these changes, TC:HDL-C and apo B decreased by 19.8% and 24.2%, respectively.

In a follow-up study[183] comparing the Portfolio diet (20.0% kcal protein: 99% as vegetable protein, 56.6% kcal CHO, 23.2% kcal total fat, 4.9% kcal SFA, 9.5% kcal MUFA, 7.9% kcal PUFA, 48 mg cholesterol/1000 kcal, and 37.2 g fiber/1000 kcal) to a Step II diet (19.6% kcal protein: 30% as vegetable protein, 58.8% kcal CHO, 21.6% kcal total fat, 4.4% kcal SFA, 8.5% kcal MUFA, 7.5% kcal PUFA, 34 mg cholesterol/1000 kcal, and 26.6 g fiber/1000 kcal), TC and LDL-C levels decreased by 26.6% and 35.0% ($p < 0.001$), respectively, on the Portfolio diet but by only 9.9% and 12.1% ($p < 0.001$), respectively, on the Step II diet. Consistent with the change in TC and LDL-C levels, TC:HDL-C and apo B decreased 20.8% and 26.7%, respectively, following the Portfolio diet compared with a reduction of only 2.6% and 8.1%, respectively, when following the Step II diet ($p < 0.001$). In addition, TG levels decreased 6.3% following consumption of the Portfolio diet but increased 4.9% when following the Step II diet. Neither diet affected HDL-C or apo A-I levels.

In another study,[184] the magnitude of cholesterol reduction observed following the Portfolio diet was similar to low-dose statin therapy. TC and LDL-C levels decreased by 21.9% and 28.6%, respectively, ($p < 0.001$, from baseline) on the Portfolio diet, by 23.3% and 30.9%, respectively, ($p < 0.001$, from baseline) on lovastatin treatment, but by only 6.3% and 8.0%, respectively, ($p = 0.002$, from baseline) on the vegetable-rich control diet. Likewise, TC:HDL-C and apo B decreased by 17.1% and 22.8%, respectively, following consumption of the Portfolio diet and by 21.6% and 26.6% on statin treatment ($p < 0.005$, compared with control diet). None of the diets affected HDL-C levels. These results suggest that when several interventions are employed concurrently, diet can produce favorable effects on the lipid profile that are similar in magnitude to statin therapy.

Lifestyle Heart Program

The Lifestyle Heart Trial evaluated patients with previous CHD who were randomized to either a usual-care group or an intensive lifestyle change group.[185] The intervention consisted of a very-low-fat vegetarian diet high in complex-carbohydrates (15–20% kcal protein, 70–75% kcal CHO, 10% kcal total fat [PUFA:SFA > 1] and 5 mg/day cholesterol), moderate aerobic exercise, stress management training, smoking cessation, and group psychosocial support. After one year on the program, significant reductions occurred in TC, LDL-C, and apo B levels by 27.6%, 39.8%, and 23.2%, respectively (all ps < 0.005). HDL-C levels decreased non-significantly by 9.6%, while TG levels non-significantly increased by 13.4%. The benefits of reducing these CVD risk factors were seen after five years when the experimental group experienced significant reductions in average percent diameter stenosis (–3.1% vs. +11.8%, $p = 0.001$) and angina (–91% vs. +186%, $p < 0.001$) and experienced significantly fewer cardiac events than the control group (25 vs. 45, $p < 0.001$).

Mediterranean Diet

The dietary patterns characteristic of the Mediterranean region have been extensively studied to determine why inhabitants of this area have decreased rates of coronary disease. Diet composition varies in this region but tends to emphasize fruits, vegetables, breads, cereals, potatoes, beans, nuts, olive oil, and seeds. Other common characteristics of Mediterranean-style diets include dairy products (mainly cheese and yogurt), fish, poultry, and wine consumed in low to moderate amounts, eggs consumed zero to four times per week, and minimal consumption of red meat.

The Seven Countries Study stimulated interest in the Mediterranean diet when it was reported that the 15-year mortality rate from CHD in Southern Europe was two to three times lower than that in Northern Europe or the United States; yet the mean serum TC values were similar.[186] Other epidemiologic studies, such as the ATTICA Study,[187,188] have shown that factors, other than lipids (i.e., physical activity, education, and markers of inflammation and coagulation), contribute to reduced mortality from CHD. The majority of study participants lived in areas surrounding Athens and had elevated TC and LDL-C levels, while one-fifth of the subjects had low HDL-C levels.

In the Lyon Diet Heart Study,[189] a randomized, single-blind secondary prevention trial, subjects consumed a Western diet or an experimental diet rich in ALA (30.5% kcal total fat, 8.3% kcal SFA, 12.9% kcal 18:1, 3.6% kcal 18:2, 0.81% kcal 18:3, and 217 mg/day cholesterol). This Mediterranean-type diet was rich in whole grains, root vegetables and green vegetables, fish, fruits at least once daily, and low in red meat (replaced with poultry). Margarine that had a fatty acid profile similar to that of olive oil, except that it was higher in linoleic acid and more so in α-linolenic acid, was supplied by the study to replace butter and cream. Rapeseed and olive oils were used exclusively for salads and food preparation. After two years on the experimental diet or Western diet, TC, LDL-C, HDL-C, TG, apo B, and apo A-I levels were unchanged. Although both groups had similar lipids, lipoproteins, blood pressure, BMI, and smoking status, subjects consuming the ALA-rich Mediterranean diet had a 50–70% lower risk of recurrent coronary events.

The Indo-Mediterranean Diet Heart Study,[190] another secondary prevention trial incorporating a diet rich in ALA, showed beneficial effects on blood lipids, lipoproteins, as well as recurrent coronary events. In this study, the experimental group was instructed to consume a diet rich in ALA consisting of 400–500 g of fruits, vegetables, and nuts, 400–500 g of whole grains, and three to four servings of mustard seed or soybean oil daily; while the control group was counseled on the Step I diet. After 2 years, TC, LDL-C, and TG levels decreased in the experimental group by 12.2%, 17.6%, and 19.6%, respectively; and by 3.1%, 4.2%, and 5.9%, respectively, in the control group ($p < 0.0001$ at 2 years between groups). HDL-C levels increased 2.6% in the experimental group only ($p = 0.0288$). Like the Lyon Diet Heart Study, subjects consuming the ALA-rich Mediterranean diet had significantly fewer total cardiac events than the control group (39 vs. 76, $p < 0.001$).

While epidemiologic evidence and some clinical trial evidence does not show a beneficial effect of the Mediterranean diet on lipids and lipoproteins, there is some clinical evidence that demonstrates a beneficial effect. Therefore, further studies are needed to determine the underlying mechanism(s) for the reduction in coronary events in coronary patients consuming a diet characteristic of the Mediterranean region.

Dietary Approaches to Stop Hypertension (DASH) Diet

In a secondary analysis of the Dietary Approaches to Stop Hypertension (DASH) trial,[136] a trial designed to compare the effects of three dietary patterns on blood pressure, the effect of the DASH diet on blood lipids was assessed. Subjects consumed a control diet high in saturated fat and low in dietary fiber (15% kcal protein, 52% kcal CHO, 37% kcal total fat, 13% kcal SFA, 14% kcal MUFA, 7% kcal PUFA, 188 mg/day cholesterol), a fruit and vegetable diet with a similar macronutrient profile but high in dietary fiber (29.9 g/day), or a DASH diet emphasizing fruits, vegetables, and low-fat dairy products (18% kcal protein, 58% kcal CHO, 27% kcal total fat, 7% kcal SFA, 10% kcal MUFA, 8% kcal PUFA, 141 mg/day cholesterol, 29.7 g/day fiber). Following the DASH diet, TC, LDL-C, and HDL-C levels decreased significantly compared with the control group (7.3%, 9.0%, and 7.5%, respectively, $p < 0.0001$), while non-significant reductions occurred in the fruit and vegetable group (1.9%, 1.5%, and 0.4%, respectively). TC:HDL-C and TG levels were unaffected in subjects on the DASH diet.

Different dietary patterns have different effects on lipids and lipoproteins. Some diets, like the Lifestyle Heart, also show beneficial effects on CHD events. There are many strategies for diet modification to reduce risk of heart disease. The optimal dietary pattern is selected in a way that favorably affects the lipid and lipoprotein profile, body weight, and long-term adherence.

Effects of Weight Loss Diets on Lipids and Lipoproteins

The weight loss diet debate has been ongoing for many years. For some individuals low-fat diets achieve the most weight loss; while for others, moderate-fat or low-carbohydrate diets do. Although initial weight loss associated with different dietary plans is promising, the ability to maintain a lower weight over an extended period of time defines successful weight loss.

Low-Fat Diets

The Pritikin Program, a lifestyle intervention program that includes a high-complex-carbohydrate, high-fiber (35–40 g/1000 kcal), low-fat (< 10% total calories) and low-cholesterol (< 25 mg/day) diet and exercise component, reduced weight, TC, and TG by 5%, 21%, and 50%, respectively.[191] However, this weight reduction diet was associated with a 14.6% decrease in HDL-C levels. When assessing the effects of a low-fat, reduced-calorie diet on weight and lipids over 10 weeks,[192] mean body weight declined by 0.62 ± 0.47 kg/week during the first 5 weeks and 0.43 ± 0.43 kg/week during the second 5 weeks. Likewise, TC, LDL-C, and apo B levels decreased by 15%, 23%, and 23%, respectively, during the 10-week low-fat, reduced-calorie diet. However, TG levels increased 22% and HDL-C levels decreased 18%, causing TC:HDL-C to increase. Thus, while low-fat diets can achieve desired weight loss and reduce TC and LDL-C levels, they also may exacerbate the hypertriglyceridemic response associated with high-carbohydrate, low-fat diets.[129] Therefore, when employing a low-fat diet to elicit weight loss, especially in individuals with hypertriglyceridemia, it is important to replace simple carbohydrates with complex carbohydrates and increase dietary fiber to blunt the hypertriglyceridemic response associated with high-carbohydrate, low-fat diets.[128]

Moderate-Fat Diets with MUFA

Although low-fat diets result in weight loss and lower TC and LDL-C levels, they also are associated with increases in TG levels, decreases in HDL-C levels, and adherence problems. Several studies have shown that moderate-fat diets promote weight loss,[193–195] lower TG levels,[194,195] maintain HDL-C levels,[195] and improve diet adherence[193] and weight maintenance.[193,195]

When comparing a high-carbohydrate weight loss diet with a moderate-MUFA fat weight loss diet in a controlled clinical setting, TC levels (~ 7%) and weight (~ 8%) were significantly reduced following both diets; however, the only moderate-MUFA fat diet significantly lowered LDL-C (8.2%, $p < 0.02$) and TG levels (21.9%, $p < 0.05$).[194] An innovative controlled feeding study by Pelkman et al.[195] compared the effects of a low-fat diet (28% kcal total fat, 7.2% kcal MUFA) vs. a moderate-fat diet (32% kcal total fat, 14.2% kcal MUFA) during 6 weeks of controlled weight loss followed by 4 weeks of weight maintenance. At the end of the weight loss period, both diet groups lost equal amounts of weight (moderate-fat diet group, 7.2 ± 0.29 kg; low-fat diet group, 6.5 ± 0.34 kg; $p > 0.10$). In addition, TC, LDL-C, TG, apo A-I, and apo B levels significantly declined during weight loss in both diet groups (all *ps* < 0.05). However, individuals following the low-fat diet experienced significant reductions in HDL-C (12.1%, $p < 0.05$), while those on the moderate-fat diet maintained HDL-C levels and had significant reductions in TC:HDL-C (10.9%, $p < 0.05$). During the weight maintenance period, TG rebounded to above-baseline levels, while HDL-C remained lower than baseline levels in the low-fat diet group only. While these results suggest that a moderate-fat weight-loss diet decreases CVD risk by favorably affecting the lipid profile, other studies conclude that low-fat diets rich in fiber are as effective for weight loss and do not cause unfavorable alterations in plasma lipids.[196] Gerhard et al.[196] found that a low-fat *ad libitum* diet (20% kcal total fat, 8% kcal MUFA) and a moderate-fat *ad libitum* diet (40% kcal total fat, 26% kcal MUFA) reduced TC and LDL-C similarly (low-fat diet, 9.6% and 10.2%, respectively, and moderate-fat diet, 10.2% and 7.5%, respectively). However, only the low-fat diet significantly decreased weight (1.53 kg, $p < 0.001$).

High-Protein Diets

While several studies show some beneficial effects of energy-restricted, high-protein diets on total weight loss and the blood lipid profile,[197–203] others do not.[201,204] In a recent study, researchers reported that a 6-month very-low-carbohydrate-diet program, similar to the Atkins diet (carbohydrate intake < 25 g/day), led to a sustained weight loss (10.3%, $p < 0.02$) with improvements in the lipid profile (decreased TC by 5%, LDL-C by 7% and TG levels by 43% and increased HDL by 19%, all *ps* < 0.02).[200] Layman et al.[198,199] determined that increasing the proportion of protein to carbohydrate in the diet has beneficial effects on body composition and blood lipids. Subjects were randomized to either a carbohydrate (CHO) group (diet with a CHO/protein ratio of 3.5 [68 g protein/day]) or a protein group (diet with a CHO/protein ratio of 0.4 [125 g protein/day]). The diets were isoenergetic (1700 kcal/day) and provided similar amounts of fat (~ 50 g/day). Both groups had significant reductions in TC (16.15 mg/dl for protein group and 20.00 mg/dl for CHO group; $p < 0.05$), while only the protein group experienced significant reductions in TG (10 mg/dl; $p < 0.05$). These findings agree with other studies of high-protein, weight-loss diets, which have also shown improvements in LDL-C particle size and in postprandial blood-lipid profile.[197]

These results are somewhat surprising and need to be confirmed in long-term studies. More importantly, these markedly improved lipid profiles can be attributed to the substantial simultaneous weight loss and little is known what occurs when weight loss plateaus. A few studies have shown that when subjects enter weight maintenance, lipids rebound and adverse effects on blood lipids persist with time.[195,205] In support of these studies, Anderson et al.[202] performed a computer analysis, based on the composition of the recommended diets, to predict the effects of staying on these diets to maintain weight with an energy intake of 2000 calories per day. The results of the analysis suggest that increases in fatty acid content, increases in dietary cholesterol and the reduction in soluble fiber implemented in the Atkins diet would raise serum cholesterol values 9%, 19%, and 2%, respectively. Since every 1% increase in serum cholesterol values are estimated to increase the risk of cardiovascular disease 2–3%,[206] long-term use of the Atkins diet might increase the risk of cardiovascular disease by > 50%.

Early work assessing the effects of a high-protein, low-carbohydrate weight loss diet on lipids and lipoproteins showed that LDL-C levels increased from baseline by 23% ($p < 0.01$), while TG levels decreased by 45% ($p < 0.01$).[203] In a multicenter study, Foster et al.[201] found that 12 weeks of weight loss therapy utilizing the Atkins diet resulted in a greater weight loss (4%) in 63 non-diabetic subjects when compared with a conventional diet. At three months, individuals following the Atkins diet experienced significant increases in TC (+ 5%) and LDL-C (+ 9%) vs. the group on the conventional diet (– 10% and – 15%, respectively); however, by the end of the study the levels were similar between groups.

Although research has shown that low-fat diets, moderate-fat diets, and high-protein diets can promote weight loss due to reduced total calorie intake, they differentially affect lipid metabolism. Selecting a weight loss diet depends on an individual's need to lose weight, motivation, and preference for a specific diet. The available evidence suggests that there is a range of fat intake that can be used for successful weight loss diets. However, the long-term effects of high-protein, low-carbohydrate diets on health and disease prevention are unknown.

Emerging Lipid and Lipoprotein CVD Risk Factors Affected by Diet

In addition to the major lipid and lipoprotein CVD risk factors, other emerging lipid risk factors have been identified. These include LDL particle size, HDL particle size, postprandial TG, and lipoprotein (a).

Diet Effects on LDL Particle Size

LDL subpopulations have been defined on the basis of a number of characteristics, including particle density, size (particle diameter), charge, and chemical composition.[207] The diameter of the most prominent LDL subclass has been identified and is referred to as LDL peak particle diameter (PPD), which generally ranges from 22 to 28 nm. Individuals with a predominance of larger, more buoyant LDL (LDL-I or II) with a peak diameter >25.5 nm have been defined as pattern or phenotype A, whereas those with a higher proportion of smaller, more dense LDL (LDL-III or IV) with a peak diameter < 25.5 nm are referred to as pattern or phenotype B.[23,208,209] The size of LDL particles confers an independent risk of coronary disease.[210,211] Individuals with predominantly small LDL particles (pattern B) experience greater CHD risk than those with larger LDL particles (pattern A).[212–215] About 30–35% of adult men and 15–25% of postmenopausal women have LDL pattern B, while the prevalence is much lower in men less than 20 years old and in premenopausal women (5–10%).[23,216] Even though there is a genetic basis for LDL particle size,[217] dietary factors also[218, 219] have an impact. A number of studies have reported changes in LDL particle size in response to different dietary interventions, including, changes in macronutrient composition, type of dietary fat, type and amount of dietary fiber, and a combination of multiple dietary factors that achieve maximal LDL-C reduction (Table 11.4).

The Effects of a Changing Macronutrient Profile on LDL Particle Size

Effects of High-Fat, Moderate-Fat Diets

Cross-sectional population analyses[220] have demonstrated an association between reduced LDL particle size and a low-fat, high-carbohydrate diet. Several clinical studies have been conducted to evaluate the effects of total fat and carbohydrate on the change in LDL particle size. Krauss and Dreon,[221] using a crossover design, studied 105 normolipidemic men who were instructed to consume a high-fat diet (46% kcal total fat, 39% kcal CHO, 16.2% kcal protein) and a low-fat diet (24% kcal total fat, 60% kcal CHO, 16.1% kcal protein) for 6 weeks. LDL-C was reduced on the low-fat diet in subjects with either pattern A or B phenotype; however, individuals with pattern B exhibited a twofold greater reduction than those with pattern A. Importantly, on the high-fat diet, 87 subjects showed LDL subclass pattern A and only 18 subjects had pattern B; however, when subjects switched to the low-fat diet, 36 subjects (41% of pattern A) converted to pattern B while all subjects with pattern B (when consuming high-fat diet) retained the classification. In another study, using a very-low-fat diet (about 10.4% kcal total fat, 75.7% kcal CHO, 14.5% kcal protein) compared with subject's habitual diet (about 31.8% kcal total fat, 52.1% kcal CHO, 14.0% kcal protein), Dreon et al.[222] found that 26 subjects remained in phenotype A, whereas 12 subjects changed into the denser phenotype B. Collectively, progressive reductions in dietary fat and increases in carbohydrate increase the proportion of subjects that convert from phenotype A to phenotype B.

Effects of High-Protein, Low-Carbohydrate Diets

Dumesnil et al.[166] evaluated the effects of a moderate carbohydrate restricted diet on LDL particle size. In this study, 12 subjects were randomly assigned to a Step I diet (15% kcal protein, 55% kcal CHO and 30% kcal total fat) or

TABLE 11.4

Effects of High-Fat, Low-Carbohydrate Diets vs. Low-Fat, High-Carbohydrate Diets on LDL Phenotype and Particle Size

Study	High-Fat, Low-Carbohydrate Diet				Low-Fat, High-Carbohydrate Diet				% of Subjects Who Switched from phA to phB When on the Low-Fat, High-CHO Diet (%, *n*)
	Total fat, SFA, CHO, P (% energy)	Subjects (*n*) PhA	Subjects (*n*) PhB	LDL Particle Size (nm)	Total Fat, SFA, CHO, P (% energy)	Subjects (*n*) PhA	Subjects (*n*) PhB	LDL Particle Size (nm)	
Krauss et al.[221]	46, 18, 39, 16	87	18	phA: 26.8 phB: 25.3	24, 6, 59, 16	51	54	phA: 26.5* phB: 25.1	41%, 36
Dreon et al.[222]	31.8, 10.8, 52.1, 14.0	38	0	26.62	10.4, 2.7, 75.7, 14.5	26	12	26.05**	32%, 12
Sharman et al.[197]	61, 25, 8, 30	10	2	phB: 26.16	25, 12, 59, 15	7	5	phB: 25.28***	30%, 3
Sharman et al.[249]	63, 22.3, 8, 28	11	4	27.0	23, 7.7, 56, 20	6	9	26.4***	45%, 5
Volek et al.[250]	60, 20.8, 10, 29	[a]	[a]	27.6	19, 5.6, 62, 17	[a]	[a]	27.2	[a]

SFA, saturated fatty acids; CHO, carbohydrate; P, protein; phA, phenotype A; phB, phenotype B.

Significantly different from high-fat, low-carbohydrate diet: $^{*}p < 0.0001$, $^{**}p < 0.001$, $^{***}p \leq 0.05$.

[a] Data not reported.

a diet that was moderately restricted in carbohydrate (31% kcal protein, 37% kcal CHO and 32% kcal total fat). The latter diet significantly increased ($p < 0.05$) LDL peak particle diameter.

Three studies[197,249,250] have evaluated the effects of diets with a greater restriction in dietary carbohydrate (8 to 10% kcal CHO) on LDL particle size. All diets were high in protein (29–30% kcal) rather than fat. These studies reported a significant increase in peak LDL particle diameter in subjects on the low-carbohydrate diet. In the Sharman et al., 2004 study,[249] there were increases or no changes in LDL particle size for pattern A subjects, whereas there were pronounced increases in LDL particle size for pattern B subjects during the very-low-carbohydrate high-protein diet.

Other Dietary Interventions – Type of Fat, Dietary Fiber, and Multiple Dietary Strategies

In a cross-section study with 291 men conducted in Sweden, Sjogren et al.[223] reported that individual fatty acids (C4:0–C10:0 and C14:0) typically found in dairy products were associated with fewer small dense LDL particles when assessed over tertile of LDL particle size. Dreon et al.[224] reported a positive correlation between SFA content (specifically, C14:0 and C16:0) and LDL peak particle diameter in men following a high-fat, high-SFA diet (46% and 18% kcal, respectively) versus a low-fat diet (24% and 6% kcal, respectively); however, there was no association of MUFA or PUFA with LDL particle size. Kratz et al.[225] reported that unsaturated fat reduced LDL particle size relative to SFA. However, Rivellese et al.[78] reported neither MUFA or SFA affected LDL particle size. Increases in LDL particle size from baseline have been reported with supplementation with 4 g of highly purified fish oil[226] and with 0.95 g EPA + 0.68 g DHA,[227] whereas some studies reported no effect of n-3 fatty acids on LDL particle size.[228,229]

With respect to dietary fiber, Davey et al.[140] examined the effects of large servings (14 g/day of dietary fiber) of oat cereal or wheat cereal on LDL size. Subjects with pattern A phenotype ($n = 5$) had a significant reduction in LDL size (from 21.0 ± 0.2 to 20.8 ± 0.2 nm; $p = 0.05$) in the oat group as did subjects in the wheat group ($n = 8$) (from 21.1 ± 0.1 to 20.5 ± 0.3 nm; $p = 0.05$). However, when examining subjects with pattern B phenotype ($n = 12$), oat cereal produced significant decreases in small LDL-C concentrations (from 2.41 ± 0.39 to 1.92 ± 0.38 mmol/L; $p = 0.05$), while the wheat cereal produced significant increases in small LDL-C concentrations (from 0.13 ± 0.1 to 1.23 ± 0.5 mmol/L; $p = 0.05$) and in particle concentration (1385 ± 89 to 1746 ± 137 nmol/L; $p = 0.01$). The effects of soy protein and plant sterols/stanols on LDL particle size also have been examined. Desroches et al.[230] reported that consumption of soy protein was associated with a larger LDL particle size compared with animal protein. Unesterified plant sterols and stanols (both 1.8g/day) did not change LDL peak particle diameter or the small dense LDL levels.[231] Lamarche et al.[232] examined the effects of combining plant sterols (1 g/1000 kcal), soybean proteins (23 g/1000 kcal), viscous fiber (9 g/1000 kcal) and nuts (almond 15 g/1000 kcal) in a very low SFA diet on LDL particle size. This dietary pattern reduced serum concentration of all LDL fractions: large LDL-$C_{>26.0\ nm}$ (– 0.57 mmol/L, $p < 0.0001$), medium LDL-$C_{25.5–26.0\ nm}$ (– 0.23 mmol/L, $p < 0.0001$) and small LDL-$C_{<25.5\ nm}$ (– 0.45, $p < 0.01$).

HDL Particle Size

Based on the NCEP-ATP III Guidelines,[233] HDL-C levels are > 40 mg/dl for men and > 50 mg/dl for women. The anti-atherogenic property of HDL-C is due to its role in the reverse transport of cholesterol from arterial wall cells to the liver and steroidogenic organs.[234] While a majority of the HDL particles contain apolipoprotein A-1, there are distinct differences in the quantitative and qualitative content of the lipid fraction, apolipoproteins, enzymes, and lipid transfer proteins associated with different HDL subclasses. These HDL subclasses are characterized by the differences in their shape, density, size, charge and anti-atherogenicity,[235] and consequently differ widely in their functional properties. One of the most common classifications of HDL-C is based on differential precipitation, which classifies HDL particles based on their density, with HDL_2 representing a less dense particle and HDL_3 a more dense subclass of particles.[236] Other classifications, based on particle size, identify five subpopulations of HDL-C using gradient gel electrophoresis. These subpopulations include HDL_{2b}, HDL_{2a}, HDL_{3a}, HDL_{3b}, HDL_{3c}.[236]

Despite epidemiologic evidence from the Physicians' Health Study, which indicated that HDL_3 levels were the strongest predictor of a reduction in the risk of myocardial infarction,[237] the less dense larger HDL_2 particle is considered the most cardioprotective subpopulation, due to its effect on both reverse cholesterol transport and the reduction of serum TG levels.[238] In addition, small HDL particle size has been associated with the metabolic syndrome, including the high plasma TG levels, low HDL-C concentrations, visceral adiposity, and hyperinsulinemia.[239]

A strong body of evidence indicates that variations in total dietary fat intake affect HDL heterogeneity. In a study evaluating the effects of replacing dietary fat with carbohydrates, individuals consumed a low-fat diet (24% kcal) and a high-fat diet (46% kcal) in a randomized 2-period crossover design study.[240] Following the consumption of the low-fat diet individuals had significantly decreased levels of HDL_{3a}, HDL_{2a}, and HDL_{2b}. Levels of HDL_{2b} were reduced significantly more in those individuals who exhibited LDL subclass pattern A, compared with those who had pattern B phenotype. The results of this study therefore indicate that a low-fat diet elicits unfavorable changes in HDL subclasses, and that these adverse effects are more prominent in individuals with LDL subclass pattern A. Whereas these results are representative of drastic reductions in total fat levels, they are not reflective of smaller changes in total fat intake typical of average food consumption patterns.

The Dietary Effects on Lipoproteins and Thrombogenic Activity (DELTA) Study was a multicenter controlled feeding study that evaluated the effects of a stepwise reduction in total and saturated fat on lipids and lipoproteins in healthy individuals.[34] The three diets used were: (1) average American diet (AAD; 34.3% kcal total fat, 15.0% kcal SFA, 12.8% kcal MUFA, and 6.5% kcal PUFA), (2) a Step I diet (28.6% kcal total fat, 9.0% kcal SFA, 12.9% kcal MUFA, and 6.7% kcal PUFA), and (3) a low-fat diet (25.3% kcal total fat, 6.1% kcal SFA, 12.4% kcal MUFA, and 6.7% kcal PUFA). Following a reduction in total and saturated fat, HDL-C concentrations were decreased and TG levels were increased. Given this general effect on plasma lipids, further analyses were conducted to determine whether the stepwise reduction in total and saturated fat would influence primarily the larger cardioprotective HDL subpopulations.[241] As a result of the stepwise reduction in total and saturated fat, there were significant reductions ($p < 0.001$) in the larger, less dense HDL subpopulations (HDL_2 and HDL_{2b}).[241] Although HDL_3 concentrations followed a similar pattern in subjects on the three test diets, the reductions in HDL_2 (17.2%) were greater than the reductions in HDL_3 (5.7%). In addition, the concentrations of these larger HDL subpopulations were significantly correlated with serum TG levels during all of the test diets ($r = -0.45$; $p < 0.0001$ for low-fat diet), such that as HDL_2 concentrations decreased TG levels increased. These decreases in large HDL particles were accompanied by a reduction in LDL-C and apo B concentrations. This led the investigators to speculate that reductions in these larger HDL subpopulations may not be harmful if they are coupled with reductions in LDL-C.

One of the major strengths of the study conducted by Berglund et al.[241] was the use of two different and independent methods (stepwise precipitation procedure and lipid staining) to assess HDL subpopulation changes, which yielded similar results. In addition, because of the large and varied subject population (men and women, African Americans and non-African Americans, pre- and post-menopausal women, and younger and older men), findings from this study are applicable to the general population. Therefore, while the dietary changes employed in the present study may be prudent for a large segment of the population, they will primarily affect the most anti-atherogenic HDL subpopulations. These reductions in large HDL particles may not be as harmful if they are accompanied by a simultaneous decrease in the atherogenic LDL subpopulation. While it is important to examine the parallel reductions in LDL and HDL subpopulations, the increase observed in TG levels with a low-fat diet approach cannot be ignored.

While research has consistently shown a reduction in fasting TG levels with marine sources of n-3 fatty acids, their effects on different HDL subpopulations are inconsistent. In a study conducted by Subbaiah and colleagues,[242] 14 hypercholesterolemic individuals received a fish oil supplement containing 7.5 g n-3 fatty acids per day, in addition to a background Step I diet. Following 30 days of supplementation, plasma TG levels were significantly decreased by 58% ($p < 0.005$), when compared with baseline levels. In addition, there was a 41% increase in HDL_2 concentrations

($p < 0.005$), a 46% increase in the HDL_2/HDL_3 ratio ($p < 0.001$), and a 14% decrease in the LDL/HDL ratio ($p < 0.005$). These results indicate that supplementation with marine n-3 fatty acids may have a further impact on the reduction of CVD risk via an increase in the cardioprotective HDL-C subclasses.

An increasingly popular strategy for the treatment of low HDL-C levels is to increase physical activity. Thomas et al.[243] designed a study to examine the effects of combining exercise with n-3 fatty acid supplementation on lipoprotein subclasses and associated enzymes. Ten healthy, physically active men were given a supplementation of 4 g/day of EPA and DHA for 4 weeks. Following 4 weeks of supplementation, total HDL-C and HDL_2 concentrations were significantly higher ($p < 0.05$) and fasting TG levels were significantly decreased (26%; $p < 0.05$). Subjects also completed an acute exercise session before and after supplementation. As a result of an acute exercise session, total HDL-C, HDL_3-C, and LDL-C levels were increased. The combination treatment of n-3 fatty acid supplementation and exercise resulted in an additive effect on both HDL_3-C levels and LDL-C concentrations. The results, therefore, indicate that the combined treatment of marine-based n-3 fatty acids and physical activity has beneficial affects on fasting levels of the cardioprotective HDL_2 subpopulation. Further research is needed to determine the chronic impact of the observed increase in HDL_3-C levels and LDL-C following an acute bout of exercise on cardiovascular disease risk.

The results of the research to date indicate that low-fat diets appear to adversely affect cardioprotective subclasses of HDL-C, and elicit an increase in fasting TG levels. In addition, preliminary research suggests that supplementation of marine-based n-3 fatty acids may have a positive impact on these larger less dense HDL particles. Thus, a moderate-fat diet, rich in n-3 fatty acids is recommended for the treatment of low HDL-C levels. This dietary strategy also will be effective in reducing levels of elevated fasting TG levels in the presence of low HDL-C.

Postprandial TG

There is growing evidence that an elevated TG level is an independent risk factor for CVD. ATP III recommends treating an elevated TG level ($\geq$ 150 mg/dl).[233] In addition, the delayed clearance of postprandial lipemia is an independent risk factor for coronary heart disease.[244] Abnormal transport and metabolism of postprandial TG-rich lipoproteins are linked to atherosclerosis in the coronary and carotid arteries.[139] At a given amount of dietary fat, postprandial lipids are cleared more slowly in individuals who have a higher baseline TG level. A delayed clearance of these atherogenic TG-rich lipoproteins is thought to create a metabolic milieu that results in the promotion of atherogenesis. Thus, a dietary pattern that reduces fasting and postprandial plasma TG may decrease the accumulation of atherogenic, TG-rich lipoproteins resulting in decreased risk for atherosclerosis.

A number of studies have been conducted to assess postprandial TG clearance with respect to n-3 fatty acids. Most studies have been done with fish-derived n-3 fatty acids and have shown increased postprandial lipid clearance,[245] driven by the potent hypotriglyceridemic effect of n-3 fatty acids. A study conducted in physically active males illustrated that the supplementation of 4.0 g of n-3 fatty acids/day for 5 weeks decreased postprandial TG area under the curve (AUC) by 42%.[246] When a single bout of exercise (1-h treadmill run) was completed 12 h prior to the high-fat test challenge, the reduction in the postprandial TG AUC elicited by n-3 fatty acid supplementation was significantly enhanced (– 58%), beyond that of the effects seen with n-3 fatty acid supplementation alone.

A recent study[247] compared the effects of α-linolenic acid (ALA) and EPA + DHA on several cardiovascular disease risk factors, including postprandial blood lipid concentrations. The study was a placebo-controlled parallel arm design involving 150 moderately hypercholesterolemic individuals. Subjects were randomly assigned to receive one of five interventions: (1) 0.8 g EPA + DHA/day, (2) 1.7 g EPA + DHA/day, (3) 4.5 g ALA/day, (4) 9.5 g ALA/day, and (5) n-6 fatty acid control. A postprandial fat challenge was completed at baseline and following 6 months of treatment. While the decrease in fasting TG levels following the supplementation of 1.7 g/day EPA + DHA (– 7.7%) was significantly different ($p < 0.05$) from the supplementation of 9.5 g/day ALA (10.9%), there were no treatment differences on the postprandial response to a standard fat load. This lack of effect could possibly be explained by the restricted range of baseline TG levels for the study subjects and the fact that comparisons were made to a n-6 fatty acid control, rather than to a standardized SFA load.

A controlled feeding study was conducted in 26 healthy men to evaluate the effects of n-3 fatty acids, n-6 fatty acids, and saturated fatty acids on postprandial TG, hemostatic factors and blood lipids and lipoproteins.[248] For the first 3 weeks all subjects consumed a diet high in SFA (30% kcal total fat, 16% kcal SFA, 8% kcal MUFA, 4% kcal PUFA). Immediately following this diet period, subjects were randomized to either a high n-3 diet (approximately 5 g/day EPA and DHA) or a high n-6 diet (approximately 5 g/day linoleic acid) for 3 weeks in a crossover design, with an 8-week washout period between diets. Both diets contained 30% kcal total fat, 8% kcal SFA, 14% kcal MUFA, 6% kcal PUFA. At the end of each diet period, subjects participated in a postprandial fat challenge that reflected the diet period that they had just completed. Following these challenges, postprandial TG levels were greatest on the n-6, lowest on the n-3 diet ($p < 0.001$), and intermediary on the SFA diet. In addition, fasting TG levels were lowest following the n-3 diet. This study lends further support to the database that demonstrates a potent hypotriglyceridemic effect of n-3 fatty acids in both the fasting and postprandial state.

Very few studies have been conducted to evaluate the effects of different dietary patterns on postprandial TG response. In a recent study,[249] the effects of a hypoenergetic very-low-carbohydrate (< 10% kcal as carbohydrate) and a hypoenergetic low-fat diet (< 30% kcal as total fat) on fasting blood lipids and postprandial lipemia were studied in overweight men. Subjects consumed the two diets in a randomized, crossover design for two consecutive 6-week periods. An oral fat tolerance test (86% kcal total fat, 11% kcal carbohydrate, 3% kcal protein) was completed at baseline and at the conclusion of each of the test diet periods. Postprandial TG levels were significantly reduced following the consumption of both test diets, compared with baseline, with the greatest reduction following the very-low-carbohydrate diet (– 34%). These results indicate that short-term use of a hypocaloric very-low-carbohydrate diet has beneficial effects on postprandial TG levels. This effect likely is mediated by the reduction in fasting TG levels and a beneficial effect on other components of the metabolic syndrome, including small dense LDL-C particles, markers of insulin resistance and the TG:HDL-C ratio. In several other studies, similar postprandial TG-lowering was observed in normal weight, normolipidemic men (– 29%) following a ketogenic diet (61% kcal total fat, 8% kcal carbohydrate, 30% kcal protein),[197] and women (– 31%) following an isoenergetic very-low-carbohydrate diet (60% kcal total fat, 10% kcal carbohydrate, 30% kcal protein),[250] independent of weight loss.

In summary, supplementation with marine sources of n-3 fatty acids elicits a beneficial reduction on postprandial TG levels. This effect likely is mediated by the potent hypotriglyceridemic properties of marine n-3 fatty acids in the fasting state. In addition, the use of a very-low-carbohydrate diet may be an effective means for eliciting a reduction in postprandial TG levels, and may have additional beneficial effects on risk factors associated with the metabolic syndrome. In conclusion, the reduction observed in fasting and postprandial plasma TG decreases atherogenic, TG-rich lipoproteins, resulting in a decreased risk for atherosclerosis. Further research is warranted to develop dietary patterns that will lead to the optimization of both fasting and postprandial TG levels.

Lipoprotein (a)

Lipoprotein (a) [Lp(a)] is a LDL-modified particle found almost exclusively in primates. It is composed of an LDL moiety with the apolipoprotein B-100 attached to an apolipoprotein (a) (apo(a), a plasminogen-like protein) by a disulfide bridge.[251] Elevated Lp(a) has been identified as a powerful risk factor for the development of CHD.[252–254] The concentration of Lp(a) is largely controlled by the apo(a) gene, with Lp(a) levels being inversely associated with the size of apo(a).[255–257] Population studies have noted that African-Americans generally have higher levels of Lp(a) than other groups, including Caucasians and Asians;[258–260] however, the reasons for this remain unknown.

Although the level of Lp(a) is primarily genetically determined, several studies have observed changes in Lp(a) with dietary manipulation. SFA appear superior to other fatty acids in decreasing Lp(a) concentrations. A study (n = 58) that investigated the effects of *trans* fatty acid consumption in amounts typical of Western diets found that a diet high in SFA (16.2% kcal) significantly reduced Lp(a) levels by 8–11% compared with diets high in oleic acid (16.7% kcal), moderate in *trans* fatty acids (3.8% to kcal), and high in *trans* fat (6.6% total calories).[261] Likewise, Nestel et al.[42] reported that 3 weeks of consumption of *trans* fatty acids at 7% of calories produced a 19% reduction in Lp(a) when palmitic acid replaced elaidic acid (18:1 *trans*). These findings are consistent with previous reports which have shown that the saturated fatty acids, lauric, myristic, and palmitic acids, resulted in lower levels of Lp(a) than oleic acid,[262] and that substitution of butter for either partially hydrogenated safflower or partially hydrogenated fish oil resulted in lower Lp(a) concentrations.[263] The DELTA study (n = 103) observed a stepwise increase in Lp(a) concentrations (15.5, 17.0, and 18.2 mg/dl, $p < 0.01$) as dietary SFA was reduced from 15% to 9.0% to 6.1%, respectively.[34] As the amount of SFA decreased in the diets, the amount of stearic acid increased, which has been shown to increase Lp(a).[264,265] However, when compared with a diet rich in stearic acid (9.3% kcal), a diet high in *trans* fat (8.7% kcal) increases Lp(a) significantly more (10% vs. 30%, respectively).[43] A study in healthy young women (n = 25) examined the effect of a high SFA diet (38.2% kcal total fat, 22.7% kcal SFA) on Lp(a) in direct comparison with a low SFA diet (19.7% kcal total fat, 10.5% kcal SFA) with no change in the PUFA to SFA ratio (0.14 and 0.17, respectively).[266] Compared with a diet high in MUFA and PUFA (38.2% kcal total fat, 2.4% kcal SFA, PUFA:SFA = 1.9) both the higher SFA diets decreased Lp(a), with the highest level of SFA reducing it the most (13.3%, $p < 0.001$). Furthermore, the concentrations of total and LDL-C were similar between the two higher SFA diets.[267] A 3-month intervention in obese African Americans (n = 105) that included both diet (total fat kcal 25.3%, SFA kcal 7.1%) and exercise components (45–60 min of treadmill exercise three times per week) increased Lp(a) levels 35%, while improving other factors (decreasing total and LDL-C, TG, and BMI, and increasing HDL-C).[268]

The use of n-3 PUFA to modify Lp(a) levels has received less attention. In hypertriglyceridemic patients, fish oil has been shown to reduce Lp(a) concentrations.[269] The combination of a high dose (12 g/day) of fish oil (8.5 g of omega-3 fatty acids) and a low-fat (30% kcal total fat) low-calorie diet resulted in a 14% reduction in plasma Lp(a) levels in one study.[270] However, several studies could find no Lp(a)-lowering effect of n-3 fatty acids.[248,271] Dietary soy protein has also been shown to modestly increase Lp(a) compared with casein;[272] however, this effect is eliminated after alcohol extraction of soy protein.[273] In addition, diets high in fruits and vegetables do not appear to attenuate the rise in Lp(a) associated with low-SFA diets.[274]

New evidence also suggests that Lp(a) is differentially affected by specific individual dietary fatty acids in the postprandial state.[275] After 16 young normolipidemic men consumed a meal rich in *trans* fat, Lp(a) levels did not significantly change over 8 h. However, test meals with stearic acid produced significantly higher Lp(a) levels at 4 h postprandially, followed by palmitic, oleic, or linoleic acid. Acute changes in Lp(a) following a fat load have not been consistently shown, however.[276,277]

Science-Based Dietary Guidelines for Health

Several agencies and organizations such as the National Academies,[22] the National Institutes of Health/National Heart, Lung and Blood Institute,[6] the U.S. Departments of Agriculture/Health and Human Services,[278,279] the American Heart Association,[175,280] and the American Diabetes Association,[281] have reviewed the scientific literature and developed recommendations for the prevention and treatment of coronary disease. Overall, the recommendations made for macronutrients, micronutrients, and other dietary constituents by these groups are comparable (Table 11.5). The recommendations for dietary fat intake (ranging between 20% and 35% of calories) and protein intake (between 10% and 35% of calories) are similar among agencies. Likewise, total carbohydrate intake comprises the remainder of the macronutrient component of the diet. Specific recommendations highlight decreasing SFA and *trans* fat intake and to consume adequate amounts of unsaturated fatty acids, including linoleic acid and α-linolenic acid. Importantly, all recommendations advise achieving and maintaining a healthy weight and participating in regular physical activity.

Summary

The evolution of our understanding of the role that diet plays in modifying lipid and lipoprotein risk factors for CVD is impressive. For many years, the research focus was on studying how diet affected established risk factors. It is clear that saturated and unsaturated fatty acids, as well as dietary cholesterol, affect the traditional lipid and lipoprotein CVD risk factors. More recent research has resulted in a growing recognition that diet affects new lipid and lipoprotein risk factors for CVD such as LDL and HDL size, lipoprotein (a), and postprandial lipids and lipoproteins. In addition, contemporary research has identified some dietary factors and strategies that affect both established and emerging risk factors. These include *trans* fatty acids, soluble fiber, n-3 fatty acids, glycemic load, and the total diet approach, which incorporates nutrient-based and food-based dietary interventions. Interventions that target multiple dietary strategies are expected to have the greatest impact on reducing total CVD risk. Because LDL-C remains the dominant lipid risk factor for CVD interventions, a primary goal is to integrate multiple dietary strategies that maximally lower LDL-C (Table 11.6).

TABLE 11.5

Current Recommendations and Guidelines for Macronutrients[a]

	NAS DRIs[22]	American Diabetes Association[281]	NHLBI NCEP-ATP III[6]	USDA Dietary Guidelines 2005[278]	AHA Dietary Guidelines[175,280]
Total fat	20–35%	< 30%	25–35%	Choose fats wisely for good health, 20–35%	< 30%
SFA	Low as possible	< 10% < 7%[b]	< 7%	< 10% < 7%[b]	< 10% < 7%[b]
MUFA	Remaining fatty acids to achieve total fat	–	Up to 20%	Remaining fatty acids to achieve total fat	Unsaturated for SFA
PUFA	5–10%	~ 10%	Up to 10%	5–10%	Unsaturated for SFA
Linoleic acid (n-6 PUFA)	5–10%	–	–	5–10%	–
Linolenic acid	0.6–1.2%	2 to 3 servings of fish/week	–	0.6–1.2%	2 servings of fatty fish/week
1 g/day EPA & DHA for coronary patients					
EPA & DHA (n-3 PUFA)	Up to 10% can be consumed as EPA + DHA				
Trans fat	Low as possible	Minimize intake	Keep intake low	Low as possible	*Trans* fat + SFA < 10%
Cholesterol (mg/day)	Low as possible	< 300 < 200[b]	< 200	< 300 < 200[b]	< 300
Carbohydrate	45–65%	60–70% from carbohydrates plus MUFA	50–60%	Choose carbohydrates wisely for good health, 45–65%	≥ 6 servings, include 3 servings whole grains
Protein	10–35%	≤ 20%	15%	10–35%, 2–3 servings	50–100 g/day
Fiber (g/day)	21–38	–	20–30	≥ 3 servings/day of whole grains	> 25

NAS DRIs, National Academy of Science Dietary Reference Intakes; NHLBI NCEP-ATP III, National Heart Lung and Blood Institute, National Cholesterol Education Program-Adult Treatment Panel III; USDA, United States Department of Agriculture; AHA, American Heart Association; SFA, saturated fat; MUFA, monounsaturated fat; PUFA, polyunsaturated fat; EPA, Eicosapentanoic acid; DHA, Docosahexanoic acid.

[a] Values are expressed as % of calories unless indicated otherwise.

[b] For individuals at high risk.

TABLE 11.6

Components of the Optimal Diet for LDL Cholesterol Reduction

Dietary Component	Reduction in LDL-C
Reduced saturated and *trans* fat (< 7% calories)	8–10%
Reduced dietary cholesterol (< 200 mg/day)	3–5%
Viscous fiber (5–10 g/day)	3–5%
Plant sterol/stanol esters (2 g/day)	6–15%
Soy protein (25 g/day)	5%
Weight reduction (– 10 lb)	5–8%
Cumulative Estimate	30–48%

Source: Adapted from: National Cholesterol Education Program. NIH Publication No. 02-5215, 1993; Jenkins, D.J. et al., *Curr Opin Lipidol*, 11, 49, 2000.

Based on an extensive database as discussed herein, the "optimal diet" will provide a cornucopia of foods and nutrients that represent dietary patterns that target multiple CVD risk factors.[282,283] Overall, a diet that is very low in saturated and *trans* fatty acids and cholesterol, rich in vitamins and minerals, controlled in calories, high in dietary fiber, moderate in unsaturated fats including n-3 fatty acids, and low in simple carbohydrates will improve the lipid and lipoprotein profile the most. As our knowledge base increases, it is likely that we will continue to evolve science-based dietary recommendations that will target a growing number of risk factors. With this, implementation of multiple dietary strategies will elicit unprecedented reductions in CVD risk as the result of targeting a growing number of lipid and lipoprotein risk factors for CVD. The consequence of this will be to accelerate the decline of CVD as an important cause of mortality and morbidity in the population.

References

1. Macheboeufm, M., Recherches sur les phosphoaminolipides et les sterids du serum et du plasma sanguins. II. Etude physiochimique de la fraction proteidique la plus riche en phospholipids et in sterides, *Bull Soc Chim Biol*, 11, 485, 1929.
2. Olson, R.E., Discovery of the lipoproteins, their role in fat transport and their significance as risk factors, *J Nutr*, 128, 439S, 1998.
3. Gofman, J.W., Lindgren, F.T., Elliot, H., Ultracentrifugal studies of lipoproteins of human serum, *J Biol Chem*, 179, 973, 1949.
4. Fredrickson, D.S., Levy, R.I., and Lees, R.S., Fat transport in lipoproteins–an integrated approach to mechanisms and disorders, *N Engl J Med*, 276, 34, 1967.
5. Alaupovic, P., The concept of apolipoprotein-defined lipoprotein families and its clinical significance, *Curr Atheroscler Rep*, 5, 459, 2003.

6. National Cholesterol Education Program, Detection, Evaluation, and Treatment of High Blood Cholesterol in Adults (Adult Treatment Panel III): Final report. Bethesda, MD: National Institutes of Health, National Heart, Lung and Blood Institute, 1993. NIH Publication No. 02-5215.
7. Ginsberg, H.N. et al., Reduction of plasma cholesterol levels in normal men on an American Heart Association step 1 diet or a step 1 diet with added monounsaturated fat, *N Engl J Med,* 322, 574, 1990.
8. Berry, E.M. et al., Effects of diets rich in monounsaturated fatty acids on plasma lipoproteins–the Jerusalem Nutrition Study. II. Monounsaturated fatty acids vs carbohydrates, *Am J Clin Nutr,* 56, 394, 1992.
9. Baggio, G. et al., Olive-oil-enriched diet: effect on serum lipoprotein levels and biliary cholesterol saturation, *Am J Clin Nutr,* 47, 960, 1988.
10. Grundy, S.M. et al., Comparison of monounsaturated fatty acids and carbohydrates for reducing raised levels of plasma cholesterol in man, *Am J Clin Nutr,* 47, 965, 1988.
11. Colquhoun, D.M. et al., Comparison of the effects on lipoproteins and apolipoproteins of a diet high in monounsaturated fatty acids, enriched with avocado, and a high-carbohydrate diet, *Am J Clin Nutr,* 56, 671, 1992.
12. Mensink, R.P. et al., Effects of monounsaturated fatty acids v. complex carbohydrates on serum lipoproteins and apoproteins in healthy men and women, *Metabolism,* 38, 172, 1989.
13. Mensink, R.P. and Katan, M.B., Effect of monounsaturated fatty acids versus complex carbohydrates on high-density lipoproteins in healthy men and women, *Lancet,* 1, 122, 1987.
14. Grundy, S.M., Comparison of monounsaturated fatty acids and carbohydrates for lowering plasma cholesterol, *N Engl J Med,* 314, 745, 1986.
15. Kris-Etherton, P.M. et al., High-monounsaturated fatty acid diets lower both plasma cholesterol and triacylglycerol concentrations, *Am J Clin Nutr,* 70, 1009, 1999.
16. Lefevre, M. et al., Is carbohydrate or monounsaturated fatty acids the preferred replacement for saturated fatty acids to reduce CAD risk in subjects with low HDL, high triglycerides and/or high insulin?, *Am J Clin Nutr,* submitted.
17. Lerman-Garber, I. et al., Effect of a high-monounsaturated fat diet enriched with avocado in NIDDM patients, *Diabetes Care,* 17, 311, 1994.
18. Lopez-Segura, F. et al., Monounsaturated fatty acid-enriched diet decreases plasma plasminogen activator inhibitor type 1, *Arterioscler Thromb Vasc Biol,* 16, 82, 1996.
19. Jansen, S. et al., Plasma lipid response to hypolipidemic diets in young healthy non-obese men varies with body mass index, *J Nutr,* 128, 1144, 1998.
20. Sacks, F.M. and Katan, M., Randomized clinical trials on the effects of dietary fat and carbohydrate on plasma lipoproteins and cardiovascular disease, *Am J Med,* 113 Suppl 9B, 13S, 2002.
21. Mensink, R.P. and Katan, M.B., Effect of dietary fatty acids on serum lipids and lipoproteins. A meta-analysis of 27 trials, *Arterioscler Thromb,* 12, 911, 1992.
22. National Academy of Sciences and the Institutes of Medicine. Dietary Reference Intakes: Energy, Carbohydrate, Fiber, Fat, Fatty Acids, Cholesterol, Protein, and Amino Acids, Washington, DC, 2002.
23. Austin, M.A. et al., Atherogenic lipoprotein phenotype. A proposed genetic marker for coronary heart disease risk, *Circulation,* 82, 495, 1990.
24. Keys, A., Coronary heart disease in seven countries, *Circulation,* 41, I1, 1970.

25. Posner, B.M. et al., Dietary lipid predictors of coronary heart disease in men. The Framingham Study, *Arch Intern Med,* 151, 1181, 1991.
26. Hu, F.B. et al., Dietary fat intake and the risk of coronary heart disease in women, *N Engl J Med,* 337, 1491, 1997.
27. Kromhout, D. et al., Dietary saturated and trans fatty acids and cholesterol and 25-year mortality from coronary heart disease: the Seven Countries Study, *Prev Med,* 24, 308, 1995.
28. Keys, A., Anderson, J.T., Grande, F., Serum cholesterol response to changes in the diet. IV. Particular saturated fatty acids in the diet, *Metabolism,* 14, 776, 1965.
29. Hegsted, D.M. et al., Quantitative effects of dietary fat on serum cholesterol in man, *Am J Clin Nutr,* 17, 281, 1965.
30. Mattson, F.H. and Grundy, S.M., Comparison of effects of dietary saturated, monounsaturated, and polyunsaturated fatty acids on plasma lipids and lipoproteins in man, *J Lipid Res,* 26, 194, 1985.
31. Grundy, S.M. and Vega, G.L., Plasma cholesterol responsiveness to saturated fatty acids, *Am J Clin Nutr,* 47, 822, 1988.
32. Clarke, R. et al., Dietary lipids and blood cholesterol: quantitative meta-analysis of metabolic ward studies, *BMJ,* 314, 112, 1997.
33. Hegsted, D.M. et al., Dietary fat and serum lipids: an evaluation of the experimental data, *Am J Clin Nutr,* 57, 875, 1993.
34. Ginsberg, H.N. et al., Effects of reducing dietary saturated fatty acids on plasma lipids and lipoproteins in healthy subjects: the DELTA Study, protocol 1, *Arterioscler Thromb Vasc Biol,* 18, 441, 1998.
35. Yu, S. et al., Plasma cholesterol-predictive equations demonstrate that stearic acid is neutral and monounsaturated fatty acids are hypocholesterolemic, *Am J Clin Nutr,* 61, 1129, 1995.
36. Muller, H., Kirkhus, B., and Pedersen, J.I., Serum cholesterol predictive equations with special emphasis on trans and saturated fatty acids. An analysis from designed controlled studies, *Lipids,* 36, 783, 2001.
37. Mensink, R.P. et al., Effects of dietary fatty acids and carbohydrates on the ratio of serum total to HDL cholesterol and on serum lipids and apolipoproteins: a meta-analysis of 60 controlled trials, *Am J Clin Nutr,* 77, 1146, 2003.
38. Oomen, C.M. et al., Association between trans fatty acid intake and 10-year risk of coronary heart disease in the Zutphen Elderly Study: a prospective population-based study, *Lancet,* 357, 746, 2001.
39. Willett, W.C. et al., Intake of trans fatty acids and risk of coronary heart disease among women, *Lancet,* 341, 581, 1993.
40. Hu, F.B., Manson, J.E., and Willett, W.C., Types of dietary fat and risk of coronary heart disease: a critical review, *J Am Coll Nutr,* 20, 5, 2001.
41. Mauger, J.F. et al., Effect of different forms of dietary hydrogenated fats on LDL particle size, *Am J Clin Nutr,* 78, 370, 2003.
42. Nestel, P. et al., Plasma lipoprotein lipid and Lp[a] changes with substitution of elaidic acid for oleic acid in the diet, *J Lipid Res,* 33, 1029, 1992.
43. Aro, A. et al., Stearic acid, trans fatty acids, and dairy fat: effects on serum and lipoprotein lipids, apolipoproteins, lipoprotein(a), and lipid transfer proteins in healthy subjects, *Am J Clin Nutr,* 65, 1419, 1997.
44. Sundram, K. et al., Trans (elaidic) fatty acids adversely affect the lipoprotein profile relative to specific saturated fatty acids in humans, *J Nutr,* 127, 514S, 1997.

45. Judd, J.T. et al., Dietary cis and trans monounsaturated and saturated FA and plasma lipids and lipoproteins in men, *Lipids,* 37, 123, 2002.
46. Ascherio, A. and Willett, W.C., Health effects of trans fatty acids, *Am J Clin Nutr,* 66, 1006S, 1997.
47. Mensink, R.P. and Katan, M.B., Effect of dietary trans fatty acids on high-density and low-density lipoprotein cholesterol levels in healthy subjects, *N Engl J Med,* 323, 439, 1990.
48. de Roos, N., Schouten, E., and Katan, M., Consumption of a solid fat rich in lauric acid results in a more favorable serum lipid profile in healthy men and women than consumption of a solid fat rich in trans-fatty acids, *J Nutr,* 131, 242, 2001.
49. Dyerberg, J. et al., Effects of trans- and n-3 unsaturated fatty acids on cardiovascular risk markers in healthy males. An 8 week dietary intervention study, *Eur J Clin Nutr,* 58, 1062, 2004.
50. Lichtenstein, A.H. et al., Effects of different forms of dietary hydrogenated fats on serum lipoprotein cholesterol levels, *N Engl J Med,* 340, 1933, 1999.
51. Gillman, M.W. et al., Inverse association of dietary fat with development of ischemic stroke in men, *JAMA,* 278, 2145, 1997.
52. Artaud-Wild, S.M. et al., Differences in coronary mortality can be explained by differences in cholesterol and saturated fat intakes in 40 countries but not in France and Finland. A paradox, *Circulation,* 88, 2771, 1993.
53. Kris-Etherton, P.M. and Yu, S., Individual fatty acid effects on plasma lipids and lipoproteins: human studies, *Am J Clin Nutr,* 65, 1628S, 1997.
54. Kris-Etherton, P., Effects of replacing saturated fat (SFA) with monounsaturated fat (MUFA) or carbohydrates (CHO) on plasma lipids and lipoproteins in individuals with markers for insulin resistance, *FASEB J,* 10, 1996.
55. Garg, A., High-monounsaturated-fat diets for patients with diabetes mellitus: a meta-analysis, *Am J Clin Nutr,* 67, 577S, 1998.
56. Caggiula, A.W. and Mustad, V.A., Effects of dietary fat and fatty acids on coronary artery disease risk and total and lipoprotein cholesterol concentrations: epidemiologic studies, *Am J Clin Nutr,* 65, 1597S, 1997.
57. Riemersma, R.A., Wood, D.A., Butler, S., Elton, R.A., et al., Linoleic acid content in adipose tissue and coronary heart disease, *Br Med J (Clin Res Ed),* 292, 1423, 1986.
58. Kark, J.D. et al., Adipose tissue n-6 fatty acids and acute myocardial infarction in a population consuming a diet high in polyunsaturated fatty acids, *Am J Clin Nutr,* 77, 796, 2003.
59. Dayton, S. et al., Controlled trial of a diet high in unsaturated fat for prevention of atherosclerotic complications, *Lancet,* 2, 1060, 1968.
60. Leren, P., The Oslo diet-heart study. Eleven-year report, *Circulation,* 42, 935, 1970.
61. Turpeinen, O. et al., Dietary prevention of coronary heart disease: the Finnish Mental Hospital Study, *Int J Epidemiol,* 8, 99, 1979.
62. Frantz, I.D., Jr. et al., Test of effect of lipid lowering by diet on cardiovascular risk. The Minnesota Coronary Survey, *Arteriosclerosis,* 9, 129, 1989.
63. Gardner, C.D. and Kraemer, H.C., Monounsaturated versus polyunsaturated dietary fat and serum lipids. A meta-analysis, *Arterioscler Thromb Vasc Biol,* 15, 1917, 1995.
64. Harris, W.S., N-3 fatty acids and serum lipoproteins: human studies, *Am J Clin Nutr,* 65, 1645S, 1997.

65. Kromhout, D., Bosschieter, E.B., and de Lezenne Coulander, C., The inverse relation between fish consumption and 20-year mortality from coronary heart disease, *N Engl J Med*, 312, 1205, 1985.
66. Ascherio, A. et al., Dietary fat and risk of coronary heart disease in men: cohort follow up study in the United States, *BMJ*, 313, 84, 1996.
67. G.-P. Investigators, Dietary supplementation with n-3 polyunsaturated fatty acids and vitamin E after myocardial infarction: results of the GISSI-Prevenzione trial. Gruppo Italiano per lo Studio della Sopravvivenza nell'Infarto miocardico, *Lancet*, 354, 447, 1999.
68. Calder, P.C., N-3 Fatty acids and cardiovascular disease: evidence explained and mechanisms explored, *Clin Sci (Lond)*, 107, 1, 2004.
69. Harris, W.S., Fish oils and plasma lipid and lipoprotein metabolism in humans: a critical review, *J Lipid Res*, 30, 785, 1989.
70. Roche, H.M. and Gibney, M.J., Postprandial triacylglycerolaemia: the effect of low-fat dietary treatment with and without fish oil supplementation, *Eur J Clin Nutr*, 50, 617, 1996.
71. Svensson, M. et al., The effect of n-3 fatty acids on plasma lipids and lipoproteins and blood pressure in patients with CRF, *Am J Kidney Dis*, 44, 77, 2004.
72. Thomas, T.R. et al., Effects of omega-3 fatty acid supplementation and exercise on low-density lipoprotein and high-density lipoprotein subfractions, *Metabolism*, 53, 749, 2004.
73. Sucic, M., Katica, D., and Kovacevic, V., Effect of dietary fish supplementation on lipoprotein levels in patients with hyperlipoproteinemia, *Coll Antropol*, 22, 77, 1998.
74. Sirtori, C.R. et al., One-year treatment with ethyl esters of n-3 fatty acids in patients with hypertriglyceridemia and glucose intolerance: reduced triglyceridemia, total cholesterol and increased HDL-C without glycemic alterations, *Atherosclerosis*, 137, 419, 1998.
75. Davidson, M.H. et al., Effects of docosahexaenoic acid on serum lipoproteins in patients with combined hyperlipidemia: a randomized, double-blind, placebo-controlled trial, *J Am Coll Nutr*, 16, 236, 1997.
76. Kestin, M. et al., N-3 fatty acids of marine origin lower systolic blood pressure and triglycerides but raise LDL cholesterol compared with n-3 and n-6 fatty acids from plants, *Am J Clin Nutr*, 51, 1028, 1990.
77. Sanchez-Muniz, F.J. et al., Small supplements of N-3 fatty acids change serum low density lipoprotein composition by decreasing phospholipid and apolipoprotein B concentrations in young adult women, *Eur J Nutr*, 38, 20, 1999.
78. Rivellese, A.A. et al., Effects of dietary saturated, monounsaturated and n-3 fatty acids on fasting lipoproteins, LDL size and post-prandial lipid metabolism in healthy subjects, *Atherosclerosis*, 167, 149, 2003.
79. Theobald, H.E. et al., LDL cholesterol-raising effect of low-dose docosahexaenoic acid in middle-aged men and women, *Am J Clin Nutr*, 79, 558, 2004.
80. McGee, D.L. et al., Ten-year incidence of coronary heart disease in the Honolulu Heart Program. Relationship to nutrient intake, *Am J Epidemiol*, 119, 667, 1984.
81. Shekelle, R.B. et al., Diet, serum cholesterol, and death from coronary heart disease. The Western Electric study, *N Engl J Med*, 304, 65, 1981.
82. Pietinen, P. et al., Intake of fatty acids and risk of coronary heart disease in a cohort of Finnish men. The Alpha-Tocopherol, Beta-Carotene Cancer Prevention Study, *Am J Epidemiol*, 145, 876, 1997.

83. Ginsberg, H.N. et al., Increases in dietary cholesterol are associated with modest increases in both LDL and HDL cholesterol in healthy young women, *Arterioscler Thromb Vasc Biol,* 15, 169, 1995.
84. Ballesteros, M.N. et al., Dietary cholesterol does not increase biomarkers for chronic disease in a pediatric population from northern Mexico, *Am J Clin Nutr,* 80, 855, 2004.
85. Herron, K.L. et al., Pre-menopausal women, classified as hypo- or hyperresponders, do not alter their LDL/HDL ratio following a high dietary cholesterol challenge, *J Am Coll Nutr,* 21, 250, 2002.
86. Herron, K.L. et al., Men classified as hypo- or hyperresponders to dietary cholesterol feeding exhibit differences in lipoprotein metabolism, *J Nutr,* 133, 1036, 2003.
87. Rimm, E.B. et al., Vegetable, fruit, and cereal fiber intake and risk of coronary heart disease among men, *JAMA,* 275, 447, 1996.
88. Wolk, A. et al., Long-term intake of dietary fiber and decreased risk of coronary heart disease among women, *JAMA,* 281, 1998, 1999.
89. Pietinen, P. et al., Intake of dietary fiber and risk of coronary heart disease in a cohort of Finnish men. The Alpha-Tocopherol, Beta-Carotene Cancer Prevention Study, *Circulation,* 94, 2720, 1996.
90. Pereira, M.A. et al., Dietary fiber and risk of coronary heart disease: a pooled analysis of cohort studies, *Arch Intern Med,* 164, 370, 2004.
91. Bazzano, L.A. et al., Dietary fiber intake and reduced risk of coronary heart disease in US men and women: the National Health and Nutrition Examination Survey I. Epidemiologic Follow-up Study, *Arch Intern Med,* 163, 1897, 2003.
92. Liu, S. et al., A prospective study of dietary fiber intake and risk of cardiovascular disease among women, *J Am Coll Cardiol,* 39, 49, 2002.
93. Jacobs, D.R., Jr. et al., Is whole grain intake associated with reduced total and cause-specific death rates in older women? The Iowa Women's Health Study, *Am J Public Health,* 89, 322, 1999.
94. Liu, S. et al., Whole-grain consumption and risk of coronary heart disease: results from the Nurses' Health Study, *Am J Clin Nutr,* 70, 412, 1999.
95. Jacobs, D.R. et al., Fiber from whole grains, but not refined grains, is inversely associated with all-cause mortality in older women: the Iowa Women's Health Study, *J Am Coll Nutr,* 19, 326S, 2000.
96. Mozaffarian, D. et al., Cereal, fruit, and vegetable fiber intake and the risk of cardiovascular disease in elderly individuals, *JAMA,* 289, 1659, 2003.
97. Anderson, J.W. et al., Whole grain foods and heart disease risk, *J Am Coll Nutr,* 19, 291S, 2000.
98. Jacobs, D.R., Jr. et al., Whole-grain intake may reduce the risk of ischemic heart disease death in postmenopausal women: the Iowa Women's Health Study, *Am J Clin Nutr,* 68, 248, 1998.
99. Fraser, G.E. et al., A possible protective effect of nut consumption on risk of coronary heart disease. The Adventist Health Study, *Arch Intern Med,* 152, 1416, 1992.
100. Fraser, G.E., Associations between diet and cancer, ischemic heart disease, and all-cause mortality in non-Hispanic white California Seventh-Day Adventists, *Am J Clin Nutr,* 70, 532S, 1999.
101. Liu, S. et al., Is intake of breakfast cereals related to total and cause-specific mortality in men?, *Am J Clin Nutr,* 77, 594, 2003.

102. Liu, S. et al., Whole grain consumption and risk of ischemic stroke in women: a prospective study, *JAMA*, 284, 1534, 2000.
103. Ascherio, A. et al., A prospective study of nutritional factors and hypertension among US men, *Circulation*, 86, 1475, 1992.
104. Montonen, J. et al., Whole-grain and fiber intake and the incidence of type 2 diabetes, *Am J Clin Nutr*, 77, 622, 2003.
105. He, J. et al., Oats and buckwheat intakes and cardiovascular disease risk factors in an ethnic minority of China, *Am J Clin Nutr*, 61, 366, 1995.
106. Fung, T.T. et al., Association between dietary patterns and plasma biomarkers of obesity and cardiovascular disease risk, *Am J Clin Nutr*, 73, 61, 2001.
107. McKeown, N.M. et al., Whole-grain intake is favorably associated with metabolic risk factors for type 2 diabetes and cardiovascular disease in the Framingham Offspring Study, *Am J Clin Nutr*, 76, 390, 2002.
108. Fung, T.T. et al., Whole-grain intake and the risk of type 2 diabetes: a prospective study in men, *Am J Clin Nutr*, 76, 535, 2002.
109. Jenkins, D.J. et al., Soluble fiber intake at a dose approved by the US Food and Drug Administration for a claim of health benefits: serum lipid risk factors for cardiovascular disease assessed in a randomized controlled crossover trial, *Am J Clin Nutr*, 75, 834, 2002.
110. Onning, G. et al., Consumption of oat milk for 5 weeks lowers serum cholesterol and LDL cholesterol in free-living men with moderate hypercholesterolemia, *Ann Nutr Metab*, 43, 301, 1999.
111. Dubois, C. et al., Chronic oat bran intake alters postprandial lipemia and lipoproteins in healthy adults, *Am J Clin Nutr*, 61, 325, 1995.
112. Lupton, J.R., Robinson, M.C., and Morin, J.L., Cholesterol-lowering effect of barley bran flour and oil, *J Am Diet Assoc*, 94, 65, 1994.
113. Kestin, M. et al., Comparative effects of three cereal brans on plasma lipids, blood pressure, and glucose metabolism in mildly hypercholesterolemic men, *Am J Clin Nutr*, 52, 661, 1990.
114. Anderson, J.W. et al., Lipid responses of hypercholesterolemic men to oat-bran and wheat-bran intake, *Am J Clin Nutr*, 54, 678, 1991.
115. Zhang, J.X. et al., Effect of oat bran on plasma cholesterol and bile acid excretion in nine subjects with ileostomies, *Am J Clin Nutr*, 56, 99, 1992.
116. Glore, S.R. et al., Soluble fiber and serum lipids: a literature review, *J Am Diet Assoc*, 94, 425, 1994.
117. Tillotson, J.L. et al., Relation of dietary fiber to blood lipids in the special intervention and usual care groups in the Multiple Risk Factor Intervention Trial, *Am J Clin Nutr*, 65, 327S, 1997.
118. Slavin, J.L. et al., Plausible mechanisms for the protectiveness of whole grains, *Am J Clin Nutr*, 70, 459S, 1999.
119. Anderson, J.W. et al., Cholesterol-lowering effects of psyllium intake adjunctive to diet therapy in men and women with hypercholesterolemia: meta-analysis of 8 controlled trials, *Am J Clin Nutr*, 71, 472, 2000.
120. Brown, L. et al., Cholesterol-lowering effects of dietary fiber: a meta-analysis, *Am J Clin Nutr*, 69, 30, 1999.
121. Ripsin, C.M. et al., Oat products and lipid lowering. A meta-analysis, *JAMA*, 267, 3317, 1992.
122. Aller, R. et al., Effect of soluble fiber intake in lipid and glucose levels in healthy subjects: a randomized clinical trial, *Diabetes Res Clin Pract*, 65, 7, 2004.

123. Behall, K.M., Scholfield, D.J., and Hallfrisch, J., Diets containing barley significantly reduce lipids in mildly hypercholesterolemic men and women, *Am J Clin Nutr,* 80, 1185, 2004.
124. Behall, K.M., Scholfield, D.J., and Hallfrisch, J., Lipids significantly reduced by diets containing barley in moderately hypercholesterolemic men, *J Am Coll Nutr,* 23, 55, 2004.
125. Li, J. et al., Effects of barley intake on glucose tolerance, lipid metabolism, and bowel function in women, *Nutrition,* 19, 926, 2003.
126. Keogh, G.F. et al., Randomized controlled crossover study of the effect of a highly beta-glucan-enriched barley on cardiovascular disease risk factors in mildly hypercholesterolemic men, *Am J Clin Nutr,* 78, 711, 2003.
127. Program, L.R.C., The Lipid Research Clinics Coronary Primary Prevention Trial results I: reduction in incidence of coronary heart disease., *JAMA,* 251, 365, 1984.
128. Anderson, J.W., Dietary fiber prevents carbohydrate-induced hypertriglyceridemia, *Curr Atheroscler Rep,* 2, 536, 2000.
129. Parks, E.J. and Hellerstein, M.K., Carbohydrate-induced hypertriacylglycerolemia: historical perspective and review of biological mechanisms, *Am J Clin Nutr,* 71, 412, 2000.
130. Parks, E.J. et al., Effects of a low-fat, high-carbohydrate diet on VLDL-triglyceride assembly, production, and clearance, *J Clin Invest,* 104, 1087, 1999.
131. Mittendorfer, B. and Sidossis, L.S., Mechanism for the increase in plasma triacylglycerol concentrations after consumption of short-term, high-carbohydrate diets, *Am J Clin Nutr,* 73, 892, 2001.
132. Hudgins, L.C., Effect of high-carbohydrate feeding on triglyceride and saturated fatty acid synthesis, *Proc Soc Exp Biol Med,* 225, 178, 2000.
133. Cullen, P., Evidence that triglycerides are an independent coronary heart disease risk factor, *Am J Cardiol,* 86, 943, 2000.
134. Hokanson, J.E. and Austin, M.A., Plasma triglyceride level is a risk factor for cardiovascular disease independent of high-density lipoprotein cholesterol level: a meta-analysis of population-based prospective studies, *J Cardiovasc Risk,* 3, 213, 1996.
135. Austin, M.A., Epidemiology of hypertriglyceridemia and cardiovascular disease, *Am J Cardiol,* 83, 13F, 1999.
136. Obarzanek, E. et al., Effects on blood lipids of a blood pressure-lowering diet: the Dietary Approaches to Stop Hypertension (DASH) Trial, *Am J Clin Nutr,* 74, 80, 2001.
137. Chandalia, M. et al., Beneficial effects of high dietary fiber intake in patients with type 2 diabetes mellitus, *N Engl J Med,* 342, 1392, 2000.
138. Garg, A., Grundy, S.M., and Unger, R.H., Comparison of effects of high and low carbohydrate diets on plasma lipoproteins and insulin sensitivity in patients with mild NIDDM, *Diabetes,* 41, 1278, 1992.
139. Ginsberg, H.N., New perspectives on atherogenesis: role of abnormal triglyceride-rich lipoprotein metabolism, *Circulation,* 106, 2137, 2002.
140. Davy, B.M. et al., High-fiber oat cereal compared with wheat cereal consumption favorably alters LDL-cholesterol subclass and particle numbers in middle-aged and older men, *Am J Clin Nutr,* 76, 351, 2002.
141. King, D.E., Egan, B.M., and Geesey, M.E., Relation of dietary fat and fiber to elevation of C-reactive protein, *Am J Cardiol,* 92, 1335, 2003.

142. Ajani, U.A., Ford, E.S., and Mokdad, A.H., Dietary fiber and C-reactive protein: findings from national health and nutrition examination survey data, *J Nutr,* 134, 1181, 2004.
143. Jenkins, D.J. et al., Glycemic index of foods: a physiological basis for carbohydrate exchange, *Am J Clin Nutr,* 34, 362, 1981.
144. Wolever, T.M. et al., The glycemic index: methodology and clinical implications, *Am J Clin Nutr,* 54, 846, 1991.
145. Pelkman, C.L., Effects of the glycemic index of foods on serum concentrations of high-density lipoprotein cholesterol and triglycerides, *Curr Atheroscler Rep,* 3, 456, 2001.
146. DECODE Study Group, Glucose tolerance and mortality: comparison of WHO and American Diabetes Association diagnostic criteria. Diabetes epidemiology: collaborative analysis of diagnostic criteria in Europe, *Lancet,* 354, 617, 1999.
147. de Vegt, F. et al., Hyperglycaemia is associated with all-cause and cardiovascular mortality in the Hoorn population: the Hoorn Study, *Diabetologia,* 42, 926, 1999.
148. Levitan, E.B. et al., Is nondiabetic hyperglycemia a risk factor for cardiovascular disease? A meta-analysis of prospective studies, *Arch Intern Med,* 164, 2147, 2004.
149. Esposito, K. et al., Regression of carotid atherosclerosis by control of postprandial hyperglycemia in type 2 diabetes mellitus, *Circulation,* 110, 214, 2004.
150. Tropeano, A.I. et al., Glucose level is a major determinant of carotid intima-media thickness in patients with hypertension and hyperglycemia, *J Hypertens,* 22, 2153, 2004.
151. Lee, I.K., Kim, H.S., and Bae, J.H., Endothelial dysfunction: its relationship with acute hyperglycaemia and hyperlipidemia, *Int J Clin Pract Suppl,* 59, 2002.
152. Ceriello, A. et al., Meal-induced oxidative stress and low-density lipoprotein oxidation in diabetes: the possible role of hyperglycemia, *Metabolism,* 48, 1503, 1999.
153. Stout, R.W., Hyperinsulinemia and atherosclerosis, *Diabetes,* 45 Suppl 3, S45, 1996.
154. Steiner, G. and Lewis, G.F., Hyperinsulinemia and triglyceride-rich lipoproteins, *Diabetes,* 45 Suppl 3, S24, 1996.
155. Foster-Powell, K., Holt, S.H., and Brand-Miller, J.C., International table of glycemic index and glycemic load values: 2002, *Am J Clin Nutr,* 76, 5, 2002.
156. Schulze, M.B. et al., Glycemic index, glycemic load, and dietary fiber intake and incidence of type 2 diabetes in younger and middle-aged women, *Am J Clin Nutr,* 80, 348, 2004.
157. Liu, S. et al., A prospective study of dietary glycemic load, carbohydrate intake, and risk of coronary heart disease in US women, *Am J Clin Nutr,* 71, 1455, 2000.
158. Salmeron, J. et al., Dietary fiber, glycemic load, and risk of NIDDM in men, *Diabetes Care,* 20, 545, 1997.
159. Liu, S. et al., Dietary glycemic load assessed by food-frequency questionnaire in relation to plasma high-density-lipoprotein cholesterol and fasting plasma triacylglycerols in postmenopausal women, *Am J Clin Nutr,* 73, 560, 2001.
160. Frost, G. et al., Glycaemic index as a determinant of serum HDL-cholesterol concentration, *Lancet,* 353, 1045, 1999.
161. Ford, E.S. and Liu, S., Glycemic index and serum high-density lipoprotein cholesterol concentration among US adults, *Arch Intern Med,* 161, 572, 2001.

162. Buyken, A.E. et al., Glycemic index in the diet of European outpatients with type 1 diabetes: relations to glycated hemoglobin and serum lipids, *Am J Clin Nutr,* 73, 574, 2001.
163. Miller, J.C., Importance of glycemic index in diabetes, *Am J Clin Nutr,* 59, 747S, 1994.
164. Jenkins, D.J. et al., Low-glycemic index diet in hyperlipidemia: use of traditional starchy foods, *Am J Clin Nutr,* 46, 66, 1987.
165. Wolever, T.M. et al., Beneficial effect of low-glycemic index diet in overweight NIDDM subjects, *Diabetes Care,* 15, 562, 1992.
166. Dumesnil, J.G. et al., Effect of a low-glycaemic index–low-fat–high protein diet on the atherogenic metabolic risk profile of abdominally obese men, *Br J Nutr,* 86, 557, 2001.
167. Luscombe, N.D., Noakes, M., and Clifton, P.M., Diets high and low in glycemic index versus high monounsaturated fat diets: effects on glucose and lipid metabolism in NIDDM, *Eur J Clin Nutr,* 53, 473, 1999.
168. Wolever, T.M. and Mehling, C., High-carbohydrate-low-glycaemic index dietary advice improves glucose disposition index in subjects with impaired glucose tolerance, *Br J Nutr,* 87, 477, 2002.
169. Heilbronn, L.K., Noakes, M., and Clifton, P.M., The effect of high- and low-glycemic index energy restricted diets on plasma lipid and glucose profiles in type 2 diabetic subjects with varying glycemic control, *J Am Coll Nutr,* 21, 120, 2002.
170. Jarvi, A.E. et al., Improved glycemic control and lipid profile and normalized fibrinolytic activity on a low-glycemic index diet in type 2 diabetic patients, *Diabetes Care,* 22, 10, 1999.
171. Sloth, B. et al., No difference in body weight decrease between a low-glycemic-index and a high-glycemic-index diet but reduced LDL cholesterol after 10-wk ad libitum intake of the low-glycemic-index diet, *Am J Clin Nutr,* 80, 337, 2004.
172. Frost, G.S. et al., A prospective randomised trial to determine the efficacy of a low glycaemic index diet given in addition to healthy eating and weight loss advice in patients with coronary heart disease, *Eur J Clin Nutr,* 58, 121, 2004.
173. Brand-Miller, J. et al., Low-glycemic index diets in the management of diabetes: a meta-analysis of randomized controlled trials, *Diabetes Care,* 26, 2261, 2003.
174. Opperman, A.M. et al., Meta-analysis of the health effects of using the glycaemic index in meal-planning, *Br J Nutr,* 92, 367, 2004.
175. Krauss, R.M. et al., AHA Dietary Guidelines: revision 2000: a statement for healthcare professionals from the Nutrition Committee of the American Heart Association, *Circulation,* 102, 2284, 2000.
176. Koh, K.K. et al., Vascular effects of step I diet in hypercholesterolemic patients with coronary artery disease, *Am J Cardiol,* 92, 708, 2003.
177. Ginsberg, H.N. et al., Effects of increasing dietary polyunsaturated fatty acids within the guidelines of the AHA step 1 diet on plasma lipid and lipoprotein levels in normal males, *Arterioscler Thromb,* 14, 892, 1994.
178. Lichtenstein, A.H. et al., Efficacy of a Therapeutic Lifestyle Change/step 2 diet in moderately hypercholesterolemic middle-aged and elderly female and male subjects, *J Lipid Res,* 43, 264, 2002.
179. Walden, C.E. et al., Lipoprotein lipid response to the National Cholesterol Education Program step II diet by hypercholesterolemic and combined hyperlipidemic women and men, *Arterioscler Thromb Vasc Biol,* 17, 375, 1997.

180. Yu-Poth, S. et al., Effects of the National Cholesterol Education Program's step I and step II dietary intervention programs on cardiovascular disease risk factors: a meta-analysis, *Am J Clin Nutr,* 69, 632, 1999.
181. Li, Z. et al., Men and women differ in lipoprotein response to dietary saturated fat and cholesterol restriction, *J Nutr,* 133, 3428, 2003.
182. Jenkins, D.J. et al., A dietary portfolio approach to cholesterol reduction: combined effects of plant sterols, vegetable proteins, and viscous fibers in hypercholesterolemia, *Metabolism,* 51, 1596, 2002.
183. Jenkins, D.J. et al., The effect of combining plant sterols, soy protein, viscous fibers, and almonds in treating hypercholesterolemia, *Metabolism,* 52, 1478, 2003.
184. Jenkins, D.J. et al., Effects of a dietary portfolio of cholesterol-lowering foods vs lovastatin on serum lipids and C-reactive protein, *JAMA,* 290, 502, 2003.
185. Ornish, D. et al., Intensive lifestyle changes for reversal of coronary heart disease, *JAMA,* 280, 2001, 1998.
186. Keys, A. et al., The diet and 15-year death rate in the Seven Countries Study, *Am J Epidemiol,* 124, 903, 1986.
187. Panagiotakos, D.B. et al., The associations between leisure-time physical activity and inflammatory and coagulation markers related to cardiovascular disease: the ATTICA Study, *Prev Med,* 40, 432, 2005.
188. Panagiotakos, D.B. et al., Status and management of blood lipids in Greek adults and their relation to socio-demographic, lifestyle and dietary factors: the ATTICA Study. Blood lipids distribution in Greece, *Atherosclerosis,* 173, 353, 2004.
189. de Lorgeril, M. et al., Mediterranean alpha-linolenic acid-rich diet in secondary prevention of coronary heart disease, *Lancet,* 343, 1454, 1994.
190. Singh, R.B. et al., Effect of an Indo-Mediterranean diet on progression of coronary artery disease in high risk patients (Indo-Mediterranean Diet Heart Study): a randomised single-blind trial, *Lancet,* 360, 1455, 2002.
191. Rosenthal, M.B. et al., Effects of a high-complex-carbohydrate, low-fat, low-cholesterol diet on levels of serum lipids and estradiol, *Am J Med,* 78, 23, 1985.
192. Lichtenstein, A.H. et al., Short-term consumption of a low-fat diet beneficially affects plasma lipid concentrations only when accompanied by weight loss. Hypercholesterolemia, low-fat diet, and plasma lipids, *Arterioscler Thromb,* 14, 1751, 1994.
193. McManus, K., Antinoro, L., and Sacks, F., A randomized controlled trial of a moderate-fat, low-energy diet compared with a low fat, low-energy diet for weight loss in overweight adults, *Int J Obes Relat Metab Disord,* 25, 1503, 2001.
194. Colette, C. et al., Exchanging carbohydrates for monounsaturated fats in energy-restricted diets: effects on metabolic profile and other cardiovascular risk factors, *Int J Obes Relat Metab Disord,* 27, 648, 2003.
195. Pelkman, C.L. et al., Effects of moderate-fat (from monounsaturated fat) and low-fat weight-loss diets on the serum lipid profile in overweight and obese men and women, *Am J Clin Nutr,* 79, 204, 2004.
196. Gerhard, G.T. et al., Effects of a low-fat diet compared with those of a high-monounsaturated fat diet on body weight, plasma lipids and lipoproteins, and glycemic control in type 2 diabetes, *Am J Clin Nutr,* 80, 668, 2004.
197. Sharman, M.J. et al., A ketogenic diet favorably affects serum biomarkers for cardiovascular disease in normal-weight men, *J Nutr,* 132, 1879, 2002.

198. Layman, D.K. et al., A reduced ratio of dietary carbohydrate to protein improves body composition and blood lipid profiles during weight loss in adult women, *J Nutr,* 133, 411, 2003.
199. Layman, D.K. et al., Increased dietary protein modifies glucose and insulin homeostasis in adult women during weight loss, *J Nutr,* 133, 405, 2003.
200. Westman, E.C. et al., Effect of 6-month adherence to a very low carbohydrate diet program, *Am J Med,* 113, 30, 2002.
201. Foster, G.D. et al., A randomized trial of a low-carbohydrate diet for obesity, *N Engl J Med,* 348, 2082, 2003.
202. Anderson, J.W., Konz, E.C., and Jenkins, D.J., Health advantages and disadvantages of weight-reducing diets: a computer analysis and critical review, *J Am Coll Nutr,* 19, 578, 2000.
203. Larosa, J.C. et al., Effects of high-protein, low-carbohydrate dieting on plasma lipoproteins and body weight, *J Am Diet Assoc,* 77, 264, 1980.
204. Brinkworth, G.D. et al., Long-term effects of a high-protein, low-carbohydrate diet on weight control and cardiovascular risk markers in obese hyperinsulinemic subjects, *Int J Obes Relat Metab Disord,* 28, 661, 2004.
205. Kwiterovich, P.O., Jr. et al., Effect of a high-fat ketogenic diet on plasma levels of lipids, lipoproteins, and apolipoproteins in children, *JAMA,* 290, 912, 2003.
206. Manson, J.E. et al., The primary prevention of myocardial infarction, *N Engl J Med,* 326, 1406, 1992.
207. Krauss, R.M., Blanche, P.J., Detection and quantitation of LDL subfractions, *Curr Opin Lipidol,* 3, 377, 1992.
208. Austin, M.A. and Krauss, R.M., Genetic control of low-density-lipoprotein subclasses, *Lancet,* 2, 592, 1986.
209. Austin, M.A., Hokanson, J.E., and Edwards, K.L., Hypertriglyceridemia as a cardiovascular risk factor, *Am J Cardiol,* 81, 7B, 1998.
210. Lamarche, B. et al., A prospective, population-based study of low density lipoprotein particle size as a risk factor for ischemic heart disease in men, *Can J Cardiol,* 17, 859, 2001.
211. Koba, S. et al., Remarkably high prevalence of small dense low-density lipoprotein in Japanese men with coronary artery disease, irrespective of the presence of diabetes, *Atherosclerosis,* 160, 249, 2002.
212. Austin, M.A. et al., Low-density lipoprotein subclass patterns and risk of myocardial infarction, *JAMA,* 260, 1917, 1988.
213. Stampfer, M.J. et al., A prospective study of triglyceride level, low-density lipoprotein particle diameter, and risk of myocardial infarction, *JAMA,* 276, 882, 1996.
214. Gardner, C.D., Fortmann, S.P., and Krauss, R.M., Association of small low-density lipoprotein particles with the incidence of coronary artery disease in men and women, *JAMA,* 276, 875, 1996.
215. Lamarche, B. et al., Small, dense low-density lipoprotein particles as a predictor of the risk of ischemic heart disease in men. Prospective results from the Quebec Cardiovascular Study, *Circulation,* 95, 69, 1997.
216. Campos, H. et al., LDL particle size distribution. Results from the Framingham Offspring Study, *Arterioscler Thromb,* 12, 1410, 1992.
217. Austin, M.A. et al., Inheritance of low density lipoprotein subclass patterns in familial combined hyperlipidemia, *Arteriosclerosis,* 10, 520, 1990.
218. Arisaka, O. et al., Characterization of low-density lipoprotein subclasses in children, *Metabolism,* 46, 146, 1997.

219. Williams, P.T. et al., Changes in lipoprotein subfractions during diet-induced and exercise-induced weight loss in moderately overweight men, *Circulation,* 81, 1293, 1990.
220. Campos, H. et al., Nutrient intake comparisons between Framingham and rural and Urban Puriscal, Costa Rica. Associations with lipoproteins, apolipoproteins, and low density lipoprotein particle size, *Arterioscler Thromb,* 11, 1089, 1991.
221. Krauss, R.M. and Dreon, D.M., Low-density-lipoprotein subclasses and response to a low-fat diet in healthy men, *Am J Clin Nutr,* 62, 478S, 1995.
222. Dreon, D.M. et al., A very low-fat diet is not associated with improved lipoprotein profiles in men with a predominance of large, low-density lipoproteins, *Am J Clin Nutr,* 69, 411, 1999.
223. Sjogren, P. et al., Milk-derived fatty acids are associated with a more favorable LDL particle size distribution in healthy men, *J Nutr,* 134, 1729, 2004.
224. Dreon, D.M. et al., Change in dietary saturated fat intake is correlated with change in mass of large low-density-lipoprotein particles in men, *Am J Clin Nutr,* 67, 828, 1998.
225. Kratz, M. et al., Dietary mono- and polyunsaturated fatty acids similarly affect LDL size in healthy men and women, *J Nutr,* 132, 715, 2002.
226. Suzukawa, M. et al., Effects of fish oil fatty acids on low density lipoprotein size, oxidizability, and uptake by macrophages, *J Lipid Res,* 36, 473, 1995.
227. Baumstark, M.W. et al., Influence of n-3 fatty acids from fish oils on concentration of high- and low-density lipoprotein subfractions and their lipid and apolipoprotein composition, *Clin Biochem,* 25, 338, 1992.
228. Lu, G., Windsor, S.L., and Harris, W.S., Omega-3 fatty acids alter lipoprotein subfraction distributions and the *in vitro* conversion of very low density lipoproteins to low density lipoproteins, *J Nutr Biochem,* 10, 151, 1999.
229. Li, Z. et al., Fish consumption shifts lipoprotein subfractions to a less atherogenic pattern in humans, *J Nutr,* 134, 1724, 2004.
230. Desroches, S. et al., Soy protein favorably affects LDL size independently of isoflavones in hypercholesterolemic men and women, *J Nutr,* 134, 574, 2004.
231. Charest, A. et al., Unesterified plant sterols and stanols do not affect LDL electrophoretic characteristics in hypercholesterolemic subjects, *J Nutr,* 134, 592, 2004.
232. Lamarche, B. et al., Combined effects of a dietary portfolio of plant sterols, vegetable protein, viscous fibre and almonds on LDL particle size, *Br J Nutr,* 92, 657, 2004.
233. Executive Summary of the Third Report of the National Cholesterol Education Program (NCEP) Expert Panel on Detection, Evaluation, and Treatment of High Blood Cholesterol in Adults (Adult Treatment Panel III), *JAMA,* 285, 2486, 2001.
234. von Eckardstein, A., Nofer, J.R., and Assmann, G., High density lipoproteins and arteriosclerosis. Role of cholesterol efflux and reverse cholesterol transport, *Arterioscler Thromb Vasc Biol,* 21, 13, 2001.
235. von Eckardstein, A., Huang, Y., and Assmann, G., Physiological role and clinical relevance of high-density lipoprotein subclasses, *Curr Opin Lipidol,* 5, 404, 1994.
236. Silverman, D.I., Ginsburg, G.S., and Pasternak, R.C., High-density lipoprotein subfractions, *Am J Med,* 94, 636, 1993.
237. Stampfer, M.J. et al., A prospective study of cholesterol, apolipoproteins, and the risk of myocardial infarction, *N Engl J Med,* 325, 373, 1991.

238. Miller, N.E., Associations of high-density lipoprotein subclasses and apolipoproteins with ischemic heart disease and coronary atherosclerosis, *Am Heart J*, 113, 589, 1987.
239. Pascot, A. et al., Reduced HDL particle size as an additional feature of the atherogenic dyslipidemia of abdominal obesity, *J Lipid Res*, 42, 2007, 2001.
240. Williams, P.T., Dreon, D.M., and Krauss, R.M., Effects of dietary fat on high-density-lipoprotein subclasses are influenced by both apolipoprotein E isoforms and low-density-lipoprotein subclass patterns, *Am J Clin Nutr*, 61, 1234, 1995.
241. Berglund, L. et al., HDL-subpopulation patterns in response to reductions in dietary total and saturated fat intakes in healthy subjects, *Am J Clin Nutr*, 70, 992, 1999.
242. Subbaiah, P.V. et al., Effects of dietary supplementation with marine lipid concentrate on the plasma lipoprotein composition of hypercholesterolemic patients, *Atherosclerosis*, 79, 157, 1989.
243. Thomas, T.R. et al., Effects of exercise and n-3 fatty acids on postprandial lipemia, *J Appl Physiol*, 88, 2199, 2000.
244. Parks, E.J., Recent findings in the study of postprandial lipemia, *Curr Atheroscler Rep*, 3, 462, 2001.
245. Roche, H.M. and Gibney, M.J., Effect of long-chain n-3 polyunsaturated fatty acids on fasting and postprandial triacylglycerol metabolism, *Am J Clin Nutr*, 71, 232S, 2000.
246. Smith, B.K. et al., Exercise plus n-3 fatty acids: additive effect on postprandial lipemia, *Metabolism*, 53, 1365, 2004.
247. Finnegan, Y.E. et al., Plant- and marine-derived n-3 polyunsaturated fatty acids have differential effects on fasting and postprandial blood lipid concentrations and on the susceptibility of LDL to oxidative modification in moderately hyperlipidemic subjects, *Am J Clin Nutr*, 77, 783, 2003.
248. Sanders, T.A. et al., Influence of n-6 versus n-3 polyunsaturated fatty acids in diets low in saturated fatty acids on plasma lipoproteins and hemostatic factors, *Arterioscler Thromb Vasc Biol*, 17, 3449, 1997.
249. Sharman, M.J. et al., Very low-carbohydrate and low-fat diets affect fasting lipids and postprandial lipemia differently in overweight men, *J Nutr*, 134, 880, 2004.
250. Volek, J.S. et al., An isoenergetic very low carbohydrate diet improves serum HDL cholesterol and triacylglycerol concentrations, the total cholesterol to HDL cholesterol ratio and postprandial pipemic responses compared with a low fat diet in normal weight, normolipidemic women, *J Nutr*, 133, 2756, 2003.
251. Berglund, L. and Ramakrishnan, R., Lipoprotein(a): an elusive cardiovascular risk factor, *Arterioscler Thromb Vasc Biol*, 2004.
252. Cantin, B. et al., Is lipoprotein(a) an independent risk factor for ischemic heart disease in men? The Quebec Cardiovascular Study, *J Am Coll Cardiol*, 31, 519, 1998.
253. Nguyen, T.T. et al., Predictive value of electrophoretically detected lipoprotein(a) for coronary heart disease and cerebrovascular disease in a community-based cohort of 9936 men and women, *Circulation*, 96, 1390, 1997.
254. Bostom, A.G. et al., Elevated plasma lipoprotein(a) and coronary heart disease in men aged 55 years and younger. A prospective study, *JAMA*, 276, 544, 1996.

255. Gavish, D., Azrolan, N., and Breslow, J.L., Plasma Ip(a) concentration is inversely correlated with the ratio of Kringle IV/Kringle V encoding domains in the apo(a) gene, *J Clin Invest,* 84, 2021, 1989.
256. Nachman, R.L. et al., Lipoprotein(a) in diet-induced atherosclerosis in nonhuman primates, *Arterioscler Thromb,* 11, 32, 1991.
257. Kraft, H.G. et al., The apolipoprotein (a) gene: a transcribed hypervariable locus controlling plasma lipoprotein (a) concentration, *Hum Genet,* 90, 220, 1992.
258. Paultre, F. et al., High levels of Lp(a) with a small apo(a) isoform are associated with coronary artery disease in African American and white men, *Arterioscler Thromb Vasc Biol,* 20, 2619, 2000.
259. Barkley, R.A. et al., Lack of genetic linkage evidence for a trans-acting factor having a large effect on plasma lipoprotein[a] levels in African Americans, *J Lipid Res,* 44, 1301, 2003.
260. Marcovina, S.M. et al., Differences in Lp[a] concentrations and apo[a] polymorphs between black and white Americans, *J Lipid Res,* 37, 2569, 1996.
261. Clevidence, B.A. et al., Plasma lipoprotein (a) levels in men and women consuming diets enriched in saturated, cis-, or trans-monounsaturated fatty acids, *Arterioscler Thromb Vasc Biol,* 17, 1657, 1997.
262. Mensink, R.P. et al., Effect of dietary cis and trans fatty acids on serum lipoprotein[a] levels in humans, *J Lipid Res,* 33, 1493, 1992.
263. Almendingen, K. et al., Effects of partially hydrogenated fish oil, partially hydrogenated soybean oil, and butter on serum lipoproteins and Lp[a] in men, *J Lipid Res,* 36, 1370, 1995.
264. Tholstrup, T. et al., Effect of fats high in individual saturated fatty acids on plasma lipoprotein[a] levels in young healthy men, *J Lipid Res,* 36, 1447, 1995.
265. Hornstra, G. et al., A palm oil-enriched diet lowers serum lipoprotein(a) in normocholesterolemic volunteers, *Atherosclerosis,* 90, 91, 1991.
266. Muller, H. et al., A diet rich in coconut oil reduces diurnal postprandial variations in circulating tissue plasminogen activator antigen and fasting lipoprotein (a) compared with a diet rich in unsaturated fat in women, *J Nutr,* 133, 3422, 2003.
267. Muller, H. et al., The serum LDL/HDL cholesterol ratio is influenced more favorably by exchanging saturated with unsaturated fat than by reducing saturated fat in the diet of women, *J Nutr,* 133, 78, 2003.
268. Randall, O.S. et al., Response of lipoprotein(a) levels to therapeutic life-style change in obese African-Americans, *Atherosclerosis,* 172, 155, 2004.
269. Beil, F.U. et al., Dietary fish oil lowers lipoprotein(a) in primary hypertriglyceridemia, *Atherosclerosis,* 90, 95, 1991.
270. Herrmann, W., Biermann, J., and Kostner, G.M., Comparison of effects of n-3 to n-6 fatty acids on serum level of lipoprotein(a) in patients with coronary artery disease, *Am J Cardiol,* 76, 459, 1995.
271. Gries, A. et al., Influence of dietary fish oils on plasma Lp(a) levels, *Thromb Res,* 58, 667, 1990.
272. Nilausen, K. and Meinertz, H., Lipoprotein(a) and dietary proteins: casein lowers lipoprotein(a) concentrations as compared with soy protein, *Am J Clin Nutr,* 69, 419, 1999.
273. Meinertz, H., Nilausen, K., and Hilden, J., Alcohol-extracted, but not intact, dietary soy protein lowers lipoprotein(a) markedly, *Arterioscler Thromb Vasc Biol,* 22, 312, 2002.

274. Silaste, M.L. et al., Changes in dietary fat intake alter plasma levels of oxidized low-density lipoprotein and lipoprotein(a), *Arterioscler Thromb Vasc Biol,* 24, 498, 2004.
275. Tholstrup, T. and Samman, S., Postprandial lipoprotein(a) is affected differently by specific individual dietary fatty acids in healthy young men, *J Nutr,* 134, 2550, 2004.
276. Pfaffinger, D. et al., Relationship between apo[a] isoforms and Lp[a] density in subjects with different apo[a] phenotype: a study before and after a fatty meal, *J Lipid Res,* 32, 679, 1991.
277. Hoppichler, F. et al., Lipoprotein(a) is increased in triglyceride-rich lipoproteins in men with coronary heart disease, but does not change acutely following oral fat ingestion, *Atherosclerosis,* 122, 127, 1996.
278. Dietary Guidelines for Americans 2005, U.S. Department of Health and Human Services, U.S. Department of Agriculture. www.healthierus.gov/dietaryguidelines.
279. Nutrition and Your Health: Dietary Guidelines for Americans, 5th ed., USDA Home and Garden Bulletin No. 232, 2000.
280. Kris-Etherton, P.M., Harris, W.S., and Appel, L.J., Fish consumption, fish oil, omega-3 fatty acids, and cardiovascular disease, *Circulation,* 106, 2747, 2002.
281. American Diabetes Association., Evidence-based nutrition principles and recommendations for the treatment and prevention of diabetes and related complications, *Diabetes Care,* 26, S51.
282. Jenkins, D.J. et al., Viscous and nonviscous fibres, nonabsorbable and low glycaemic index carbohydrates, blood lipids and coronary heart disease, *Curr Opin Lipidol,* 11, 49, 2000.
283. Hu, F.B. and Willett, W.C., Optimal diets for prevention of coronary heart disease, *JAMA,* 288, 2569, 2002.

12

Physical Activity, Exercise, Blood Lipids, and Lipoproteins

J. Larry Durstine and Andrea C. Summer

CONTENTS

Introduction 265
Endurance Exercise Training 266
    Lipids 266
    Lipoproteins and Lipids 266
    Apolipoproteins 270
Resistance Exercise Training 271
Postprandial Lipemia 272
Exercise-Induced Mechanisms for Changes in Lipid and Lipoprotein Metabolism 272
Physical Activity or Physical Inactivity 273
Clinical Application 274
Conclusions 275
References 275

Introduction

The impact of regular exercise on plasma lipids and lipoproteins in recent years has been more clearly defined in regard to the interactions between lipids, lipoproteins, apolipoproteins (apo), and lipoprotein enzymes; and the influence of various genetic and environmental factors such as aging, body fat distribution, dietary composition, and cigarette smoking status.[1–4] The purpose of this review is to summarize present information regarding the exercise training impact on lipid and lipoprotein concentrations.

Endurance Exercise Training

Lipids

Cross-sectional and longitudinal exercise training studies usually report lower plasma triglyceride concentrations but not always.[5,6] Large plasma triglyceride reductions after exercise training are often reported for previously inactive individuals with higher baseline concentrations,[6,7] whereas subjects with low initial triglyceride concentrations demonstrate small triglyceride reductions after exercise training[8–10] (Figure 12.1). Neither cross-sectional nor longitudinal exercise training studies support an exercise-induced change in plasma cholesterol concentration[6–10] (Figure 12.2). When reduced plasma cholesterol levels are reported after exercise training, these reductions were not related to either the initial cholesterol concentrations or the exercise training program length.[11,12] Rather, a reduction in plasma cholesterol is associated with reductions in body weight, percentage body fat, and dietary fat[1,11–13] (see Table 12.1).

Lipoproteins and Lipids

The effect that a single exercise session has on postprandial lipoproteins and lipids is greater than and different from that attributable to exercise training[14–16] and dietary energy deficiencies.[14,17] Chylomicron and very low-density lipoproteins (VLDL) are usually lower after exercise training.[1,10]

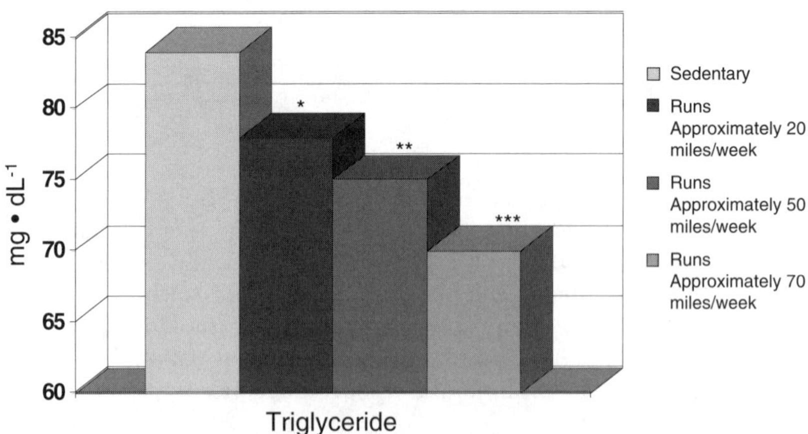

FIGURE 12.1
As the volume of exercise training is increased, the greater is the reduction in triglyceride concentration.

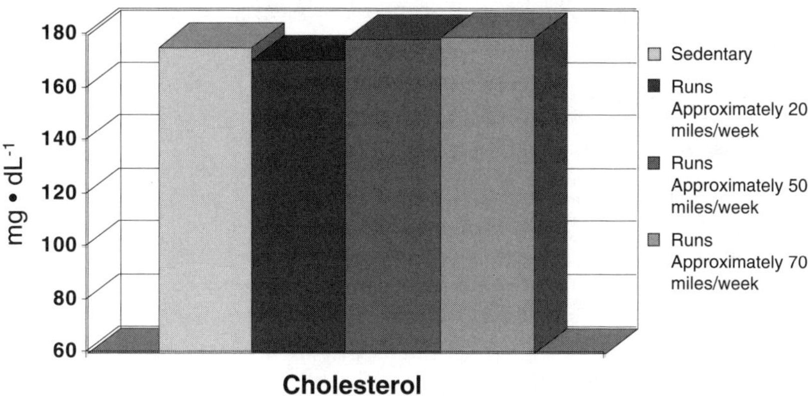

FIGURE 12.2
Exercise training has little impact on blood cholesterol. Note that even the group running 70 miles per week did not have altered cholesterol concentrations.

Plasma low-density lipoprotein cholesterol (LDL-C), a powerful coronary artery disease (CAD) risk predictor, is elevated in individuals with diets high in fat content, especially saturated fats.[14] LDL-C concentrations are not usually lower after aerobic exercise training,[6,7,9,10,12,18] though lower LDL-C levels are reported.[14] LDL particles are also categorized according to size. Each size having a different CAD risk (e.g., the smaller, denser LDL particle directly correlates with CAD incidences and may depend on elevated triglyceride concentrations).[19] Exercise training may impact these LDL particles differently. Williams et al.[20,21] found no change in small LDL particles after 1 year of exercise training in overweight men while hypercholesterolemic men (cholesterol > 240 mg/dl) have reduced triglyceride and small LDL size particles with increased physical activity levels.[22] Overweight subjects completing 6 months of jogging (~ 20 miles per week at 65–80% of their cardiovascular capacity)[23] and after 8 months of regular exercise[24] exhibited greater LDL particle sizes along with lower LDL concentrations. Beard et al.[25] demonstrated mean LDL particle size increases with 3 weeks of diet and brisk walking. Cholesterol concentrations decreased in the more dense LDL subfractions and increased in the less-dense LDL fractions, and the change was correlated with reductions in triglyceride concentrations. A 3-month atherosclerosis treatment program that included regular moderate-intensity exercise did not alter LDL particle size in 25 coronary artery disease patients.[26] However, the intervention was shown to increase the antioxidant content and reduce oxidative susceptibility of LDL particles.

Plasma lipoprotein (a) [Lp(a)], an LDL subfraction containing the apolipoprotein apo(a)[27], is highly homologous with plasminogen. As a result, the

TABLE 12.1

Lipid, Lipoprotein, Lipoprotein Enzymes and Transfer Protein Changes Associated with Exercise

	After Regular Exercise Participation
Lipid/Lipoprotein	
Triglyceride	Decreases of 4 to 37% Approximate mean change of 24%
Cholesterol	No change[a]
LDL-C	No change[a]
Lp(a)	No change
HDL-C	Increases of 4 to 18% Approximate mean change of 8%
Enzyme	
LPL	
Activity	Increased
Mass	
HL	
Activity	No change or reduced (may be reduced with weight loss)
Mass	No information
LCAT	
Activity	Increased/No change
Mass	No information
CETP	
Activity	No change/Increased
Mass	Increased

LPL, lipoprotein lipase; HL, hepatic lipase; LCAT, lecithin:cholesterol acyltransferase; CETP, cholesteryl ester transfer protein.

[a] No change if body weight and diet do not change (see text).

apo(a) portions of Lp(a) compete with plasminogen for binding sites on fibrin, inhibiting fibrinolysis.[27] Moreover, Lp(a) concentrations greater than 30 mg/dl have the same negative CAD effects as LDL-C and inhibit thrombolysis.[27] Lp(a) is an inherited trait and does not appear to change following regular physical activity participation.[2,27–30]

Exercise training longer than 12 weeks is more likely to increase plasma high-density lipoprotein (HDL-C)[1,2,10,31] (Figure 12.3) but not always.[32] These chances are usually present in a dose-dependent manner and are associated with increased energy expenditure.[1,2] Several factors deserve consideration when evaluating the impact of regular exercise participation and include the exercise training volume measured by kcal expended during the exercise training program, body weight and composition changes, dietary changes, and the length of the exercise intervention program. Exercise-induced increases in HDL-C range from 4% to 22%, while the absolute HDL-C increases are more uniform and range from 2 to 8 mg/dl. The initial HDL-C level and HDL-C change are important considerations with an inverse

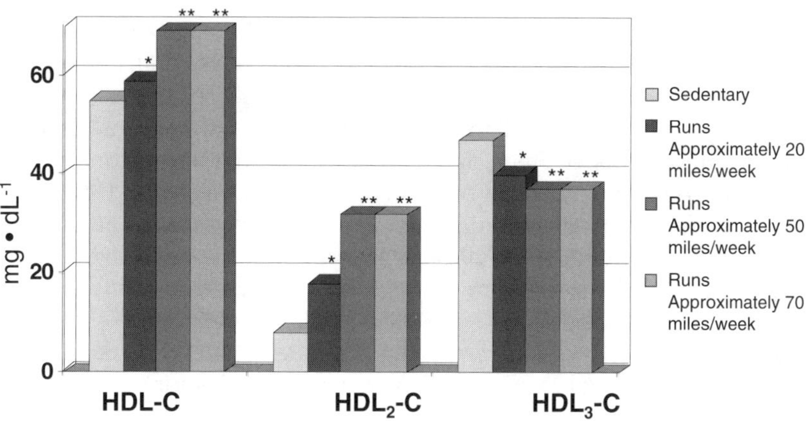

FIGURE 12.3
Exercise training is associated with increased HDL-C, and the increase in HDL-C is associated with an increase in the HDL_2-C.

correlation,[33] a greater change with higher initial HDL-C levels[34] and no relationship[7] being reported. Significant correlations have been established between distance run per week, the time spent in exercise training and HDL-C change.[6] Collectively these data provide support for a strong relationship between increased exercise training volume and HDL-C increases.[1,2] Wood et al.[9] observed an inverse relationship between body fat change and HDL-C change, but the addition of distance run per week did not improve the ability to predict HDL-C change. Maintaining body weight and body fat during exercise training resulted in HDL-C increases of 8 mg/dl[7] and 3 mg/dl,[35] whereas weight-loss programs using caloric restriction alone or caloric restriction with exercise training rendered body weight and percentage body fat decreases in both groups while HDL-C increased.[36] These findings support the finding that exercise training without altered body weight and/or composition can increase HDL-C, and this increase is augmented by body fat loss. This is especially true for men with elevated triglyceride and abdominal obesity.[37] Crouse et al.[38] reported elevated HDL-C and HDL_2-C during the 24–48 h time period immediately after a single exercise session, while the overall effect after the exercise training intervention was an increased HDL_2-C and a decreased HDL_3-C. HDL_2-C is usually increased after exercise training,[7,10,39] while HDL-$_3$C is reduced.[39] The HDL_{3b} particle is directly related to CAD risk, while HDL_{2a} and HDL_{2b} are associated with reduced CAD risk. Williams et al.[40] observed an increased HDL_{2b} and decreased HDL_{3b} after a 1-year exercise training-program (see Table 12.1).

Apolipoproteins

Apolipoproteins and exercise training have been reviewed.[1,41,42] Essentially increased apo A-I levels are observed[7,10,40] but not always.[9,12] Whether apo B levels decrease[12,43] or not,[8,9,10,12] apo B changes following exercise training usually parallel LDL-C changes. Wood et al.[9] found no overall change in apo B after 1 year of exercise training, but did find a significant inverse correlation between distance run and change in apo B levels. Although no differences in current and former runners were reported,[8] higher apo E concentrations were observed in young but not older runners.[44] Lower apo E levels after exercise have been found. Tanabe et al.[45] reported changes after exercise training in men, but not women. Taimela et al.[46] reported in a cross-sectional study of 1500 subjects between the ages of 9 and 24 evidence that leisure-time physical activity has a great effect on lipoprotein profiles of apo E_2 individuals, a lesser effect on apo E_3 subjects, with no effect on apo E_4 subjects. Data from longitudinal studies, however, may provide more direct evidence of a possible interaction between apo E polymorphism and exercise training. Nonetheless, St-Amand et al.[47] observed in men a significant interaction between physical activity, lipids and lipoproteins, and apo E phenotypes.

An inverse relationship between maximal oxygen consumption ($\dot{V}O_{2max}$) and triglyceride levels for individuals heterozygous for apo E_2 or homozygous for apo E_3 was observed but not for apo E_4 phenotypes. Plasma LDL-C levels were inversely associated with $\dot{V}O_{2max}$ only in women homozygous for apo E_3, whereas $\dot{V}O_{2max}$ was positively associated with plasma HDL_2-C only in men and women who were apo E_3 homozygotes. Though not statistically significant, post-heparin LPL activity was increased in apo E_2 subjects. Recently, Hagberg et al.[48] reported decreased triglyceride concentrations that were significantly greater in apo E_2 and E_3 groups while HDL-C increases were greater in only the apo E_2 subjects. Thompson et al.[49] examined prospectively the impact of the apo E genotyope on lipoprotein responses to exercise in healthy normolipidemic subjects following 6 months of exercise training. The results of this study demonstrated that apo E polymorphisms affect the lipid response to exercise training. Specifically, reductions in LDL-C/HDL-C and total cholesterol/HDL-C ratio were greater in apo E_3 homozygotes producing significantly greater reductions with exercise training in common markers of CAD risk. Thus, one of apo E's major functions might be to facilitate triglyceride clearance. Apo E_2 has a low affinity for the apo E receptor and in the homozygous form can produce marked hyperlipidemia. Hence, this information suggests that exercise training is most effective at reducing plasma triglyceride while increasing HDL-C and LPL activity in those persons who have an impaired ability to clear triglycerides or the subjects having apo E_2 phenotype. Thereby, increased HDL-C may be limited by the presence of the apo E_2 gene when subjects are sedentary (see Table 12.1).

Leon et al.,[50] on the other hand, found that Apo E polymorphism was not associated with $\dot{V}O_{2max}$ levels in the sedentary state nor after exercise training. Nevertheless, VLDL, cholesterol, and triglyceride levels were significantly higher in persons with the apo E_2 and apo E_4 in white men only.

Resistance Exercise Training

Compared with endurance training literature, considerably less information exists supporting resistance training as a modifier of plasma lipids and lipoprotein-lipids.[51] Present resistance exercise studies are often contradictory, with some showing positive benefits of resistance exercise on the lipid profile,[52–54] while others find no benefit.[55–57] Inter-study variations in methodologies can contribute to the many study outcome differences. Although it is unlikely that differences between studies can be attributed to any single reason, several possibilities exist with the leading candidate being variation in the exercise volume (caloric expenditure) completed during resistance exercise. It may simply be that the caloric threshold for inducing lipid and lipoprotein changes is typically not reached with resistance training. Indeed, a concern with the methodology from many resistance exercise studies is the lack of proper volume quantification and the failure to include a proper non-exercise control group. Training studies reviewed here meet the following requirements: (1) resistance exercise training groups met at least three times a week, (2) training routines were composed of exercises designed to train the major muscle groups of the body, performed in one to three sets, at least six repetitions per set with 15 to 120 s rest between sets, and (3) resistance training lasted from 8 weeks to 22 months.

Generally, triglyceride concentrations are not altered by resistance exercise training[53,55,57,58] even when initial triglyceride levels were elevated.[56] In contrast, decreased triglyceride concentrations after resistance training are reported in elderly women.[54] and after moderate-intensity, high-volume training.[59] Plasma cholesterol,[56,60] LDL-C,[60] and apo B-100 concentrations[61] were usually not altered following resistance training when total body mass, lean body mass, and percentage body fat were not changed.[56,57,60,61] However, decreased body fat percentage and an increase in lean body mass after resistance exercise training[53] are associated with a decrease in plasma cholesterol and LDL-C concentrations. Both LDL-C and total cholesterol have been shown to be reduced after circuit resistance training.[59] In the most published studies, HDL-C concentrations are unresponsive to resistance training,[56,60] yet increases have been reported.[54] When resistance exercise is combined with aerobic exercise, results are conflicting; HDL-C was variously reported to be increased[62] or unchanged[57] after training. Following a single resistance exercise session, triglyceride is reduced and HDL-C increased, although the changes appear to be volume dependent.[63]

Postprandial Lipemia

Exaggerated postprandial lipemia, a comparatively prolonged elevated blood triglyceride concentration after a meal, is associated with atherosclerosis. Exercise completed within 24 h before a high-fat meal reduces postprandial lipemia.[64] This triglyceride reduction is found after jogging,[65] exercise cycling,[66] and resistance exercise.[63,67] Current evidence indicates that the magnitude of the reduction is primarily related to total energy expended during the preceding exercise session(s), whether the exercise is performed all at once or intermittently.[64,68–70] Neither exercise intensity nor duration effect postprandial lipemia independent of total energy expenditure.[64] Yet to be clarified are subject characteristics that may influence the magnitude of the response, such as training status, gender, obesity, and existing atherosclerosis. Furthermore, the mechanism responsible for reduced postprandial lipemia is not well-defined, but is likely related to increased lipoprotein lipase (LPL) activity in the hours after an exercise session.[65,66]

To summarize, reduced postprandial lipemia is found when exercise precedes a meal by up to 24 h. The magnitude of the effect is related to the exercise volume performed. A measurable, beneficial effect on circulating lipids and lipoprotein-lipids may be expected by untrained persons after a single exercise session where 350 kcal are expended, whereas trained individuals may require 800 kcal or more to elicit comparable changes. Under these circumstances, the beneficial changes in lipid and lipoprotein-lipid concentrations after exercise are similar in magnitude to those reported after the completion of a longitudinal exercise training program. Since blood lipids and lipoprotein lipids are associated with coronary artery disease, the changes induced by a single exercise session can be expected to reduce the risk of this disease. In order for these beneficial lipid and lipoprotein-lipid changes to be maintained, exercise must be performed on a regular basis, optimally every other day.

Exercise-Induced Mechanisms for Changes in Lipid and Lipoprotein Metabolism

Intravenous heparin injections and muscle and adipose tissue biopsy samples are used to measure LPL activity. High-intensity exercise sessions and high energy expenditure that deplete intramuscular triglyceride stores are needed to increase muscle LPL synthesis and release (Table 12.1).[26,71] Increased plasma post-heparin LPL activity (PHLPL) is usually not found until 4 to 18 h post-exercise,[72,73] is reported for endurance athletes,[74] and is increased after exercise training,[75,76] though not always.[5,7,77,78] Ethnic PHLPL differences exist with higher PHLPL values in white males, but not in black males after 20 weeks of endurance training.[75] Increases in PHLPL were recently related to endothelial lipase genotype.[79]

Seip and Semenkovich[71] have reviewed the molecular explanations for the exercise impact on LPL gene expression. In essence, a transient rise in LPL messenger RNA (mRNA) is present by the fifth day of exercise, while 5–13 consecutive days of exercise training were needed to increase skeletal muscle LPL mRNA, LPL mass, and total LPL enzyme activity.[76,80] Nevertheless, adipose tissue LPL mRNA, protein mass and enzyme activity remained unchanged.[77,80] Rat white skeletal muscle used during voluntary running had elevated LPL mass, total LPL activity, and heparin-releasable LPL activity with no change in either white or red muscle not recruited during voluntary exercise.[78,81] Thus, exercised white skeletal muscle intrinsically results in elevated LPL activity by pretranslational mechanisms, and an increase in LPL expression during exercise training likely requires local contractile activity.

An inverse association exists between resting HL activity and HDL_2-C while HL is directly related to HDL_3-C.[82] In general, no changes in resting HL activity are reported between inactive and active individuals,[74] and a single exercise session results in no significant HL activity changes.[73,80,83–86] Low CETP activity may provide an anti-atherogenic effect by slowing hepatic HDL_2 catabolism and decreasing the amount of plasma cholesterol-rich particles.[81,87] Elevated plasma CETP activity is found in physically active individuals,[5,82] while decreased CETP activity following exercise training is reported.[77,85,86] In addition, LCAT activity is increased in physically active men,[82,87] but not post-exercise training.[5,20,75]

Physical Activity or Physical Inactivity

Up to this point our discussion has centered around the positive impact of regular exercise participation on lipid and lipoprotein metabolism, which can result in a reduction for cardiovascular disease risk. On the other hand, it is also known that physical inactivity and lower cardiovascular fitness are clearly associated with increased heart disease risk.[88] The question that comes to mind concerns the potential for just everyday physical activity, not including planned exercise programming, and the likelihood for beneficial improvement in blood lipid and lipoprotein levels and reduced heart disease risk. Presently, the existing data are conflicting. In the past some published reviews have suggested that LDL-C and HDL-C are positively influenced by physical activity,[89,90] whereas others[3,4] indicate that physical activity has little effect on LDL-C and only small positive effects on HDL-C. However, several studies have reported that moderate-intensity physical activity is associated with positive blood lipid and lipoprotein changes.[91–94] Finally, multiple studies have reported that the volume of physical activity or exercise performed, regardless of intensity, is an important predictor of HDL-C change.[2–4,41,95,96] Present information does support some positive modification in blood lipids and lipoproteins for people maintaining an active lifestyle. To maximize the benefits, a person must lead a very active lifestyle. The current literature is not clear in this area.

Another way to look at the benefits of physical activity on blood lipids and lipoproteins is to understand how the body adapts to physical inactivity. Hamilton et al.[97] recently proposed a relatively new concept he has termed "Inactivity Physiology." He suggests that some health-related proteins like lipoprotein-lipase are regulated by different metabolic processes over the physical activity continuum, and this different regulation process is highly sensitive to physical inactivity. Essentially, physical inactivity could elicit a physically inactive pathway that in turn would generate a powerful regulation process that can inhibit lipoprotein-lipase. There is evidence that physical inactivity does develop a biological inhibitory signal that reduces lipoprotein-lipase activity, and that this process may be independent of lipoprotein-lipase messenger RNA.[98,99] However, much more work in this area is needed before conclusive statements can be made.

Clinical Application

Current treatment guidelines for the medical management of plasma lipids and lipoproteins are provided by the National Cholesterol Education Program Adult Treatment Panel III (NCEP).[100] Combining these guidelines with an individual risk assessment estimated from Framingham Study data is one clinical approach to hyperlipidemia management.[101] Pharmacologic therapy is the primary therapy for reducing lipid and lipoprotein levels since it is highly effective and generally well tolerated.[102] Considered adjunctive to pharmacologic therapy are secondary therapies such as reduced dietary fat intake, weight loss, and exercise interventions. These therapies are extremely important, but are greatly limited by patient compliance. Some patients achieve these desired lipid levels by these interventions, but in clinical practice this is unfortunately the exception and not the rule. Daily exercise programs are recommended for all patients with lipid disorders because exercise can profoundly decrease plasma triglyceride and improve glucose intolerance that contribute to dyslipidemia. Finally, when incorporating physical activity or exercise programming as an intervention, it must be borne in mind that the volume of physical activity or exercise completed is a key in determining whether a positive impact on blood lipid and lipoprotein levels will be observed. In order for these intervention programs to contribute to lipid management and optimize blood lipids and lipoproteins, the volume of physical activity or exercise training completed must be greater than

1200–1500 kcal of energy expenditure each week. The daily energy expenditure should be approximately 200 kcal.

Conclusions

Current information supports the favorable impact of exercise training on the lipid and lipoprotein profile. Regarding hyperlipidemic disorders, the primary intervention is pharmacological while diet modification, weight loss, and exercise, though important, are considered adjunctive therapies. Because much is known about the exercise training-induced plasma lipid and lipoprotein modifications as well as the responsible mechanisms for these changes, we are now better able to develop a comprehensive medical management plan that optimizes pharmacological and adjunctive therapies. Present scientific investigations are focusing on the molecular basis for lipid and lipoprotein change as a result of various interventions (e.g., knowing a person's apo E genotype). Information from these studies will provide a better understanding as to why some individuals respond to exercise, while others do not. Another research concern is the interactive effects between regular exercise participation and pharmacological inventions. This knowledge coupled with available lipid intervention information, such as diet modification and weight loss, can aid in optimizing individual medical management for special lipid disorders.

References

1. Durstine, J.L., and Thompson, P.D., Cardiology clinics: exercise in secondary prevention and cardiac rehabilitation, 19(3):471; 2001.
2. Durstine, J.L., Grandjean, P.W., Davis, P.G., Ferguson, M.A., Alderson, N.L., and DuBose, K.D., The effects of exercise training on serum lipids and lipoproteins: a quantitative analysis, *Sports Med.*, 31:1033; 2001.
3. Durstine, J.L., and Haskell, W.L., Effects of exercise training on plasma lipids and lipoproteins, *Exerc. Sports Sci. Rev.*, 22:477; 1994.
4. Leon, A.S., and Sanchez, O.A., Response of blood lipids to exercise training alone or combined with dietary intervention, *Med. Sci. Sports Exerc.*, 33(6):S502; 2001.
5. Grandjean, P.W., Crouse, S.F., O'Brien, B.C., Rohack, J.J., and Brown, J.A., The effects of menopausal status and exercise training on serum lipids and the activities of intravascular enzymes related to lipid transport, *Metabolism*, 47(4):377; 1998.
6. Kokkinos, P.F., Holland, J.C., Narayan, P., Colleran, J.A., Dotson, C.O., and Papademetriou, V., Miles run per week and high-density lipoprotein cholesterol levels in healthy, middle-aged men, *Arch. Intern. Med.*, 155:415; 1995.

7. Thompson, P.D., Yurgalevitch, S.M., Flynn, M.M., Zmuda, J.M., Spannaus-Martin, D., Saritelli, A., Bausserman, L., and Herbert, P.N., Effect of prolonged exercise training without weight loss on high-density lipoprotein metabolism in overweight men, *Metabolism*, 46:217; 1997.
8. Marti, B., Suter, E., Riesen, W.F., Tschopp, A., Wanner, H.U., and Gutzwiller, F., Effects of long-term, self-monitored exercise on the serum lipoprotein and apolipoprotein profile in middle-aged men, *Atherosclerosis*, 81:19; 1990.
9. Wood, P.D., Haskell, W.L., Blair, S.N., Williams, P.T., Krauss, R.M., Lindgren, F.T., Albers, J.J., Ho, P.H., and Farquhar, J.W., Increased exercise level and plasma lipoprotein concentrations: a one-year randomized, controlled study in sedentary middle-aged men, *Metabolism*, 32(1):31; 1983.
10. Leon, A.S., Rice, T., Mandel, S., Després, J-P., Bergeron, J., Gagnon, J., Rao, D.C., Skinner, J.S., Wilmore, J.H., and Bouchard, C., Blood lipid response to 20 weeks of supervised exercise in a large biracial population, *Metabolism*, 49(4):513; 2000.
11. Kiens, B., Jörgenson, I., Lewis, S., Jensen, G., Lithell, H., Vessby, B., Hoe, S., and Schnohr, P., Increased plasma HDL-cholesterol and apo A-I in sedentary middle-aged men after physical conditioning, *Eur. J. Clin. Invest.*, 10:203; 1980.
12. Després, J.-P., Moorjani, S., Tremblay, A., Poehlman, E.T., Lupien, P.J., Nadeau, A., and Bouchard, C., Heredity and changes in plasma lipids and lipoproteins after short-term exercise training in men, *Arteriosclerosis*, 8:402; 1998.
13. Seip, R.L., Moulin, P., Cocke, T., Tall, A., Kohrt, W.M., Mankowitz, K., Semenkovich, C.F., Ostlund, R., and Schonfeld, G., Exercise training decreases plasma cholesteryl ester transfer protein, *Arterioscler. Thromb. Vasc. Biol.*, 13:1359; 1993.
14. Ziogas, G.G., Thomas, T.R., and Harris, W.S., Exercise training, postprandial hypertriglyceridemia, and LDL subfraction distribution, *Med. Sci. Sports Exerc.*, 29(8):986; 1997.
15. Bøsheim, E., Knardahl, S., and Høstmark, A.T., Short-term effects of exercise on plasma very low density lipoproteins (VLDL) and fatty acids, *Med. Sci. Sports Exerc.*, 31(4):522; 1999.
16. Hardman, A.E., Lawrence, J.M., and Herd, S.L., Postprandial lipemia in endurance-trained people during a short interruption to training, *J. Appl. Physiol.*, 84(6):1895; 1998.
17. Gill, J.M., and Hardman, A.E., Postprandial lipemia: effects of exercise and restriction of energy intake compared, *Am. J. Clin. Nutr.*, 71(2):465; 2000.
18. Williams, P.T., Relationship of distance run per week to coronary heart disease risk factors in 8283 male runners: the National Runners' Health Study, *Arch. Intern. Med.* 157:191; 1997.
19. Coresh, J., and Kwiterovich, P.O., Jr., Small, dense low-density lipoprotein particles and coronary heart disease risk: a clear association with uncertain implications, *J.A.M.A.*, 276(11):914; 1996.
20. Williams, P.T., Krauss, R.M., Vranizan, K.M., and Wood, P.D., Changes in lipoprotein subfractions during diet-induced weight loss in moderately overweight men, *Circulation*, 81:1293; 1990.
21. Williams, P.T., Krauss, R.M., Vranizan, K.M., Albers, J.J., Terry, R.B., and Wood, P.D., Effects of exercise-induced weight loss on low density lipoprotein subfractions in healthy men, *Arteriosclerosis*, 9(5):623; 1989.
22. Halle, M., Berg, A., König, D., Keul, J., and Baumstark, M.W., Differences in the concentration and composition of low-density lipoprotein subfraction particles between sedentary and trained hypercholesterolemic men, *Metabolism*, 46(7):186; 1997.

23. Kraus, W.E., Houmard, J.A., Duscha, B.D., Knetzger, K.J., Wharton, M.B., McCartney, J.S., Bales, C.W., Henes, S., Samsa, G.P., Otvos, J.D., Kulkarni, K.R., and Slentz, C.A., Effects of the amount and intensity of exercise on plasma lipoproteins, *N. Engl. J. Med.*, 347(19):1483; 2002.
24. Kang, H.S., Gutin, B., Barbeau, P., Owens, S., Lemmon, C.R., Allison, J., Litaker, M.S., Le, N.A., Physical training improves insulin resistance syndrome markers in obese adolescents, *Med. Sci. Sports Exerc.*, 34(12):1920; 2002.
25. Beard, C.M., Barnard, R.J., Robbins, D.C., Ordovas, J.M., and Schaefer, E.J., Effects of diet and exercise on qualitative and quantitative measures of LDL and its susceptibility to oxidation, *Arterioscler. Thromb. Vasc. Biol.*, 16(2):201; 1996.
26. Parks, E.J., German, J.B., Davis, P.A., Frankel, E.N., Kappagoda, C.T., Rutledge, J.C., Hyson, D.A., and Schneeman, B.O., Reduced oxidative susceptibility of LDL from patients participating in an intensive atherosclerosis treatment program, *Am. J. Clin. Nutr.*, 69(4):778; 1998.
27. Israel, R.G., Sullivan, M.J., Marks, R.H., Cayton, R.S., and Chenier, T.C., Relationship between cardiorespiratory fitness and lipoprotein(a) in men and women, *Med. Sci. Sports Exerc.*, 26(4):425; 1994.
28. Szymanski, L.M., Durstine, J.L., Davis, P.G., Dowda, M., and Pate, R.R., Factors affecting fibrinolytic potential: cardiovascular fitness, body composition, lipoprotein(a), *Metabolism*, 45:1427; 1996.
29. Durstine, J.L., Davis, P.G., Ferguson, M.A., Alderson, N.L., and Trost, S.G., Effects of short-duration and long-duration exercise on lipoprotein(a), *Med. Sci. Sports Exerc.*, 33(9):1511; 2001.
30. Drowatzky, K.L., Durstine, J.L., Irwin, M.L., Moore, C.G., Davis, P.G., Hand, G.A., Gonzalez, M.F., and Ainsworth, B.E., The association between physical activity, cardiorespiratory fitness, and lipoprotein(a) concentrations in a triethnic sample of women: the Cross Cultural Activity Participation Study, *Vascul. Med.*, 6(1):15; 2001.
31. Leon, A.S., Gaskill, S.E., Bergeron, J., Gagnon, J., Rao, D.C., Skinner, J.S., Wilmore, J.H., and Bouchard, C., Variability in the response of HDL cholesterol to exercise training in the HERITAGE Family Study, *Int. J. Sports Med.*, 23:1; 2002.
32. Stefanick, M.L., Mackey, S., Sheehan, M., Ellsworth, N., Haskell, W.L., and Wood, P.D., Effects of diet and exercise in men and postmenopausal women with low levels of HDL cholesterol and high levels of LDL cholesterol, *N. Engl. J. Med.*, 339(1):12; 1998.
33. Tran, Z.V., Weltman, A., Glass, G.V., and Mood, D.P., The effects of exercise on blood lipids and lipoproteins: a meta-analysis of studies, *Med. Sci. Sports Exerc.*, 15(5):393; 1983.
34. Williams, P.T., Stefanick, M.L., Vranizan, K.M., and Wood, P.D., Effects of weight loss by exercise or by dieting on plasma high-density lipoprotein (HDL) levels in men with low, intermediate, and normal-to-high HDL at baseline, *Metabolism*, 43(7):917; 1994.
35. Thompson, P.D., Cullinane, E.M., Sady, S.P., Flynn, M.M., Bernier, D.N., Kantor, M.A., Saritelli, A.L., and Herbert, P.N., Modest changes in high-density lipoprotein concentrations and metabolism with prolonged exercise training, *Circulation*, 78(1):25; 1988.
36. Wood, P.D., Stefanick, M.L., Williams, P.T., and Haskell, W.L., The effects on plasma lipoproteins of a prudent weight-reducing diet, with or without exercise in overweight men and women, *N. Engl. J. Med.*, 325:461; 1991.

37. Couillard, C., Després, J.-P., Lamarche, B., Bergeron, J., Gagnon, J., Leon, A.S., Rao, D.C., Skinner, J.S., Wilmore, J.H., and Bouchard, C., Effects of endurance exercise training on plasma HDL cholesterol levels depend on levels of triglycerides: evidence from men of the Health, Risk Factors, Exercise Training and Genetics (HERITAGE) Family Study, *Arterioscler. Thromb. Vasc. Biol.*, 21(7):1226; 2001.
38. Crouse, S.F., O'Brien, B.C., Grandjean, P.W., Lowe, R.C., Rohack, J.J., and Green, J.S., Effects of training and single session of exercise on lipids and apolipoproteins in hypercholesterolemic men, *J. Appl. Physiol.*, 83(6):2019; 1997.
39. Durstine, J.L., Pate, R.R., Sparling, P.B., Wilson, G.E., Senn, M.D., and Bartoli, W.P., Lipid, lipoprotein, and iron status of elite women distance runners, *Int. J. Sports Med.*, 8:119; 1987.
40. Williams, P.T., Krauss, R.M., Vranizan, K.M., Albers, J.J., and Wood, P.D., Effects of weight-loss by exercise and by diet on apolipoproteins A-I and A-II and the particle-size distribution of high-density lipoproteins in men, *Metabolism*, 41(4):441; 1992.
41. Durstine, J.L., Grandjean, P.W., Cox, C.A., and Thompson, P.D., Lipids, lipoproteins, and exercise, *J. Cardiopulm. Rehabil.*, 22:385; 2002.
42. Velliquette, R.A., Durstine, J.L., Hand, G.A., Davis, P.G., and Ainsworth, B.E., Apolipoprotein E, an important protein involved in triglyceride and cholesterol homeostasis: physical activity implications, *Clin. Exerc. Physiol.*, 2(1):4; 2002.
43. Després, J.-P., Tremblay, A., Moorjani, S., Lupien, P.J., Theriault, G., Nadeau, A., and Bouchard, C., Long-term exercise training with constant energy intake: effects on plasma lipoprotein levels, *Int. J. Obes.*,14:85; 1990.
44. Tamai, T., Higuchi, M., Oida, K., Nakai, T., Miyabo, S., and Kobayashi, S., Effects of exercise on plasma lipoprotein metabolism, in *Integration of Sports Sciences*. Sato, Y., Poortmans, J., Hashimoto, I., and Oshida, Y., editors. *Med. Sports Sci.*, 37:430; 1992.
45. Tanabe, Y., Sasaki, J., Urata, H., Kiyonaga, A., Tanaka, H., Shindo, M., and Arakawa, K., Effects of mild aerobic exercise on lipid and apolipoprotein levels in patients with essential hypertension, *Japan. Heart J.* 29:199; 1988.
46. Taimela, S., Lehtimaki, T., Porkka, K.V., Rasanen, L., and Viikari, J.S., The effect of physical activity on serum total and low-density lipoprotein cholesterol concentrations varies with apolipoprotein E phenotype in male children and young adults: the Cardiovascular Risk in Young Finns Study, *Metabolism*, 45:797; 1996.
47. St.-Amand, J., Prud'homme, D., Moorjani, S., Nadeau, A., Tremblay, A., Bouchard, C., Lupien, P.J., and Després, J.-P., Apo E polymorphism and the relationships of physical fitness to plasma lipoprotein-lipid levels in men and women, *Med. Sci. Sports Exerc.*, 31:692; 1999.
48. Hagberg, J.M., Ferrell, R.E., Katzel, L.I., Dengel, D.R., Sorkin, J.D., and Goldberg, A.P., Apolipoprotein E genotype and exercise training-induced increases in plasma high-density lipoprotein (HDL)- and HDL_2-cholesterol levels in overweight men, *Metabolism*, 48:943; 1999.
49. Thompson, P.D., Tongalis, G.J., Seip, R.L., Bilbie, C., Miles, M., Zoeller, R., Visich, P., Gordon, P., Angelopoulos, T.J., Pascatello, L., Bausserman, L., and Moyna, N., Apolipoprotein E genotype and changes in serum lipids and maximal oxygen uptake with exercise training, *Metabolism*, 53(2):193; 2004.

50. Leon, A.S., Togashi, K., Rankinen, T. Després, J.-P., Rao, D.C., Skinner, J.S., Wilmore, J.H., and Bouchard, C., Association of apolipoprotein E polymorphism with blood lipids and maximal oxygen uptake in the sedentary state and after exercise training in the HERITAGE Family Study, *Metabolism*, 53:108; 2004.
51. Thompson, P.D., Crouse, S.F., Goodpaster, B., Kelley, D., Moyna, N., and Pescatello, L., The acute versus the chronic response to exercise, *Med. Sci. Sports Exerc.*, 33(6):S438; 2001.
52. Behall, K.M., Howe, J.C., Martel, G., Scott, W.H., and Dooly, C.R., Comparison of resistive to aerobic exercise training on cardiovascular risk factors of sedentary, overweight premenopausal and postmenopausal women, *Nutr. Res.*, 23:607; 2003.
53. Boyden, T.W., Pamenter, R.W., Going, S.B., Lohman, T.G., Hall, M.C., Houtkooper, L.B., Bunt, J.C., Ritenbaugh, C., and Aickin, M., Resistance exercise training is associated with decreases in serum low-density lipoprotein cholesterol levels in premenopausal women, *Arch. Intern. Med.*, 153:97; 1993.
54. Fahlman, M.M., Boardley, D., Lambert, C.P., and Flynn, M.G., Effects of endurance training and resistance training on plasma lipoprotein profiles in elderly women, *J. Gerontol. A Biol. Sci. Med. Sci.*, 57:B54; 2002.
55. Elliott, K.J., Sale, C., and Cable, N.T., Effects of resistance training and detraining on muscle strength and blood lipid profiles in postmenopausal women, *Br. J. Sports Med.*, 36:340; 2002.
56. Kokkinos, P.F., Hurley, B.F., Smutok, M.A., Farmer, C., Reece, C., Shulman, R., Charabogos, C., Patterson, J., Will, S., Devane-Bell, J., and Goldberg, A.P., Strength training does not improve lipoprotein-lipid profiles in men at risk for CHD, *Med. Sci. Sports Exerc.*, 32(10):1134; 1991.
57. LeMura, L.M., von Duvillard, S.P., Andreacci, J., Klebez, J.M., Chelland, S.A., and Russo, J., Lipid and lipoprotein profiles, cardiovascular fitness, body composition, and dieting during and after resistance, aerobic and combination training in young women, *Eur. J. Appl. Physiol.*, 82:451; 2000.
58. Prabhakaran, B., Dowling, E.A., Branch, J.D., Swain, D.P., and Leutholtz, B.C., Effects of 14 weeks of resistance training on lipid profile and body fat percentage in premenopausal women, *Br. J. Sports Med.*, 33:190; 1999.
59. Honkola, A., Forsen, T., and Eriksson, J., Resistance training improves the metabolic profile in individuals with type 2 diabetes, *Acta Diabetol.*, 34:245; 1997.
60. Smutok, M.A., Reece, C., Kokkinos, P.F., Farmer, C., Dawson, P., Shulman, R., DeVane-Bell, J., Patterson, J., Charabogos, C., Goldberg, A.P., and Hurley, B.F., Aerobic versus strength training for risk factor intervention in middle-aged men at high risk for coronary artery disease, *Metabolism*, 42:177; 1993.
61. Manning, J.M., Dooly-Manning, C.R., White, K., Kampa, I., Silas, S., Kesselhaut, M., and Ruoff, M., Effects of a resistive training program on lipoprotein-lipid levels in obese women, *Med. Sci. Sports. Exerc.*, 23(11):1222; 1991.
62. Wallace, M.B., Mills, B.D., and Browning, C.L., Effects of cross training on markers of insulin resistance hyperinsulinemia, *Med. Sci. Sports Exerc.*, 29:1170; 1997.
63. Petitt, D.S., Arngrimsson, S.A., and Cureton, K.J., Effect of resistance exercise on postprandial lipemia, *J. Appl. Physiol.*, 94:694; 2003.
64. Petitt, D.S., and Cureton, K.J., Effects of prior exercise on postprandial lipemia: a quantitative review, *Metabolism*, 52(4):418; 2003.

65. Zhang, J.Q., Smith, B., Langdon, M.M., Messimer, H.L., Sun, G.Y., Cox, R.H., James-Kracke, M., and Thomas, T.R., Changes in LPL(a) and reverse cholesterol transport variables during 24-h postexercise period, *Am. J. Physiol. Endocrinol. Metab.*, 283:E267; 2002.
66. Herd, S.L., Kiens, B., Boobis, L.H., and Hardman, A.E., Moderate exercise, postprandial lipemia, and skeletal muscle lipoprotein lipase activity, *Metabolism*, 50(7):756; 2001.
67. Thyfault, J.P., Richmond, S.R., Carper, M.J., Potteiger, J.A., and Hulver, M.W., Postprandial metabolism in resistance-trained versus sedentary males, *Med. Sci. Sports Exerc.*, 36(4):709; 2004.
68. Tsetsonis, N.V., Hardman, A.E., and Mastana, S.S., Acute effects of exercise on postprandial lipemia: a comparative study in trained and untrained middle-aged women, *Am. J. Clin. Nutr.*, 65:525; 1997.
69. Tsetsonis, N.V., and Hardman, A.E., Effects of low and moderate intensity treadmill walking on postprandial lipaemia in healthy young adults, *Eur. J. Appl. Physiol.* 73:419; 1996.
70. Gill, J.M.R, Murphy, M.H., and Hardman, A.E., Postprandial lipemia: effects of intermittent versus continuous exercise, *Med. Sci. Sports Exerc.*, 30(10):1515; 1998.
71. Seip, R.L., and Semenkovich, C.F., Skeletal muscle lipoprotein lipase: molecular regulation and physiologic effects in relation to exercise, *Exerc. Sport Sci. Rev.*, 26:191; 1998.
72. Kiens, B., and Lithell, H., Lipoprotein metabolism influenced by training-induced changes in human skeletal muscle, *J. Clin. Invest.*, 83:558; 1989.
73. Ehnholm, C., and Kuusi, T., Preparation, characterization, and measurement of hepatic lipase, *Methods Enzymol.*, 129:716; 1986.
74. Thompson, P.D., Cullinane, E.M., Sady, S.P., Flynn, M.M., Chenevert, C.B., and Herbert, P.N., High density lipoprotein metabolism in endurance athletes and sedentary men, *Circulation*, 84(1):140; 1991.
75. Bergeron, J., Couillard, C., Després, J-P., Gagnon, J., Leon, A.S., Rao, D.C., Skinner, J.S., Wilmore, J.H., and Bouchard, C., Race differences in the response of postheparin plasma lipoprotein lipase and hepatic lipase activity to endurance exercise training in men. *Atherosclerosis*, 159:399; 2001.
76. Seip, R.L., Mair, K., Cole, T.G., and Semenkovich, C.F., Induction of human skeletal muscle lipoprotein lipase gene expression by short-term exercise is transient, *Am. J. Physiol.*, 272(2):E255; 1997.
77. Seip, R.L., Angelopoulos, T.J., and Semenkovich, C.F., Exercise induces human lipoprotein lipase gene expression in skeletal muscle but not adipose tissue, *Am. J. Physiol.*, 268(2):E229; 1995.
78. Hamilton, M.T., Etienne, J., McClure, W.C., Pavey, B.S., and Holloway, A.K., Role of local contractile activity and muscle fiber type on LPL regulation during exercise, *Am. J. Physiol.*, 275(6):E1016; 1998.
79. Halverstadt, A., Phares, D.A., Ferrell, R.E., Wilund, K.R., Goldberg, A.P., and Hagberg, J.M., High-density lipoprotein-cholesterol, its subfraction, and responses to exercise training are dependent on endothelial lipase genotype, *Metabolism*, 52(11):1505; 2003.
80. Kantor, M.A., Cullinane, E.M., Sady, S.P., Herbert, P.N., and Thompson, P.D., Exercise acutely increases high density lipoprotein-cholesterol and lipoprotein lipase activity in trained and untrained men. *Metabolism*, 36(2):188; 1987.

81. Quintao, E., Is reverse cholesterol transport a misnomer for suggesting its role in the prevention of atheroma formation?, *Atherosclerosis*, 116:1; 1995.
82. Gupta, A.K., Ross, E.A., Myers, J.N., and Kashyap, M.L., Increased reverse cholesterol transport in athletes, *Metabolism*, 42(6):684; 1993.
83. Ferguson, M.A., Alderson, N.L., Trost, S.G., Essig, D.A., Burke, J.R., and Durstine, J.L., Effects of four different single exercise sessions on lipids, lipoproteins, and lipoprotein lipase, *J Appl. Physiol.*, 85(3):1169; 1998.
84. Kantor, M.A., Cullinane, E.M., Herbert, P.N., and Thompson, P.D., Acute increase in lipoprotein lipase following prolonged exercise, *Metabolism*, 33(5):454; 1984.
85. Serrat-Serrat, J., Ordonez-Llanos, J., Serra-Grima, R., Gomez-Gerique, J.A., Pellicer-Thoma, E., Payes-Romero, A., and Gonzalez-Sastre, F., Marathon runners presented lower serum cholesteryl ester transfer activity than sedentary subjects. *Atherosclerosis*, 101:43; 1993.
86. Föger, B., Wohlfarter, T., Ritsch, A., Lechleitner, M., Miller, C.H., Dienstl, A., and Patsch, J.R., Kinetics of lipids, apolipoproteins, and cholesteryl ester transfer protein in plasma after a bicycle marathon. *Metabolism*, 43(5):633; 1994.
87. Marniemi, J., Dahlstrom, S., Kvist, M., Seppanen, A., and Hietanen, E., Dependence of serum lipid and lecithin: cholesterol acyltransferase levels on physical training in young men, *Eur. J. Appl. Physiol.* 49:25; 1982.
88. Haskell, W.L., The J.B. Wolf Memorial Lecture. Health consequences of physical activity: understanding and challenges regarding dose-response, *Med. Sci. Sports Exerc.*, 26:649; 1994.
89. Wood, P.D., Physical activity, diet, and health: independent and interactive effects, *Med. Sci. Sports Exerc.*, 26:838; 1994.
90. Berg, A., Frey, I., Baumstark, M.W., Halle, M., and Keul, J., Physical activity and lipoprotein lipid disorders, *Sports Med.*, 17:6; 1994.
91. Duncan, J.J., Gordon, N.F., and Scott, C.B., Women walking for health and fitness: how much is enough, *J.A.M.A.*, 266:3295; 1991.
92. King, A.C., Haskell, W.L., Young, D.R., Oka, R.K., and Staefanick, M.L., Long term effects of varying intensities and formats of physical activity on participation rates, fitness, and lipoproteins in men and women age 50 to 65 years, *Circulation*, 91:2596; 1995.
93. Sunami, Y., Motoyama, M., Kinoshita, F., Mizooka, Y., Sueta, K., Matsunaga, A., Sasaki, J., Tanaka, H., and Shindo, M., Effects of low-intensity aerobic training on the high-density lipoprotein cholesterol concentration in healthy elderly subjects, *Metabolism*, 48:984; 1999.
94. Spate-Douglas, T., and Keyser, R.E., Exercise intensity: its effect on the high-density lipoprotein profile, *Arach. Phys. Med. Rehabil.* 80:691; 1991.
95. Kraus, W.E., Houmard, J.A., Duscha, B.D., Knetzger, K.J., Wharton, M.B., McCartney, J.S., Bales, C.W., Henes, S., Samsa, G.P., Otvos, J.D., Kulkarni, K.R., and Slentz, C.A., Effects of the amount and intensity of exercise on plasma lipoproteins, *N. Engl. J. Med.*, 347:1482; 2002.
96. Kokkinos, P.F., and Fernhall, B., Physical activity and high density lipoprotein cholesterol levels: what is the relationship? *Sports Med.*, 28:307; 1999.
97. Hamilton, M.T., Hamilton, D.G., and Zderic, T.W., Exercise physiology versus inactivity physiology: an essential concept for understanding lipoprotein lipase regulation, *Exerc. Sport Sci. Rev.*, 32(4):161; 2004.

98. Bey, L., and Hamilton, M.T., Suppression of skeletal muscle lipoprotein lipase activity during physical inactivity: a molecular reason to maintain daily low-intensity activity. *J. Physiol.*, 551:673, 2003.
99. Bey, L., Akunuri, N., Zhao, P., Hoffman, E.P., Hamilton, D.G., and Hamilton, M.T., Patterns of global gene expression in rat skeletal muscle during unloading and low-intensity ambulatory activity. *Physiol. Genomics*, 13:157; 2003.
100. Executive Summary of the Third Report of the National Cholesterol Education Program (NCEP) Expert Panel on Detection, Evaluation, and Treatment of High Blood Cholesterol in Adults (Adult Treatment Panel III), *JAMA*, 285(19):2486; 2001.
101. Wilson, P.W., D' Agostino, R.B., Levy, D., Belanger, A.M., Silbershatz, H., and Kannel, W.B., Prediction of coronary heart disease using risk factor categories, *Circulation*, 97:1837; 1998.
102. Cao, J., Savage, P., Brochu, M., and Ades, P., Prevalence of lipid-lowering therapy at cardiac rehabilitation entry: 2000 versus 1996, *J Cardiopulm. Rehabil.*, 22:80; 2002.

13

Acute Changes in Lipids and Lipoprotein-Lipids Induced by Exercise

Stephen F. Crouse

CONTENTS

Introduction 283
Acute HDL-C and HDL-C Subfraction Changes with Exercise 284
Changes in Blood Triglycerides after Exercise 285
Post-Exercise Changes in Total Cholesterol and LDL Cholesterol 290
Lipoprotein (a) after Exercise 291
Apolipoproteins and Exercise-Induced Changes 291
Mechanisms for Changes in Blood Lipids and Lipoproteins Following Exercise 292
Other Exercise Considerations for Lipid Benefit 293
Summary 294
References 295

Introduction

Under normal fed conditions in humans, lipids stored in muscle and circulating in blood are an important source of energy to perform physical exercise. The proportion of energy coming from oxidation of lipids, primarily fatty acids, during exercise is a function of the work intensity. At relatively low to moderate intensities (< 65% VO_{2max}), lipid oxidation may supply more than half of the energy required by exercise, but at higher intensities most energy is provided through oxidation of carbohydrate.[1] Regardless of the energy source during exercise, lipids are the predominant fuel oxidized during recovery from exercise. Thus an acute change in blood (and muscle) lipid concentrations is a natural consequence of the use of this energy source for the work of physical exercise. This is especially the case when the work demands of exercise can be met predominantly by aerobic means. Furthermore, metabolic, hormonal, and physiologic effects of a single session of exercise, especially intense and prolonged exercise, may take hours or days from which to fully recover. For example, muscle insulin sensitivity, glucose transport, and uptake of blood triglycerides (TG) are increased for at least several hours after a single session of exercise.[2,3] Thus, a rationale for acute changes in blood lipid concentrations is firmly based on known exercise-induced changes in fuel metabolism.

These acute blood lipid changes lasting for hours or days after exercise may be at least partly responsible for the anti-atherogenic lipid profile characteristic of physically trained persons. This hypothesis was proposed quite some time ago following observations that blood TG and total cholesterol (TC) concentrations were often lower, while high-density lipoprotein cholesterol (HDL-C) concentrations were often higher up to 44 h after exercise.[4–8] Attempts to verify these early findings have produced hundreds of studies with results that vary widely. A careful review of the related literature will show that factors that could spuriously affect the post-exercise lipid concentrations were not controlled in a majority of the published studies. There was wide inter-study variability with respect to exercise mode, intensity, duration, and volume, all factors that could impact post-exercise lipid concentrations. Often exercise-induced changes in plasma volume were not considered when reporting blood lipid concentrations. The timing of blood collection relative to the exercise session was not uniformly controlled among existing studies. Not surprisingly for human studies, inter-study variation exists with respect to such potentially confounding variables as subject age, training history, gender, menopausal status, diet, body weight, body fat, and pre-exercise blood lipid concentrations.[9,10] The acute exercise studies selected for review in this chapter include those in which the methods provide some level of control for changes in plasma volume induced by exercise (Table 13.1).

Acute HDL-C and HDL-C Subfraction Changes with Exercise

It is well documented from case-control study designs that runners show higher blood HDL-C concentrations as compared to non-runners.[9,11–13] However, in studies in which untrained subjects were trained under controlled conditions, only about half show significant improvements in HDL-C concentrations.[13] Several of the early cross-sectional and training studies did not control for the timing of the last session of exercise before blood samples were taken. Thus, it is very possible that many studies actually were measuring acute changes in HDL-C rather than a training effect. As evidence that this could be the case, several well-controlled studies have shown that HDL-C concentrations were raised by a single session of aerobic exercise. In the majority of published studies related to acute exercise and lipids, a delayed increase in blood HDL-C concentration was noted 24–72 h after exercise, and ranged from 4% to 34% over pre-exercise values.[14–21] Even individuals with high blood cholesterol may benefit from this short-term rise in blood HDL-C.[10,22,23] Some data suggest that a volume threshold exists for the HDL-C change that depends on the functional capacity of the individual. Research has shown that in trained individuals up to 1000 kcal of exercise energy expenditure is necessary to produce significant elevations in blood HDL-C concentrations, whereas 350–400 kcal energy expenditure is sufficient to elicit significant increases in less well-trained and sedentary persons.[10,15,20,21,24]

The subfractions of HDL-C identified by ultracentrifugation, namely the relatively more buoyant HDL_2-C and the denser HDL_3-C, may confer protection from cardiovascular disease. Although some differences exist in the metabolism of these lipoproteins, both have been shown to be inversely related to heart disease.[25] Studies show that both may be acutely elevated after exercise.[10,14–16,19–23,26] As with HDL-C, training status may influence the response of the HDL subfractions. However, this issue has been addressed only rarely, so conclusions are tenuous. In a study to compare the exercise response in untrained and trained men, Kantor et al.[18] reported that HDL_2-C concentration was acutely elevated in trained men following aerobic exercise, while in untrained men HDL_3-C was higher. In contrast, Crouse et al.[10] found that blood HDL_3-C, but not HDL_2-C, concentration was higher following a single session of aerobic exercise completed by men with elevated cholesterol before and after 6 months of aerobic training. In support for an acute increase in the relatively denser HDL_3-C subspecies, HDL density assayed by ultracentrifugation was reportedly reduced for up to 2 days in physically active women after aerobic exercise.[27] This finding demonstrates that there may be a shift from the less dense (HDL_2) to the more dense (HDL_3) HDL subspecies following aerobic exercise. Although several questions remain unanswered (e.g., which HDL subspecies is changed with exercise and what volume of exercise is required to produce a beneficial change), it is clear from these studies that HDL-C and HDL-C subspecies are responsive to a single session of exercise, and that the response generally results in a less atherogenic lipid profile.

Changes in Blood Triglycerides after Exercise

In addition to the beneficial effects of exercise on HDL, it is reported in the majority of controlled acute exercise studies that TG concentrations fall significantly after a single session of aerobic exercise. This beneficial fall in circulating TG persists for up to 72 h.[10,14–16,19–23] The acute effect does not appear to depend on an individual's training experience, intensity, or mode of aerobic exercise. There have been relatively few well-controlled studies

TABLE 13.1

Acute Exercise Studies Selected for Review

First Author, Year[ref #]	Subject	Timing	TC	TG	VLDL-C	LDL-C	HDL-C	HDL2-C	HDL3-C	APO A-I	APO A-II	APO B	APO E	LPLa	HTGLa	LCATa	CETPa	CETPm
Bounds, 2000[14]	14, m, 28, t, 50.2	pre-exercise	160	113	nr	89	48	13.5	35	nr	nr	nr	nr	nr	nr	nr	nr	nr
		IPE	–5.1*	–14.1	nr	ns	1.6	ns	0	nr	nr	nr	nr	nr	nr	nr	nr	nr
		+24 h	0.5	–16.4*	nr	ns	10.5*	ns	7.7*	nr	nr	nr	nr	nr	nr	nr	nr	nr
		+48 h	–3.1	–25.9*	nr	ns	8.1*	ns	2.2	nr	nr	nr	nr	nr	nr	nr	nr	nr
Crouse, 1997[10]	26, m, 47, t, 42.9	pre-exercise	251	163	nr	171	46	10.9	36.4	135	nr	95	nr	nr	nr	nr	nr	nr
		IPE	–3.2*	3.7	nr	–0.6	0	–13.8	0.5	–2.2	nr	–2.1	nr	nr	nr	nr	nr	nr
		+24 h	0	–9.8*	nr	5.3*	6.5*	6.4	5.8*	3.0*	nr	4.2*	nr	nr	nr	nr	nr	nr
		+48 h	1.6*	–6.8*	nr	5.9*	4.4*	14.7*	3.6*	0.7	nr	1.1	nr	nr	nr	nr	nr	nr
Crouse, 1995[22]	39, m, 46, ut, 31	pre-exercise	254	177	nr	173	45	6.2	38.5	141	nr	99	nr	nr	nr	nr	nr	nr
		IPE	–4.7*	–5.7	nr	–4.1*	–2.2	ns	–2.9	ns	nr	0	nr	nr	nr	nr	nr	nr
		+24 h	1.2	–18.6*	nr	5.8*	6.7*	ns	8.3*	ns	nr	9.1*	nr	nr	nr	nr	nr	nr
		+48 h	4.7*	–14.7*	nr	8.1*	8.9*	ns	7.0*	ns	nr	9.1*	nr	nr	nr	nr	nr	nr
Davis, 1992[33]	10, m, 28, t, 62	–24 h	150	85	14	80	57	12	45	111	40	78	nr	nr	nr	nr	nr	nr
		pre-exercise	ns	ns	ns	ns	ns	ns	ns	ns	ns	ns	nr	nr	nr	nr	nr	nr
		IPE	ns	ns	ns	ns	ns	ns	ns	ns	ns	ns	nr	nr	nr	nr	nr	nr
		+1 h	ns	ns	ns	ns	ns	ns	ns	ns	ns	ns	nr	nr	nr	nr	nr	nr
		+24 h	ns	ns	ns	ns	ns	ns	ns	ns	ns	ns	nr	nr	nr	nr	nr	nr
		+48 h	ns	ns	ns	ns	ns	ns	ns	ns	ns	ns	nr	nr	nr	nr	nr	nr
		+72 h	ns	ns	ns	ns	ns	ns	ns	ns	ns	ns	nr	nr	nr	nr	nr	nr
Ferguson, 1998[15]	11, m, 26, t, 56.2	–24 h	166	101	20	101	45	14	31	nr	nr	nr	nr	13.1	19.5	nr	nr	nr
		pre-exercise	169	110	22	105	42	14	28	nr	nr	nr	nr	nr	nr	nr	nr	nr
		IPE	–6.5	1	0	–18.1*	21.4*	28.6*	17.9	nr	nr	nr	nr	–8.4	–15.4	nr	nr	nr
		+24 h	–4.7	–36.4*	–36.4*	–11.4*	28.6*	35.7*	25.0*	nr	nr	nr	nr	48.9*	–4.6	nr	nr	nr

		+48 h	–3	–20*	–22.7*	–10.5	23.8*	42.9*	14.3	nr	nr	nr	nr	47.3*	–18	nr	nr	nr
Ferguson, 2003[24]	11, m, 27, t, 56.2	–24 h	166	101	20	101	45	14	31	nr	nr	nr	nr	nr	nr	nr	nr	nr
		pre-exercise	4.37	1.24	0.57	2.72	1.09	0.36	0.72	nr	nr	nr	nr	nr	nr	nr	nr	nr
		During Ex 1	–4.81	–3.23	–8.77	–9.56	9.17	–5.56	18.06	nr	nr	nr	nr	nr	nr	nr	nr	nr
		During Ex 2	–6.41*	–5.65	–5.26	–15.44*	9.17	0.00	15.28	nr	nr	nr	nr	nr	nr	nr	nr	nr
		During Ex 3	–5.26	–6.45	–5.26	–9.56	4.59	–13.89	15.28	nr	nr	nr	nr	nr	nr	nr	nr	nr
		During Ex 4	–8.47*	–1.61	–5.26	–16.18*	6.42	–5.56	11.11	nr	nr	nr	nr	nr	nr	nr	nr	nr
		During Ex 5	–7.78*	–4.03	0	–15.44	6.42	0.00	15.28	nr	nr	nr	nr	nr	nr	nr	nr	nr
		IPE	–6.41	0.81	0	–18.38*	21.1*	30.56*	18.06	nr	nr	nr	nr	nr	nr	nr	nr	nr
Foger, 1994[16]	8, m, 34, t, nr	–48 h	224	132	nr	130	67	12	55	144	53	77	nr	nr	nr	nr	109	1.23
		+24	–33*	–69*	nr	–38*	–9	8	–13	–24*	–25*	–31*	nr	nr	nr	nr	–25	–31*
		+48	–1	–18*	nr	–18*	33*	92*	20*	20*	25*	3	nr	nr	nr	nr	6	–15*
		+72	2	–5	nr	–12*	34*	150*	11	23*	19*	3	nr	nr	nr	nr	8	–10
		+120	4	17	nr	–3	15	83*	0	19*	19*	5	nr	nr	nr	nr	10	–5
		+192	1	19	nr	–5	6	42*	–2	10*	19*	8	nr	nr	nr	nr	10	1
Goodyear, 1990[17]	12, f, 25, t, 53	–24 h	197	49	nr	115	72	nr	nr	nr	nr	nr	nr	nr	nr	nr	nr	nr
		+10 min	–5.1	159.2*	nr	–25.2*	5.6	nr	nr	nr	nr	nr	nr	nr	nr	nr	nr	nr
		+24 h	–13.2*	2.2	nr	–31.3*	15.3*	nr	nr	nr	nr	nr	nr	nr	nr	nr	nr	nr
		+72 h	–9.1*	14.3	nr	–13	–5.6	nr	nr	nr	nr	nr	nr	nr	nr	nr	nr	nr
		+120 h	–14.7*	6.1	nr	–18.3	–9.7	nr	nr	nr	nr	nr	nr	nr	nr	nr	nr	nr
Grandjean, 2000[23]	25, m, 45, ut, 33.3	–24h	217	144	nr	147	42	9	34	nr	nr	nr	nr	13.1	21.1	nr	31.4	nr
		IPE	–3.2*	–2.8	nr	–5.4	2.4	–11	2.9*	nr	nr	nr	nr	7.6	–6.6	nr	–0.3	nr
		+24 h	0.5	–11.1*	nr	–2.0	9.5*	11	8.8*	nr	nr	nr	nr	20.6*	–0.5	nr	2.9	nr
		+48 h	0	–11.1*	nr	–2.7	14.3*	11	8.8*	nr	nr	nr	nr	12.2	–3.8	nr	4.8	nr
Hughes, 1991(30)	32, f, 22, ut, 39.4	pre-exercise	167	78	nr	98	54	nr	nr	nr	nr	nr	nr	nr	nr	nr	nr	nr
		+10 min	2.7	3.0	nr	2.5	4.3	nr	nr	nr	nr	nr	nr	nr	nr	nr	nr	nr
		+1 h	0	–9.6	nr	0	2.5	nr	nr	nr	nr	nr	nr	nr	nr	nr	nr	nr
		+24 h	–1.3	–18.6*	nr	–1.0	1	nr	nr	nr	nr	nr	nr	nr	nr	nr	nr	nr
		+48 h	–2.1	–21.6*	nr	–1.0	1	nr	nr	nr	nr	nr	nr	nr	nr	nr	nr	nr

TABLE 13.1 (CONTINUED)

Acute Exercise Studies Selected for Review

First Author, Year[ref #]	Subject	Timing	TC	TG	VLDL-C	LDL-C	HDL-C	HDL2-C	HDL3-C	APO A-I	APO A-II	APO B	APO E	LPLa	HTGLa	LCATa	CETPa	CETPm
Imanura, 2000[34]	7, f, 22, ut, 36.2	−1 h	145.1	61.9	nr	78.4	53.6	37.4	15.1	116.7	25	60.4	nr	nr	nr	nr	nr	nr
		IPE	−0.14	−4.039	nr	−0.128	2.61	1.604	−1.987	3.085	1.6	−0.828	nr	nr	nr	nr	nr	nr
	30 min of exercise at 60% VO_{2max}	+.5 h	0.207	−3.716	nr	2.934	3.358	1.872	5.96	4.456	3.2	2.815	nr	nr	nr	nr	nr	nr
		+1 h	1.241	−3.231	nr	0.255	0.56	0	1.325	0.771	0.8	−0.166	nr	nr	nr	nr	nr	nr
		+2 h	−0.35	−2.908	nr	0	−0.933	−0.535	1.325	0.771	0.8	−0.497	nr	nr	nr	nr	nr	nr
		+24 h	1.103	22.132	nr	−0.51	0.933	−1.872	1.325	3.428	2.4	3.642	nr	nr	nr	nr	nr	nr
		−1 h	148.3	64.4	nr	81.4	53.3	36.5	15.2	116.9	25	62.6	nr	nr	nr	nr	nr	nr
		IPE	0.674	−7.453	nr	0.246	1.126	3.288	−3.947	2.31	−0.8	0.479	nr	nr	nr	nr	nr	nr
	60 min of exercise at 60% VO_{2max}	+.5 h	−0.41	−6.677	nr	3.194	0.188	1.918	−0.658	0.855	0.8	0	nr	nr	nr	nr	nr	nr
		+1 h	−0.14	−2.64	nr	0.246	0.563	0	0.658	−0.684	0	−0.958	nr	nr	nr	nr	nr	nr
		+2 h	1.888	−3.106	nr	−0.123	1.501	3.014	1.316	0.684	−0.4	−1.118	nr	nr	nr	nr	nr	nr
		+24 h	−0.94	−7.919	nr	−0.369	0.563	2.74	5.921	0.086	0.4	−1.438	nr	nr	nr	nr	nr	nr
Kantor, 1987[18]	11, m, 33, t, 48	−24 h	197	94	nr	126	51	18	33	nr	nr	nr	nr	8.3	13.6	nr	nr	nr
		+10 min	−2.0	−14.9	nr	−4.0*	3.9*	nr	nr	nr	nr	nr	nr	−13.4*	−2.2	nr	nr	nr
		+24 h	1.5	−6.4	nr	1.0	7.8*	nr	nr	nr	nr	nr	nr	10.8*	2.9	nr	nr	nr
		+48 h	3.6*	2.1	nr	1.6	9.8*	16.7*	3.0	nr	nr	nr	nr	1.2	5.9	nr	nr	nr
		+72 h	3.1	0.0	nr	1.6	9.8*	22.2*	3.0	nr	nr	nr	nr	8.4	8.8*	nr	nr	nr
	10, m, 32, ut, 34	−24 h	195	97	nr	136	39	11	28	nr	nr	nr	nr	8.8	15.4	nr	nr	nr
		+10 min	−3.6*	6.2	nr	−7.4*	0	nr	nr	nr	nr	nr	nr	−12.5*	−6.5	nr	nr	nr

		+24 h	1.0	8.3	nr	2.2	7.7*	nr	nr	nr	nr	nr	nr	10.2*	−3.3	nr	nr	nr
		+48 h	5.1*	13.4	nr	2.9	7.7*	−1.0	14.3*	nr	nr	nr	nr	1.1	−5.8	nr	nr	nr
		+72 h	4.1*	7.2	nr	1.5	7.7*	−1.0	14.3*	nr	nr	nr	nr	2.3	−5.2	nr	nr	nr
Sady, 1986[19]	10, m, 35, t, nr	−24 h	197	80	nr	118	63	26	38	156	32	nr	nr	10.4	12.2	nr	nr	nr
		+18 h	−4	−26*	nr	−8	10*	19*	4	0	−3	nr	nr	46*	−4	nr	nr	nr
Visich, 1996[20]	12, m, 26, t, 56.4	−24 h	164	67	nr	113	40	16	23	nr	nr	nr	nr	9.9	12.7	nr	nr	nr
		IPE	−3.8	−14.5*	nr	−3.1	−2.9	−7.1	0	nr	nr	nr	nr	nr	nr	nr	nr	nr
		+1 h	1.0	−13.2*	nr	1.4	1	0	3.3	nr	nr	nr	nr	nr	nr	nr	nr	nr
		+6 h	3.3	nr	nr	nr	2.9	7.1	3.3	nr	nr	nr	nr	2.0	−9.5	nr	nr	nr
		+24 h	3.3	−13.2*	nr	3.8	5.8*	0	11.7*	nr	nr	nr	nr	19.2*	−14.2*	nr	nr	nr
Yu, 1999[41]	22-m, 6-f, 35, t	−48 h	165	124	43.1	79	43	nr	nr	148	34	73	3.4	nr	nr	nr	nr	nr
		+15 min	−7.3*	−22.58*	−51.74*	−3.40	30.23*	nr	nr	−3.38	3.53	−12.33*	−2.94	nr	nr	nr	nr	nr

Subject information is: subject number, gender, male (m) or female (f); age in years; training status: mixed trained (mx), trained (t), untrained (ut); and VO_{2peak} (ml/kg/min). Baseline lipids and lipoprotein-lipids are given as mg/dl, then percent change from baseline. Baseline LPLa (mmol FFA/ml/h), HTGLa (mmol FFA/ml/h), $LCAT_a$ (mmol cholest/L/h), CETPa (%CE transferred/4 h), CETP mass (mg/ml).

In Crouse et al.,[10] LDL-C was reported for 50% intensity group, and HDL_2-C was reported for 80% intensity group.

* Significantly different from baseline, $p < 0.05$.

published on women. Those that exist suggest some gender differences with respect to acute TG responsiveness after exercise. In premenopausal women, it has been reported that exercise of low and high intensity resulted in an increase in TG concentration immediately following aerobic exercise.[17,28] The reason for this different response in women compared with men is not known, but it may be related to gender differences in LPL activity (discussion to follow).[29] Others have shown that despite an immediate post-exercise rise in TG concentrations in women, values may fall below pre-exercise values by 1 h and up to 48 h after exercise.[30] Thus, it can be concluded from the results of existing studies that blood TG concentrations are more resistant to change with exercise in women than in men.

As with HDL-C, there are published data to suggest that a threshold of about 350 kcal of energy must be expended before a significant change in circulating TG will occur; however, this finding is not universal. In this regard, when higher thresholds have been reported the subjects were relatively well-trained men.[15] It has also been reported that those with the highest pre-exercise TG values show the greatest post-exercise decrease.[18,22,31,32]

Post-Exercise Changes in Total Cholesterol and LDL Cholesterol

The response pattern of blood total cholesterol (TC) concentration following exercise reportedly varies from an increase to a decrease after a single session of exercise. Increased blood TC concentrations were found in untrained men with normal and high blood cholesterol for up to 48 h after a single session of aerobic exercise.[10,18,22] In contrast, post-exercise reductions in TC have been reported in men and women who were trained and untrained.[10,14,18,22,23,28] Reductions that have been reported generally do not persist for long (< 24 h), and are modest at best, ranging from 3% to 5%. Some evidence suggests that high-volume exercise (e.g., marathon) may produce TC reductions lasting up to 120 h post-exercise, especially in trained women.[16,17] In addition to these studies in which blood TC was altered, there are several published reports in which blood TC concentrations did not change after a single session of exercise.[15,19,20,30,33,34] Thus, the weight of the evidence supports the conclusion that a single session of exercise has little or no effect on circulating TC. When effects have been shown to occur at all, they were modest and short-lived.

Similar to study results with respect to blood TC, the published response to exercise of blood low-density lipoprotein cholesterol (LDL-C) concentration has been variable. In women LDL-C concentration was reportedly reduced 24 h after a single session of high-intensity, high-volume exercise.[17,28] Others report no change in this lipoprotein concentration in untrained women after more moderate amounts of aerobic exercise.[30,34] Furthermore,

LDL density, as assessed by ultracentrifugation, was not altered in either normal- or hypercholesterolemic women by a single session of aerobic exercise.[27] In support of these findings, Lamon-Fava et al.[35] reported that LDL particle size did not change in women after completion of a marathon, but increased in men. Reasons for this apparent gender effect are not known. Following intense endurance events, LDL-C concentrations in men were variously reduced from 0% to 38% for up to 72 h.[14–16,19,20] In men with high cholesterol, LDL-C concentration has been shown to increase and decrease from 5% to 8% after exercise.[22,23] Reasons for the conflicting findings are not presently known, but may be related to study differences in the volume of exercise performed, or to the training status of the subjects. While rare, some studies exist which suggest exercise may acutely produce harmful effects on lipoproteins. After long-duration, high-volume exercise (marathon), circulating LDL has been shown to be more susceptible to oxidation making it more atherogenic.[36]

Lipoprotein (a) after Exercise

Lipoprotein (a) [Lp(a)] is a modification of LDL in that the apolipoprotein B-100 of LDL is linked to a glycoprotein, apoprotein (a). An elevated blood concentration of Lp(a) is a strong risk factor for cardiovascular disease.[37,38] Several studies have been conducted to explore the effect of exercise on this lipid risk marker, since it is thought that lowering Lp(a) would reduce the risk of cardiovascular disease. Overall, Lp(a) appears to be relatively resistant to many interventions, including exercise. Lp(a) was not changed in men and women immediately after and up to 7 days after a single session of cycle ergometer or treadmill exercise.[39,40] However, Lp(a) was reduced 18% when measured 15 min after men and women completed a triathlon.[41] Thus, the weight of published evidence, although sparse, suggests that Lp(a) is unresponsive to a single session of exercise under normal circumstances, but may be reduced by exercise when the volume performed is extremely high.

Apolipoproteins and Exercise-Induced Changes

The majority of the circulating apolipoproteins A-1 and B are found in HDL and LDL, respectively. Apo A-1 is inversely and apo B directly related to CVD risk.[42] Only a very few acute exercise studies have been published to date in which apo A-1 and apo B were measured. In men with high blood cholesterol, apo B concentrations rose an average of 4–9% after a single session of exercise at a moderate intensity.[10,22] In contrast, apo B concentrations were not altered by strenuous exercise performed by well-trained men.[16]

Foger et al.[16] reported that apo A-I and A-II concentrations were reduced about 25% immediately after completion of a bicycle marathon. Subsequent measurements made during 8 days of recovery revealed that blood concentrations of these apolipoproteins rose 10–20% above pre-exercise values. In several other studies, increases in apo A-1 were minimal (e.g., 3% rise) or nonexistent following more modest amounts of exercise.[10,19,22,43] In one of the few studies published to date in which apo E was measured, there was no change in the blood concentration of this apolipoprotein after a triathlon.[41] Whether or not a single session of exercise affects blood concentrations of other circulating apolipoproteins is currently not known.

Mechanisms for Changes in Blood Lipids and Lipoproteins Following Exercise

The intravascular biotransformation and metabolism of circulating lipoproteins is regulated by a number of proteins and enzymes. The enzymes and proteins most frequently studied for their potential regulatory effects in response to exercise include endothelial-bound lipoprotein lipase (LPL), hepatic triglyceride lipase (HTGL), cholesteryl ester transfer protein (CETP), and lecithin:cholesteryl acyltransferase (LCAT).

Intravascular remodeling of several lipoproteins, notably VLDL, LDL, and HDL, is affected by CETP activity. This protein participates in the exchange of cholesterol and triglyceride among HDL and triglyceride-rich lipoproteins. If affected by the exercise stimulus, it could contribute to the modification of blood lipoprotein-lipid concentrations noted to occur after aerobic exercise. Results of a longitudinal exercise training study suggest that CETP genotype may contribute to the inter-individual differences in blood HDL subfraction changes that occur with exercise training. However, few acute exercise studies have been published in which this protein mass or activity was measured. In those that have been published results were variable, but it was generally reported that CETP activity was unchanged after a single session of exercise.[23,26] However, there is also evidence that CETP mass may be reduced up to 2 days after exercise.[16] A reduction in CETP mass could increase the proportion of the total circulating cholesterol carried in HDL, thus increasing HDL-C concentration, since a lower CETP mass would likely result in less cholesterol transferred to other lipoproteins in exchange for TG. With such a paucity of published research, it cannot be conclusively stated that there is no acute effect of exercise on CETP, but the current evidence suggests there is not.

Endothelial-bound LPL is generally accepted to be an important modulator of circulating TG concentration and, through its action on TG, a factor related to the change in HDL-C after exercise. LPL activity is acutely increased after a single session of exercise, usually reaching maximal activity by 24–48 h after exercise.[15,19,20,23,44] The peak increase in LPL is related in time to the maximal decrease in post-exercise TG concentration and the peak increase in HDL-C. Gender differences in the acute response to exercise of skeletal muscle and adipose tissue LPL activity have been reported. Three to four hours after 90 min of aerobic cycling exercise, muscle and adipose tissue LPL activity was higher in men, but unchanged from rest in women.[29] This gender-specific response, if verified by additional research, may provide a mechanistic explanation for the findings that blood TG concentration is more resistant to change after exercise in women than in men.

Hepatic triglyceride lipase activity, thought to be another important modulator of circulating lipoprotein-lipids, is generally found to be reduced or not changed for up to 72 h after exercise.[15,18–20,23] Thompson et al.[45] reported that HDL protein circulatory survival time was increased in endurance trained men compared with untrained men. A decrease in HTGL activity, if it occurs, could be at least partly responsible for a prolonged survival time for HDL in the circulation. Such an increased survival time would, in turn, result in an increase in circulating HDL concentration.

Several lines of research show the importance of LCAT activity in the reverse cholesterol transport process. LCAT activity is critical for the uptake of cholesterol from peripheral tissues by nascent HDL and HDL apolipoproteins. Such important action makes LCAT a theoretical target through which the exercise stimulus may mediate an increase in HDL-C and reverse cholesterol transport. Research efforts to measure an increase in LCAT activity after a single session of exercise have largely been unsuccessful. No change in LCAT activity has been found after a single session of exercise performed by recreational runners and untrained men. However, a large volume of exercise performed by trained men has been shown to result in increased LCAT activity.[23,46–48] Thus, a conclusion to be drawn from the published literature is that LCAT is relatively unresponsive to a single session of exercise, unless the exercise is of relatively high volume performed by trained individuals.

Other Exercise Considerations for Lipid Benefit

Aerobic exercise is generally prescribed along the dimensions of mode, frequency, intensity, duration, and volume (caloric expenditure).[49] The literature supports the conclusion that regular exercise must be performed at a frequency of every other day to maintain the beneficial acute effect. This conclusion is founded on the published literature which shows that, even after exhaustive exercise performed by trained athletes, the exercise benefit lasts only up to 3 days.[16] Further evidence to support this conclusion comes from studies in which exercise was withheld from endurance-trained athletes. Hardman et al.[50] reported that the ability to clear blood lipids after a fat meal was reduced, and blood TG, very-low density lipoprotein-cholesterol (VLDL-C), and the TC to HDL-C ratio were higher 60 h and 6.5 days after well-trained endurance athletes stopped exercising.

The studies related to exercise intensity provide results that are less conclusive. Those that do exist often yield questionable results because experimenters did not control the volume of exercise among intensity groups.[51–53] A review of these studies will show that often subjects exercised at relatively higher intensities also had a higher caloric expenditure during exercise than their lower-intensity counterparts. Since the caloric cost of exercise may affect the acute lipid response, these studies are not helpful in determining the independent effect of exercise intensity. With this in mind, there are several controlled studies published in which it was shown that the intensity at which exercise was performed did not affect the acute lipid response, as long as the caloric expenditure was equivalent.[22,33]

Some evidence exists to show that the pattern and magnitude of acute lipid changes after a single session of exercise may be altered by training. Crouse et al.[10] reported that an LDL-C increase following aerobic exercise in men with high cholesterol was no longer evident after 6 months of aerobic training. Also, training status may affect the lipid response pattern to low- or high-intensity exercise in normocholesterolemic individuals. In studies in which well-trained runners served as subjects, high intensity compared with low-intensity exercise produced relatively greater acute increases in HDL-C concentrations.[51,54] Taken as a whole, the published literature generally supports the conclusion that any effect of exercise intensity cannot be separated from the training status of those exercising, and the volume (caloric cost) of exercise performed.

Summary

Research supports the conclusion that blood lipids, lipoprotein-lipids, and lipid regulatory enzymes can be altered after a single session of aerobic exercise. The post-exercise changes are consistent with a reduction in heart and vascular disease risk. Since the benefit is lost after about 72 h, published recommendations that exercise should be performed at a frequency of every other day are justified. The intensity at which the exercise is performed is less important than the volume. Evidence demonstrates that significant acute effects occur at an exercise volume (dose) of exercise of at least 350 kcal per session and up to 1000 kcal per session; lower volumes are sufficient for moderately trained individuals, but higher volumes may be required for highly trained athletes. The mechanism through which exercise exerts this beneficial effect is not completely clear. Presently, the most likely mechanism involves an increase in LPL activity, an increase that is evident for up to 48 h after a single session of exercise. More research is necessary to understand the mechanisms responsible for the acute lipid response to exercise. Furthermore, additional studies are needed to define the optimal combination of intensity, mode, and volume of exercise that will most likely cause a measurable and risk-reducing change in blood lipid variables.

References

1. Hargreaves, M. Interactions between muscle glycogen and blood glucose during exercise. *Exerc. Sport Sci. Rev.* 1997, *25*, 21–39.
2. Jentjens, R., Jeukendrup, A.E. Determinants of post-exercise glycogen synthesis during short-term recovery. *Sports Med.* 2003, *33* (2), 117–144.
3. Mittendorfer, B., Klein, S. Physiological factors that regulate the use of endogenous fat and carbohydrate fuels during endurance exercise. *Nutr. Res. Rev.* 2003, *16* (1), 97–108.
4. Carlson, L.A., Mossfeldt, F. Acute effects of prolonged, heavy exercise on the concentration of plasma lipids and lipoproteins in man. *Acta Physiol. Scand.* 1964, *62*, 51–59.
5. Holloszy, J.O., Skinner, J.S., Toro, G., Cureton, T.K. Effects of a six month program of endurance exercise on the serum lipids of middle-aged men. *Am. J. Cardiol.* 1964, *14*, 753–759.
6. Oscai, L.B., Patterson, J.A., Bogard, D.L., Beck, R.J., Rothermel, B.L. Normalization of serum triglycerides and lipoprotein electrophoretic patterns by exercise. *Am. J. Cardiol.* 1972, *30*, 775–780.
7. Enger, S.C., Stromme, S.B., Refsum, H.E. High density lipoprotein cholesterol, total cholesterol and triglycerides in serum after a single exposure to prolonged heavy exercise. *Scand. J. Clin. Lab. Invest.* 1980, *40*, 341–345.
8. Thompson, P.D., Cullinane, E., Henderson, L.O., Herbert, P.N. Acute effects of prolonged exercise on serum lipids. *Metabolism* 1980, *29* (7), 662–665.
9. Durstine, J.L., Haskell, W.L. Effects of exercise training on plasma lipids and lipoproteins. *Exerc. Sport Sci. Rev.* 1994, *22*, 477–521.
10. Crouse, S.F., O'Brien, B.C., Grandjean, P.W., Lowe, R.C., Rohack, J.J., Green, J.S. Effects of training and a single session of exercise on lipids and apolipoproteins in hypercholesterolemic men. *J. Appl. Physiol.* 1997, *83* (6), 2019–2028.
11. Crouse, S.F., Hooper, P.L., Atterbom, H.A., Papenfuss, R.L. Zinc ingestion and lipoprotein values in sedentary and endurance-trained men. *J. Am. Med. Assoc.* 1984, *252* (6), 785–787.
12. Fang, C., Sherman, W.M., Crouse, S.F., Tolson, H. Exercise modality and selected coronary risk factors: a multivariate approach. *Med. Sci. Sports Exerc.* 1988, *20* (5), 455–462.
13. Durstine, J.L., Crouse, S.F., Moffatt, R.J. Lipids in Exercise and Sports. In *Energy-Yielding Macronutrients and Energy Metabolism in Sports Nutrition*, Driskell, J.A., Wolinsky, I., Eds., CRC Press, Boca Raton, FL, 2000, pp 87–117.
14. Bounds, R.G., Martin, S.E., Grandjean, P.W., O'Brien, B.C., Inman, C., Crouse, S.F. Diet and short term plasma lipoprotein-lipid changes after exercise in trained men. *Int. J. Sport Nutr. Exerc. Metab.* 2000, *10*, 114–127.

15. Ferguson, M.A., Alderson, N.L., Trost, S.G., Essig, D.A., Burke, J.R., Durstine, J.L. Effects of four different single exercise sessions on lipids, lipoproteins, and lipoprotein lipase. *J. Appl. Physiol.* 1998, *85* (2), 1169–1174.
16. Foger, B., Wohlfarter, T., Ritsch, A., Lechleitner, M., Miller, C.H., Dienstl, A., Patsch, J.R. Kinetics of lipids, apolipoproteins, and cholesteryl ester transfer protein in plasma after a bicycle marathon. *Metabolism* 1994, *43* (5), 633–639.
17. Goodyear, L.J., Van Houten, D.R., Fronsoe, M.S., Rocchio, M.L., Dover, E.V., Durstine, J.L. Immediate and delayed effects of marathon running on lipids and lipoproteins in women. *Med. Sci. Sports Exerc.* 1990, *22* (5), 588–592.
18. Kantor, M.A., Cullinane, E.M., Sady, S.P., Herbert, P.N., Thompson, P.D. Exercise acutely increases high density lipoprotein-cholesterol and lipoprotein lipase activity in trained and untrained men. *Metabolism* 1987, *36* (2), 188–192.
19. Sady, S.P., Thompson, P.D., Cullinane, E.M., Kantor, M.A., Domagala, E., Herbert, P.N. Prolonged exercise augments plasma triglyceride clearance. *J. Am. Med. Assoc.* 1986, *256* (18), 2552–2555.
20. Visich, P.S., Goss, F.L., Gordon, P.M., Robertson, R.J., Warty, V., Denys, B.G., Metz, K.F. Effects of exercise with varying energy expenditure on high-density lipoprotein-cholesterol. *Eur. J. Physiol.* 1996, *72*, 242–248.
21. Thompson, P.D., Crouse, S.F., Goodpaster, B., Kelley, D., Moyna, N., Pescatello, L. The acute versus the chronic response to exercise. *Med. Sci. Sports Exerc.* 2001, *33* (6 Suppl.), S438-S445.
22. Crouse, S.F., O'Brien, B.C., Rohack, J.J., Lowe, R.C., Green, J.S., Tolson, H., Reed, J.L. Changes in serum lipids and apolipoproteins after exercise in men with high cholesterol: influence of intensity. *J. Appl. Physiol.* 1995, *79* (1), 279–286.
23. Grandjean, P.W., Crouse, S.F., Rohack, J.J. Influence of cholesterol status on blood lipid and lipoprotein enzyme responses to aerobic exercise. *J. Appl. Physiol.* 2000, *89*, 472–480.
24. Ferguson, M.A., Alderson, N.L., Trost, S.G., Davis, P.G., Mosher, P.E., Durstine, J.L. Plasma lipid and lipoprotein responses during exercise. *Scand. J. Clin. Lab Invest* 2003, *63* (1), 73–79.
25. Stampfer, M.J., Sacks, F.M., Salvini, S., Willett, W.C., Hennekens, C.H. A prospective study of cholesterol, apolipoproteins, and the risk of myocardial infarction. *N. Engl. J. Med.* 1991, *325* (6), 373–381.
26. Thomas, T.R., Smith, B.K., Donahue, O.M., Altena, T.S., James-Kracke, M., Sun, G.Y. Effects of omega-3 fatty acid supplementation and exercise on low-density lipoprotein and high-density lipoprotein subfractions. *Metab. Clin. Exp.* 2004, *53* (6), 749–754.
27. Crouse, S.F., Cockrill, S.L., Grandjean, P.W., Weise, S.D., O'Brien, B.C., Rohack, J.J., Macfarlane, R.D. LDL and HDL densities after exercise in postmenopausal women with normal and high cholesterol (abstract). *Med. Sci. Sports Exerc.* 1999, *31* (5), S370.
28. Pronk, N.P., Crouse, S.F., O'Brien, B.C., Rohack, J.J. Acute effects of walking on serum lipids and lipoproteins in women. *J. Sports Med. Phys. Fitness* 1995, *35*, 50–58.
29. Perreault, L., Lavely, J.M., Kittelson, J.M., Horton, T.J. Gender differences in lipoprotein lipase activity after acute exercise. *Obes. Res.* 2004, *12* (2), 241–249.
30. Hughes, R.A., Housh, T.J., Hughes, R.J., Johnson, G.O. The effect of exercise duration on serum cholesterol and triglycerides in women. *Res. Q. Exerc. Sport* 1991, *62* (1), 98–104.

31. Cullinane, E., Lazarus, B., Thompson, P.D., Saratelli, A., Herbert, P.N. Acute effects of a single exercise session on serum lipids in untrained men. *Clin. Chim. Acta* 1981, *109*, 341–344.
32. Grandjean, P.W., Crouse, S.F., Rohack, J.J. Lipid responses to a single bout of exercise in type IIa and IIb hypercholesterolemic men (abstract). *Med. Sci. Sports Exerc.* 2000, *32* (5), S1877.
33. Davis, P.G., Bartoli, W.P., Durstine, J.L. Effects of acute exercise intensity on plasma lipids and apolipoproteins in trained runners. *J. Appl. Physiol.* 1992, *72* (3), 914–919.
34. Imamura, H., Katagiri, S., Uchid, K., Miyamoto, N., Nakano, H., Shirota, T. Acute effects of moderate exercise on serum lipids, lipoproteins and apolipoproteins in sedentary young women. *Clin. Exp. Pharmacol. Physiol* 2000, *27* (12), 975–979.
35. Lamon-Fava, S., McNamara, J.R., Farber, H.W., Hill, N.S., Schaefer, E.J. Acute changes in lipid, lipoprotein, apolipoprotein, and low-density lipoprotein particle size after an endurance triathlon. *Metabolism* 1989, *38* (9), 921–925.
36. Liu, M.-L., Bergholm, R., Makimattila, S., Lahdenpera, S., Valkonen, M., Hilden, H., Yki-Jarvinen, H., Taskinen, M.-R. A marathon run increases the susceptibility of LDL to oxidation *in vitro* and modifies plasma antioxidants. *Am. J. Physiol.* 1999, *276*, E1083-E1091.
37. Hoefler, G., Harnoncourt, F., Paschke, E., Mirti, W., Pfeiffer, K.H., Kostner, G.M. Lipoprotein Lp(a): a risk factor for myocardial infarction. *Arteriosclerosis* 1988, *8*, 398–401.
38. Seman, L.J., DeLuca, C., Jenner, J.L., Cupples, A., McNamara, J.R., Wilson, P.W.F., Castelli, W.P., Ordovas, J.M., Schaefer, E.J. Lipoprotein(a)-cholesterol and coronary heart disease in the Framingham Heart Study. *Clin. Chem.* 1999, *45* (7), 1039–1046.
39. Gruden, G., Olivetti, C., Taliano, C., Furlani, D., Gambino, R., Pagano, G., Cavallo-Perin, P. Lipoprotein(a) after acute exercise in healthy subjects. *Int. J. Clin. Lab. Res.* 1996, *26*, 140–141.
40. Hubinger, L., Mackinnon, L.T., Barber, L., McCosker, J., Howard, A., Lepre, F. Acute effects of treadmill running on lipoprotein(a) levels in males and females. *Med. Sci. Sports Exerc.* 1997, *29* (4), 436–442.
41. Yu, H.H., Ginsburg, G.S., O'Toole, M.L., Otvos, J.D., Douglas, P.S., Rifai, N. Acute changes in serum lipids and lipoprotein subclasses in triathletes as assessed by proton nuclear magnetic resonance spectroscopy. *Arterioscler. Thromb. Vasc. Biol.* 1999, *19* (8), 1945–1949.
42. Ballantyne, C.M., Hoogeveen, R.C. Role of lipid and lipoprotein profiles in risk assessment and therapy. *Am. Heart J.* 2003, *146* (2), 227–233.
43. Jafari, M., Leaf, D.A., Macrae, H., Kasem, J., O'Conner, P., Pullinger, C., Malloy, M., Kane, J.P. The effects of physical exercise on plasma prebeta-1 high-density lipoprotein. *Metabolism* 2003, *52* (4), 437–442.
44. Greiwe, J.S., Holloszy, J.O., Semenkovich, C.F. Exercise induces lipoprotein lipase and GLUT-4 protein in muscle independent of adrenergic-receptor signaling. *J. Appl. Physiol.* 2000, *89*, 176–181.
45. Thompson, P.D., Cullinane, E.M., Sady, S.P., Flynn, M.M., Chenevert, C.B., Herbert, P.N. High density lipoprotein metabolism in endurance athletes and sedentary men. *Circulation* 1991, *84*, 140–152.
46. Berger, G.M.B., Griffiths, M.P. Acute effects of moderate exercise on plasma lipoprotein parameters. *Int. J. Sports Med.* 1987, *8*, 336–341.

47. Dufaux, B., Order, U., Muller, R., Hollmann, W. Delayed effects of prolonged exercise on serum lipoproteins. *Metabolism* 1986, *35* (2), 105–109.
48. Frey, I., Baumstark, M.W., Berg, A., Keul, J. Influence of acute maximal exercise on lecithin:cholesterol acyltransferase activity in healthy adults of differing aerobic performance. *Eur. J. Appl. Physiol.* 1991, *62*, 31–35.
49. American College of Sports Medicine. *Guidelines for Exercise Testing and Prescription,* 6th ed., Lea & Febiger, Philadelphia, 2000.
50. Hardman, A.E., Lawrence, J.E.M., Herd, S.L. Postprandial lipemia in endurance-trained people during a short interruption to training. *J. Appl. Physiol.* 1998, *84* (6), 1895–1901.
51. Hicks, A.L., MacDougall, J.D., Muckle, T.J. Acute changes in high-density lipoprotein cholesterol with exercise of different intensities. *J. Appl. Physiol.* 1987, *63* (5), 1956–1960.
52. Hughes, R.A., Thorland, W.G., Housh, T.J., Johnson, G.O. The effect of exercise intensity on serum lipoprotein responses. *J. Sports Med. Phys. Fitness* 1990, *30* (3), 254–260.
53. Tsetsonis, N.V., Hardman, A.E. The influence of the intensity of treadmill walking upon changes in lipid and lipoprotein variables in healthy adults. *Eur. J. Physiol.* 1995, *70*, 329–336.
54. Gordon, P.M., Goss, F.L., Visich, P.S., Warty, V., Denys, B.J., Metz, K.F., Robertson, R.J. The acute effects of exercise intensity on HDL-C metabolism. *Med. Sci. Sports Exerc.* 1994, *26* (6), 671–677.

14

Smoking, Heart Disease, and Lipoprotein Metabolism

Robert J. Moffatt, Sarah Chelland, and Bryant A. Stamford

CONTENTS

Introduction 299
CVD and Cigarette Smoking 300
Impact of Smoking on Atherosclerosis 302
Cigarette Smoking and Lipid Metabolism 302
Triglycerides and VLDL 302
LDL 304
HDL 304
Smoking Cessation 306
Metabolic Changes after Smoking Cessation 307
Nicotine and Carbon Monoxide 308
Environmental Tobacco Smoke (ETS) 308
Conclusions 309
References 310

Introduction

Cardiovascular disease (CVD) is the leading cause of mortality and morbidity in the United States, with 1.2 million new and recurrent cases of coronary attack per year.[1] CVD can be attributed to both modifiable and non-modifiable risk factors. The non-modifiable factors are those that cannot be changed and include genetic predisposition to the disease, age, and gender. Modifiable risk factors are ones that can be altered by lifestyle intervention, and include obesity, hypertension, hypercholesterolemia, diabetes, lack of physical activity, psychological stress, and cigarette smoking.

Since the inception of the National Heart Institute and the American Heart Association in 1948 there have been several large cohort studies, which have examined the effects of the modifiable risk factors on CVD. The Framingham, Oslo, and Bogalusa Heart Studies as well as the Multiple Risk Factor Intervention Trials (MRFIT) were all designed to deeply examine the etiology of CVD and furthermore how to reduce its prevalence.[2–5] The Framingham Heart Study was among the first to reveal that the incidence of atherosclerosis is proportional to higher plasma cholesterol levels, and in fact, was among the strongest predictors of mortality.[2]

The MRFIT studies showed an independent contribution to increased mortality for cholesterol and a substantial escalation in risk when elevated cholesterol was combined with other risk factors.[5] These results are common to other epidemiological studies with diverse populations (Lipid Research Clinics, Oslo and Bogalusa Heart Studies). Eventually, investigations broadened to include examination of the various classes of lipoproteins and their contribution to CVD.[6] It was found that LDL had the strongest correlation to CVD mortality. There was an association between very low-density lipoprotein (VLDL) and CVD mortality, but it was not as strong as the relationship with low-density lipoprotein (LDL). Kostner et al.[6] also reported that high-density lipoprotein (HDL) demonstrated an inverse relationship with CVD. This information provided additional evidence and helped to solidify the connection between HDL and CVD that was originally advanced by the Framingham, Tromso and Honolulu Heart Studies of the 1970s.[7–9]

Today it is taken for granted that development of CVD is accelerated by an unfavorable plasma lipid/lipoprotein profile, and it is known that individuals with multiple lipoprotein abnormalities have a 10-year CVD risk of greater than 20%. This means that from the time CVD is established, 20 out of 100 individuals will experience their first coronary event or recurrent event within 10 years.[10] The current definition of an unfavorable lipid/lipoprotein profile[10] is LDL above 130 mg/dl, triglyceride (TG) above 150 mg/dl and total cholesterol (TC) above 200 mg/dl. In addition, HDL levels below 40 mg/dl are considered to be detrimental.

CVD and Cigarette Smoking

Historically, the death rate associated with cigarette smoking has increased steadily as smoking gradually was embraced by all segments of U.S. society. Cigarette advertisements were seen as early as 1913 and specifically targeted women, coaxing them to smoke rather than indulge in satisfying their sweet tooths.[11] From humble beginnings, cigarette advertising flourished and smoking increased in popularity. Tobacco products became more "palatable" as the former harsh tobaccos from Turkey were being replaced with milder brands. World War I helped spike the popularity of cigarettes, because cigarettes were more accessible and convenient for soldiers than a pipe, and the government provided daily rations to the soldiers free of charge.

As cigarette smoking took hold in American culture, there was no hint of health consequences for decades. The first scientific paper supporting an increased prevalence of CVD due to smoking was not until 1933 and it concluded that heavy smoking contributed to the degeneration of the arteries, including the coronary arteries.[12] The next major indicator of an association between CVD and smoking came from a Boston cardiologist named Samuel Levine,[13] who published a book providing evidence that supported death from coronary artery disease occurring prematurely in smokers compared to non-smokers. Levine indicated smoking as a major risk factor for acute myocardial infarctions. More crucial evidence was published in 1958 when Hammond and Horn[14] reported that men who smoked 20 cigarettes per day had twice the death rate due to coronary events than non-smokers. These authors later found that those men who stopped smoking decreased the mortality rate during a 12-year follow-up.[14]

Building upon these earlier studies, subsequent research has focused on two outcomes of smoking. One, an obvious starting point, is mortality rates. Data suggest that cigarette smoking is directly responsible for as many as 465,000 deaths per year, with more than 40% attributable to CVD (201,000).[11] The second is the negative physiological adaptations associated with smoking, including alteration of the lipid/lipoprotein profile. This chapter provides a review of the recent literature on cigarette smoking with particular emphasis on alterations in lipoprotein metabolism. The Lipids Research Clinic and Framingham studies have shown that there is a dose–response relationship specifically between the number of cigarettes smoked and the decline in HDL concentration.[15,16] A comprehensive meta-analysis by Craig et al.[17] examined published data from 1966 through 1987. They compared non-smokers, with *light* (1–9 cigarettes per day), *moderate* (10–19 cigarettes per day) and *heavy* (20 or more cigarettes per day) smokers. Their results showed that TC (+ 1.8% L, + 4.3% M, and + 4.5% H), TG (+ 10.7% L, + 11.5% M, and + 18.0% H), VLDL (+ 7.2% L, + 44.4% M, and 39.0% H), LDL (+ 1.1% L, + 1.4% M, and 11.0% H) increased and HDL (–4.6% L, –6.3% M, –8.9% H) decreased in a dose-dependent manner.

A smoking-induced decrease in HDL and/or increase in LDL could alter the LDL/HDL ratio to favor a more atherogenic profile. Freeman et al.[18] found that there was a significant difference in the LDL/HDL ratio between smokers (2.89 ± 1.18) compared to non-smokers (2.38 ± 0.98). This change in the LDL/HDL ratio among smokers has been subsequently shown in several study populations.[19–22]

Impact of Smoking on Atherosclerosis

The impact of smoking on the risk of major coronary events is linked to the function of the endothelial wall. The endothelial wall is made up of a single layer, monolayer, of endothelial cells that regulate blood circulation and metabolism of the vessel. Ross[23,24] suggested that injury to these cells is a critical step in initiating the atherosclerotic process. There are several factors that can directly affect the stability of the endothelial cells of the coronary vasculature.

A proposed mechanism for accelerated plaque and lesion formation due to endothelial injury is free radicals created as a result of cigarette smoking, in particular those related to increased lipid peroxidation.[25] Lipid peroxidation is responsible for the development of reactive species within the vasculature. High levels of these oxygen species can cause a modification of the LDL particle that will result in lesion formation. Oxidized LDL will cross the protective barrier and lodge itself in the endothelial wall, which stimulates a natural immune defense with macrophages, leukocytes and monocytes. This immune defense will then release paracrine factors that attract platelets to the damaged endothelial site. These platelets aggregate and create foam cells.

Research has shown that a negative correlation also exists between smoking and clotting time as a result of enhanced platelet aggregation.[26,27] Furthermore, a smoker's ability to produce nitric oxide (NO), a compound responsible for the smooth muscle dilation in the vasculature, is impaired. The result is an inability to initiate vasodilation during times of hypoxia, further complicating the smoker's physiological adaptive responses.

Mustard and Packham[28] indicated that carbon monoxide from cigarette smoke is among those factors having the greatest impact on endothelial function. Waters et al.[29] concluded that smoking will accelerate coronary progression and can produce new lesions in the arteries. Another indicator of coronary health is the size of the intima wall relative to the thickness of the cholesterol plaque. Studies have supported the finding that cigarette smoking promotes stenosis and a reduced wall-to-plaque ratio.[30–32] Furthermore, cigarette smoking promotes extensive production of fatty streaks.[33]

Cigarette Smoking and Lipid Metabolism

Triglycerides and VLDL

Chronic cigarette smokers have a perturbed TG metabolism especially at the site of the adipose tissue. Chajek-Shaul et al.[34] compared the lipid content of the adipocytes in the gluteal region of smokers and non-smokers of the same body mass index (BMI). Smokers had significantly less lipid per cell than non-smokers (0.48 ± 0.07 vs. 0.64 ± 0.16 μl/cell). The authors suggested a difference in TG metabolism between smokers and non-smokers.

A later study by Hellerstein et al.[35] examined the relationship between the thermogenic and atherogenic potential of cigarette smoke. They examined heavy smokers (> 20 cigarettes/day) held on a strict diet for 2 weeks, one week exposed to cigarette smoke and 1 week not exposed. Stable isotope diffusions were used to measure free fatty acid (FFA) flux, glycerol flux and serum FFA concentrations. As a result of smoking, plasma FFA concentration was increased by 73% and FFA flux increased by 77%. A concurrent increase in glycerol was noted and there was a threefold increase in hepatic esterification of FFA. These results suggest that cigarette smoke can provide a metabolic mechanism for atherogenesis, which can contribute to the promotion of VLDL formation and release. As already noted, VLDL was found to be positively correlated to increased risk of CVD.[36]

TG metabolism is regulated by the action of lipoprotein lipase (LPL), an enzyme also affected by smoking. Specifically, this enzyme is responsible for catalyzing TG hydrolysis and clearing TG from the blood. LPL is stimulated by insulin at the adipose tissue but suppressed by it at the muscular level. Research has been fairly consistent and suggests that LPL activity at the skeletal muscle is reduced in smokers compared to non-smokers.[34,37] It is important to note that adipose LPL activity does not appear to differ between smokers and non-smokers.[38,39]

LPL activity at the skeletal muscle provides a greater lipid clearance than at the adipose tissue, therefore an altered activity at the musculature is of great importance. A recent study by Freeman et al.[37] demonstrated a trend for lower HDL-C levels in smokers as well as higher TG, LDL, and TC levels. Furthermore, in an attempt to examine the underlying mechanisms, results of the lipid transport enzymes showed that there was a significant decrease (33%) in skeletal muscle LPL activity in smokers (3.89 ± 1.58 μmol FFA/ml per hour) compared with non-smokers (5.85 ± 2.30 μmol FFA/ml per hour). The authors concluded that the reduced LPL activity may explain the impaired TG clearance that is commonly seen in smokers due to a slower metabolism of the TG-rich chylomicrons and VLDL. This perturbation may in turn decrease the recognition of surface material by the HDL particle and further delay cholesterol clearance.

LPL at the skeletal muscle also is greatly affected by insulin, and several studies have confirmed insulin resistance among smokers.[38,40,41] Results from one study showed an inverse relationship between the amount of insulin released and the amount of LPL activity, therefore those with the greatest insulin release showed the greatest fall in LPL activity. Furthermore, Elliason et al.[38] assert that the amount of insulin released is positively correlated to the amount of nicotine consumed per day.

This can present a complicated metabolic dilemma. Cigarette smoke can create an environment that causes constant stimulation of the sympathetic nervous system, release of catecholamines, and thus release of fatty acids.

Ultimately this physiological response should stimulate LPL. However, since LPL is not stimulated, circulating TG concentration is increased. This perturbation can cause increased VLDL formation via both the decrease in LPL and insulin resistance.

LDL

The formation of excess VLDL is of significant importance because it provides the precursor for LDL formation, a major risk factor for CVD. LDL is the least affected lipoprotein by smokers.[17] However the problem, not uncovered until recently, is the impact of smoking on LDL size, altering it to become a smaller denser particle that can easily cross the endothelial barrier, lodging it into the arterial intima.[25]

Campos et al.[42] found that plasma TG concentrations are related to LDL particle size and HDL concentrations. Support for this claim comes from Griffin et al.[43] who showed a lower ratio of large-to-small LDL particles in smokers (LDL-I/III = 0.77) compared with non-smokers (LDL-I/III = 1.89). It is important to note that this disturbance was not found when corrected for TG, further suggesting that the altered TG metabolism directly influences the size and nature of the LDL particle.

A second concern regarding the impact of smoking on LDL is oxidation, which will facilitate an immune response, after it has been lodged in the arterial intima. This immune response will attract macrophages and initiate foam cell formation, the beginnings of atherosclerotic plaque. Smoking promotes this process by the abundant free radicals found in smoke. Most of these are free radicals that cause lipid peroxidation, subjecting the smokers to increased oxidative stress, as shown by elevated TBARS concentrations in smokers compared with non-smokers.[44]

The prime regulator of LDL oxidizability is the vitamin E/protein ratio of the particle.[45] Studies have revealed a difference in oxidizability associated with a low vitamin E/protein ratio.[45,46] Thus it is important to analyze the LDL particle contents to fully express the danger of oxidation.

HDL

Cigarette smoking imposes a negative impact on HDL, reducing the concentration substantially.[17] This is a highly negative consequence, because HDL is the major lipoprotein responsible for reverse cholesterol transport, a process that removes excess cholesterol from the blood and transports it to the liver for catabolism.

HDL has two important subfractions. HDL_2 and HDL_3 have different and distinct roles in HDL metabolism. HDL_2 is the larger particle ranging from 8.8 to 13 nm whereas the HDL_3 particles are smaller, ranging from 7.3 to 8.7 nm. Concentration of the HDL_3 particle seems to be positively correlated to CVD — the higher the concentration of HDL_3, the greater the atherogenic effect. The relationship between CVD and HDL_2 is negative because HDL_2 particles accumulate esterified cholesterol to transport to the liver for degradation. Smoking reduces the HDL_2 subfraction[18,39,47] while exerting a limited effect on HDL_3.[48]

HDL works in concert with three key enzymes that enable reverse cholesterol transport to occur efficiently. Lecithin cholesterol acyl-transferase (LCAT) esterifies free cholesterol in the presence of apolipoprotein (apo) A-I and promotes the movement of this esterified cholesterol into the HDL core. Cholesterol ester transfer protein (CETP) transfers esterified cholesterol from HDL to lower density particles (chylomicrons, VLDL, intermediate-density lipoproteins [IDL], LDL). Hepatic lipase (HL) is responsible for regulating the degradation rate of HDL at the liver.

McCall et al.[49] analyzed LCAT and HDL response to cigarette smoke exposure. They studied the effect of cigarette smoke on fasted plasma samples from nonsmoking volunteers. Within 1 h the smoke-exposed plasma had a 44% reduction in LCAT activity; the longer the plasma was exposed to cigarette smoke the greater was the decrease in activity, and after 6 h LCAT activity was only at 22% of the normal control. In addition, HDL apolipoproteins were cross-linking rapidly (within 1 h) after exposure to the smoke. In other words, apo A-I, which is responsible for activating LCAT, was switching with apolipoprotein A-II (apo A-II), known to deactivate LCAT. This is problematic, because the activity of LCAT is dependent upon the activation by apo A-I, which in turn governs cholesterol ester flow into the HDL core. This process "fattens" the HDL making it the larger HDL_2 particle, which can carry the cholesterol to the liver for excretion and/or catabolism. The researchers suggested that LCAT is sensitive to cigarette smoke and that this could be responsible for the changes seen in HDL-C in smokers. Other studies have shown that apo A-I concentration is 4.2% lower in smokers than non-smokers.[48,50]

Studies have shown that smoking can activate HL[38,39,51] and, as indicated above, inhibit the activity of LCAT.[37,39,48,49] The evidence on CETP is equivocal; some studies have found that CETP activity is elevated in smokers,[52] while others report decreased[18] or unchanged activity.[37] These results are also hard to interpret as the full mechanisms behind CETP activity are not yet elucidated.

Despite conflicting results, correlation analysis supports a strong negative correlation between total HDL, and HDL_2 and HL, while HDL_3 was negatively correlated with LCAT.[37] These data suggest that these enzymes are directly responsible for maintaining the balance of HDL in metabolism and that minor disruptions in the activity of these enzymes will have larger consequences.

The challenge at hand, then, is to ascertain what all of these interactions have in common and how smoking promotes the risk for CVD. What is known is that the type of HDL particle in circulation will directly influence CVD risk and that LCAT acts to facilitate the movement of cholesterol esters into the HDL core. What is more, the reverse process of taking cholesterol ester away from the HDL in exchange for TG is mediated by CETP. In addition, HL will act on the HDL_2 particles and return HDL_3 to circulation.

Smoking reduces HDL_2 and LCAT in addition to increasing or not changing the activity of CETP and HL. This suggests that even with normal CETP and HL activity, an individual will be at greater risk of CVD due to the decreased clearance of cholesterol via the HDL_2 subfraction. In addition, the movement of cholesterol esters would also be inhibited because the activity of LCAT is diminished. This combination of events leads to increased cholesterol in circulation, which can be available as substrate for other less dense particles (VLDL, LDL).

If CETP and HL were to increase along with a reduction in HDL and LCAT, metabolic problems would escalate. With more cholesterol esters in circulation and not enough LCAT activity to transport them into the HDL core, there still would be enough CETP to continuously move the esters into VLDL and LDL. In addition, with increased HL activity the cardioprotective HDL_2 particle is being broken down faster than it can be replaced, leaving an excess of HDL_3-C in circulation. Ultimately, this would result in too little HDL-C to help protect against atherosclerosis.

Smoking Cessation

The World Health Organization reaffirmed in 2000 that cigarette smoking was one of the most powerful factors contributing to CVD,[53] and thus smoking cessation is strongly recommended. Scientific evidence offers strong support for smoking cessation. Early studies[14,54] reported that those individuals who quit smoking had a substantial decrease in risk for acute myocardial infarction. Since then, many studies have shown that among all preventative interventions, the decrease in CVD and acute myocardial infarction incidence is greatest among those who stop smoking.[55] It has been observed that smoking cessation can delay the onset of atherosclerosis by 10 years when compared with individuals who continue to smoke.[56]

Research has shown is a definite adaptation period after smoking cessation before risk of CVD is diminished, and this can take from as little as 2 years to as many as 20 years.[57] Regardless of the length of the adaptation period, the risk for CVD will return to the level of those who have never smoked.[58–61]

Smoking cessation contributes to several physiologic changes that decrease the risk for CVD, including normalization of the lipid and lipoprotein profile. A recent meta-analysis[62] suggests that with smoking cessation an individual can experience an increase in HDC, but other lipids and lipoproteins (TC, LDL, TG) remain unchanged. Increases in HDL can be seen in as little as 17 days.[63] A progressive increase in HDL has been observed with sustained cessation.[64–68] These results have important implications, because an increase in HDL will alter the HDL/LDL ratio — a powerful predictor of CVD — even though the TC, LDL, and TG may not change.

Strategies that assist in efforts toward smoking cessation have received considerable attention. Studies show that administration of a nicotine patch does not alter lipid or lipoproteins.[69–71] One study, however, suggests that HDL can return to baseline on the patch.[69]

Moffatt et al. [72] examined subjects who were asked to wear a nicotine patch for the first 35 days of their cessation program, followed by 42 days without the patch. As expected HDL, HDL_2 and HDL_3 were all reduced in smokers compared with non-smokers prior to the start of the program. These differences were still present after 35 days of cessation while on the nicotine patch. Normalization of blood values were observed over the succeeding 42 days when the patch was removed, suggesting that nicotine prevents normalization of HDL and its subfractions. This effect is acute and will only persist as long as the patch is in place. Notwithstanding the negative impact of nicotine therapy during cessation, it is clearly a more desirable alternative to smoking, assuming the therapy is short-lived and that cessation will be permanent.

Metabolic Changes after Smoking Cessation

Cessation of smoking will initially result in a metabolic withdrawal syndrome that affects 80% of all smokers.[73,74] These symptoms include restlessness, irritability, anxiety, and confusion. Furthermore, weight gain, an increase in waist to hip ratio, and an increase in percent body fat due to increased caloric intake or decreased resting metabolic rate is seen after smoking cessation.[19,66,67,72,75,76]

Weight gain typically exerts a negative impact on lipids and lipoproteins. However, despite the weight gain associated with smoking cessation, HDL levels improve, progressing gradually to normal values observed in non-smokers. This suggests that smoking is a more potent mediator of the lipid and lipoprotein profile than weight gain.

Stamford et al.[67] found that following cessation from smoking, subjects increased their caloric intake by 227 kilocalories (kcal) per day, which accounted for 69% of the weight gain following cessation. This finding suggests that a substantial percentage (31%) of the weight gain could not be explained by increased kcal consumption. Stamford et al.[67] observed no chronic change in resting metabolic rate (RMR). However, numerous studies have reported acute increases in metabolism caused by smoking alone and in combination with caffeine, food intake, light physical activity, etc. that when removed would impact caloric balance.[66,77–81]

Other factors may contribute to weight gain following cessation. Oeser et al.[76] examined circulating leptin levels and the lipid profile. Leptin is known to be a powerful regulator of appetite and is thought to be altered with smoking and/or cessation. Results of their study showed, however, that 7 days of nicotine abstinence produced no differences in fasting leptin levels or plasma concentrations of glucose, insulin or free fatty acids. A limitation of this study, however, was that it only observed nicotine abstinence for 7 days.

Exercise following cessation is strongly encouraged. Niaura et al.[82] found, similar to the above studies, that smoking cessation caused an increased total caloric intake in the non-exercise group. Caloric intake did not increase in the exercise group. The exercise group also demonstrated more favorable changes in HDL and the HDL_2 subfraction.

Nicotine and Carbon Monoxide

Smoking not only exacerbates the lipid profile, it exerts its effects in several other areas of the body. Cigarettes accomplish this mainly due to their nicotine and carbon monoxide components. Nicotine is readily able to cross the blood–brain barrier and can further bind to various receptors. This binding will cause the release of acetlycholine, norepinephrine, dopamine, serotonin, and vasopressin, which promote sympathetic stimulation, feelings of fulfillment, and vasoconstriction of the arteries; in turn this can elevate heart rate and blood pressure. In addition, nicotine has a half-life of approximately 2 h, suggesting that a chronic heavy smoker (> 19 cigarettes/day) may experience these elevations during his or her sleep cycle.[83]

In addition to the nicotine delivered in cigarettes, a smoker also takes in carbon monoxide. This carbon monoxide directly contributes to coronary hypoxia. This hypoxia will manifest itself in changes that occur to the concentration of 2,3-diphosphoglycerate (2,3 DPG), an important modulator of hemoglobin's affinity for oxygen. The concentration of 2,3 DPG is found to be elevated in the blood of smokers, signifying the body's ability to attempt to compensate for the hypoxic environment created by the carbon monoxide.[84]

Environmental Tobacco Smoke (ETS)

Smoking is not only hazardous to the smoker but also to nonsmokers via environmental tobacco smoke (ETS). Research has established a link between ETS exposure and CVD,[85–90] citing that those who are chronically exposed are 1.3 times as likely to develop CVD as compared to those who have never been exposed.[86,91] Studies have also provided evidence for ETS exposure and alterations in the lipid and lipoprotein profile.[92,93] Previous research has shown that chronic ETS exposure elicits an unfavorable lipid/lipoprotein profile among various populations including hyperlipidemic children,[94] adolescents,[95] spouses,[87] and coworkers.[96]

More recent data suggest an acute effect of ETS on lipids and lipoproteins as well. An early study by Moffatt et al.[92] examined three groups of women who were either non-smokers, smokers (≥ 20 cigarettes/day for the last 5 years) or non-smoking women exposed to ETS for 6 h per day, 4 days per week for at least 6 months. Compared with nonsmokers, both smokers and ETS-exposed women showed a significant reduction in HDL, HDL_2 and apo-AI. The levels were not different between smokers and ETS-exposed women. The authors concluded that individuals who do not smoke, but who are exposed to ETS, will show similar abnormalities in the lipid/lipoprotein profile and that this can increase CVD risk.

A recent study by Moffatt et al.[93] revealed that only 6 h of ETS exposure is sufficient to reduce HDL and HDL_2 by 18% and 37%, respectively. Furthermore, HDL and HDL_2 taken 24 h post-exposure were still significantly lower, 13% and 28% respectively, compared with baseline. Exposure to cigar smoke has been shown to exert effects similar to those of cigarettes.[97] Specifically, those individuals exposed to cigar smoke, including the cigar smoker who often reports not to inhaling, for 90 min showed significant decreases in HDL and HDL_2. In addition, the TC/HDL ratio was elevated at 12 h post-cigar ETS exposure in non-smokers. Together these data suggest that all types of ETS exposure will have negative impacts on the lipid and lipoprotein profile.

Conclusions

Smoking is a major risk factor for CVD, due in part to an adverse effect on the lipid and lipoprotein profile. Similarly, ETS also exerts many of the negative influences of smoking on innocent bystanders. Smoking decreases HDL and HDL_2, while increasing levels of TC, TG and LDL. Smoking may negatively alter LDL particle size and negatively impact critical enzymes, including LCAT, CETP, and HL. Thus, reducing the number of cigarettes consumed per day is a positive step when complete cessation from smoking, clearly the preferred outcome, is not attained. With cessation, HDL begins to normalize quickly, with significant results in as little as 17 days. As cessation continues, HDL increases further.

A negative outcome is associated with smoking cessation. Although weight gain typically exerts a negative impact on lipids and lipoproteins, an increase in HDL is observed with smoking cessation in the face of weight gain, thus offering further support for cessation. Nicotine replacement therapy is helpful to patients attempting to break the addictive stranglehold of smoking. However, use of the nicotine patch or gum may interfere with the normalization of HDL. Even so, the ultimate benefits of smoking cessation on health and reduced risk of CVD would outweigh this potential outcome.

References

1. U.S. Department of Health and Human Services, Reducing Tobacco Use: A Report of the Surgeon General. U.S. Department of Health and Human Services, CDC, National Center for Chronic Disease Prevention and Health Promotion, Office on Smoking and Health, Atlanta, 2000.
2. Kannel, W.B., et al., risk factors in coronary heart disease. An evaluation of several serum lipids as predictors of coronary heart disease. The Framingham Study, *Ann Intern Med*, 61, 888, 1964.
3. Holme, I., Coronary risk factors and their possible causal role in the development of coronary heart disease: the Oslo Study, *J Oslo City Hosp*, 32, 80, 1982.
4. Srinivasan, S.R., Webber, L.S., Berenson, G.S., Lipid composition and interrelationships of major serum lipoproteins. Observations in children with different lipoprotein profiles. Bogalusa Heart Study, *Ateriosclerosis*, 2, 335, 1982.
5. MRFIT Research Group, Relationship between baseline risk factors and coronary heart disease and total mortality in the Multiple Risk Factor Intervention Trial (MRFIT), *Prev Med*, 15, 254, 1986.
6. Kostner, G.M., Apolipoproteins and lipoproteins of human plasma: significance in health and disease, *Adv Lipid Res*, 20, 1, 1983.
7. Kannel, W.B., Castelli, W.P., and Gordon, T., Cholesterol in the prediction of atherosclerotic disease, *Ann Intern Med*, 90, 85, 1979.
8. Miller, N.E., et al., The Tromso Heart-Study. High-density lipoprotein and coronary heart-disease: a prospective case-control study. *Lancet*, 1, 965, 1977.
9. Castelli, W.P., HDL cholesterol and other lipids in coronary heart disease. The cooperative lipoprotein phenotyping study, *Circulation*, 55, 767, 1977.
10. National Cholesterol Education Program, Third Report of the Expert Panel on Detection, Evaluation, and Treatment of High Blood Cholesterol in Adults (Adult Treatment Panel II). NIH Publication No. 01-3305. Department of Health and Human Services, National Institutes of Health, NHLBI, 2001.
11. U.S. Department of Health and Human Services, The Health Benefits of Smoking Cessation: A Report to the Surgeon General. Washington, D.C., Government Printing Office, Washington, DC, 1990.
12. Lewis, T., *Diseases of the Heart*, Macmillan, UK, 1933.
13. Levine, S.A., *Clinical Heart Disease*, Williams and Wilkins, Baltimore, 1950.
14. Hammond, E.C., and Horn, D., Smoking and death rates: report on forty-four months of follow-up of 187,783 men. II. Death rates by cause, *JAMA*, 166, 1294, 1958.
15. Criqui, M.H., et al., Cigarette smoking and plasma high density lipoprotein cholesterol. The Lipid Research Clinics Program Prevalence Study, *Circulation*, 62, IV70, 1980.
16. Wilson, P.W.F., Factors associated with lipoprotein cholesterol levels: the Framingham Study, *Arteriosclerosis*, 3, 273, 1983.

17. Craig, W.Y., Palomaki, G.E., and Haddow, J.E., Cigarette smoking and serum lipid and lipoprotein concentrations: an analysis of published data, *Br Med J*, 298, 784, 1989.
18. Freeman, D.J., et al., Smoking and plasma lipoproteins in man: effects on low density lipoprotein cholesterol levels and high density lipoprotein subfraction distribution, *Eur J Clin Invest*, 23, 630, 1993.
19. Green, M.S., and Harari, G., A prospective study of the effects of changes in smoking habits on blood count, serum lipids and lipoproteins, body weight and blood pressure in occupationally active men, the Israeli Cordis Study, *J Clin Epidemiol*, 48, 1159, 1995.
20. Muscat, J.E., et al., Cigarette smoking and plasma cholesterol, *Am Heart J*, 121, 141, 1991.
21. Stamford, B.A., et al., Cigarette smoking, physical activity, and alcohol consumption: relationship to blood lipids and lipoproteins in premenopausal females, *Metabolism*, 33, 585, 1984.
22. Tuomilehto, J., et al., Effects of smoking and stopping smoking on serum high density lipoprotein cholesterol levels in a representative population sample, *Prev Med*, 15, 35, 1986.
23. Ross, R., The pathogenesis of atherosclerosis: an update, *N Engl J Med*, 314, 488, 1986.
24. Ross, R., The pathogenesis of atherosclerosis: a perspective for the 1990s, *Nature*, 362, 801, 1993.
25. Pittilo, R.M., and Woolf, N., Cigarette smoking as a risk factor for atherosclerosis, *J Smoking-Related Dis*, 5, 43, 1994.
26. Blache, D., Bouthillier, D., and Davignon, J., Acute influence of smoking on platelet behviour, endothelium and plasma lipids and normalization by aspirin, *Atheroscelerosis*, 93, 179, 1992.
27. Schmidt, K.G., and Rasmussen, J.W., Acute platelet activation induced by smoking. *In vivo* and *ex vivo* studies in humans, *Thromb Haemost*, 51, 279, 1984.
28. Mustard, J.F., and Packham, The role of blood and platelets in atherosclerosis and the complications of atherosclerosis, *Thromb Diath Haemor*, 33, 444, 1975.
29. Waters, D., Effects of cigarette smoking on the angiographic evolution of coronary atherosclerosis: a Canadian Coronary Atherosclerosis Intervention Trial (CCAIT) substudy, *Circulation*, 94, 614, 1996.
30. Diexroux, A.V., et al., The relationship of active and passive smoking to carotid atherosclerosis 12–14 years later, *Prev Med*, 24, 48, 1995.
31. Howard, G,. et al., Active and passive smoking are associated with increased carotid wall thickness: the atherosclerosis risk in communities study, *Arch Intern Med*, 154, 1277, 1994.
32. Tell, G.S., et al., Relations of smoking with carotid artery wall thickness and stenosis in older adults: the cardiovascular health study, *Circulation*, 90, 2905, 1994.
33. McGill, H.C., Effects of serum lipoproteins and smoking on atherosclerosis in young men and women, *Arterioscler Thromb Vasc Biol*, 17, 95, 1997.
34. Chajek-Shaul, T., et al., Smoking depresses adipose lipoprotein lipase response to oral glucose, *Eur J Clin Invest*, 20, 299, 1990.
35. Hellerstein, M.K., et al., Effects of cigarette smoking and its cessation on lipid metabolism and energy expenditure in heavy smokers, *J Clin Invest*, 93, 265, 1994.

36. Kannel, W.B., Update on the role of cigarette smoking in coronary disease, *Am Heart J*, 101, 319, 1981.
37. Freeman, D.J., et al., The effect of smoking on post-heparin lipoprotein and hepatic lipase, cholesterol ester transfer protein and lecithin:cholesterol acyl transferase activities in human plasma, *Eur J Clin Invest*, 28, 584, 1998.
38. Eliasson, B., et al., The insulin resistance syndrome in smokers is related to smoking habits, *Arterioscler Thromb*, 14, 1946, 1994.
39. Moriguchi, E.H., et al., Effects of smoking on HDL subfractions in myocardial infarction patients: effects on lecithin cholesterol acyl transferase and hepatic lipase, *Clin Chim Acta*, 195, 139, 1990.
40. Elkels, R.S., et al., Effects of smoking on oral fat tolerance and high density lipoprotein cholesterol, *Clin Sci*, 65, 669, 1983.
41. Facchini, F.S., et al., Insulin resistance and cigarette smoking, *Lancet*, 339, 1128, 1992.
42. Campos, H., et al., Low density lipoprotein particle size and coronary heart disease, *Arterioscler Thromb*, 12, 187, 1992.
43. Griffin, B.A., et al., Role of plasma triglyceride in the regulation of plasma low density lipoprotein (LDL) subfractions: relative contribution of small dense LDL to coronary heart disease risk, *Atherosclerosis*, 106, 241, 1994.
44. van Tits, L.J., Effects of alpha-tocopherol on superoxide production and plasma intercellular adhesion molecule-1 and antibodies to oxidized LDL in chronic smokers, *Free Radic Biol Med*, 30, 1122, 2001.
45. Princen, H.M.G., et al., Supplementation with vitamin E but not beta-carotene *in vivo* protects low density lipoprotein from lipid peroxidation *in vitro*. Effect of cigarette smoking, *Arterioscler Thromb*, 12, 554, 1992.
46. Neunteufl, T., et al., Effects of vitamin E on chronic and acute endothelial dysfunction in smokers, *J Am Coll Cardiol*, 35, 277, 2000.
47. Shennan, N.M., Seed, N.M., and Wynn, V., Variation in serum lipid and lipoprotein levels associated with changes in smoking behavior in non-obese Caucasian males, *Atherosclerosis*, 58, 17, 1985.
48. Haffner, S.M., et al., Epidemiological correlates of high density lipoprotein subfractions, apolipoproteins A-I, A-II, and D and lecithin cholesterol acyl transferase. Effects of smoking, alcohol and adiposity, *Arteriosclerosis*, 5, 169, 1985.
49. McCall, M.R., et al., Modification of LCAT activity and HDL structure: new links between cigarette smoke and coronary heart disease, *Arterioscler Thromb*, 14, 248, 1994.
50. Berg, K., Borresen, A-L., and Dahlen, G., Effect of smoking on serum levels of HDL apoproteins, *Atherosclerosis*, 34, 339, 1979.
51. Kong, C., et al., Smoking is associated with increased hepatic lipase activity, insulin resistance, dyslipidemia and early atherosclerosis in type 2 diabetes, *Atherosclerosis*, 156, 373, 2001.
52. Dullart, R.P.F., et al., High plasma lipid transfer protein activities and unfavorable lipoprotein changes in cigarette smoking men, *Aterioscler Thromb*, 14, 1581, 1995.
53. Kuulasmaa, K., Estimation of contribution of changes in classic risk factors to trends in coronary event rates across WHO MONICA project populations, *Lancet*, 355, 675, 2000.
54. Doll, R., and Hill, J.B., The mortality of doctors in relation to their smoking habits, *Br Med J*, 1, 1451, 1954.

55. Killburn, K.H., Stop inhaling smoke: prevent coronary heart disease, *Arch Environ Health*, 58, 68, 2003.
56. Feeman, W.E., The role of cigarette smoking in atherosclerotic disease: an epidemiologic analysis, *J Cardio Res*, 6, 333, 1999.
57. Bolego, C., Poli, A., and Paoletti, R., Smoking and gender, *Cardiol Res*, 53, 568, 2002.
58. La Croix, A.Z., et al., Smoking mortality among older men and women in three communities, *N Engl J Med*, 324, 1619, 1991.
59. Rosenburg, L., Palmer, J.R., and Shapiro, S., Decline in the risk of myocardial infarction among women who stop smoking, *N Engl J Med*, 322, 213, 1990.
60. Tverdal, A., et al., Mortality in relation to smoking history: 13 years follow-up of 68,000 Norwegian men and women 35–49 years old, *J Clin Epidemiol*, 46, 475, 1993.
61. Wolf, P.A., Cigarette smoking as a risk factor for stroke: the Framingham Heart Study, *JAMA*, 259, 1025, 1988.
62. Maeda, K., Noguchi, Y., and Fukui, T., The effects of cessation from cigarette smoking on the lipid and lipoprotein profiles: a meta-analysis, *Prev Med*, 37, 283, 2003.
63. Moffatt, R.J., Stamford, B.A., Owens, S.J., et al., Cessation from cigarette smoking: lipoprotein changes in men and women, *J Smoking-Related Dis*, 3, 11, 1992.
64. Moffatt, R.J., Effects of cessation of smoking on serum lipids and high density lipoprotein cholesterol, *Atherosclerosis*, 74, 85, 1988.
65. Moffatt, R.J., Normalization of high density lipoprotein cholesterol following cessation from cigarette smoking, *Adv Exp Med Biol*, 267, 1990.
66. Moffatt, R.J., and Owens, S., Cessation from cigarette smoking: changes in body weight, body composition, resting metabolism and energy consumption, *Metabolism: Clin Exp*, 40, 465, 1991.
67. Stamford, B.A., et al., Effects of smoking cessation on weight gain, metabolic rate, caloric consumption and blood lipids, *Am J Clin Nutr*, 43, 486, 1986.
68. Stubbe, I., Eskilsson, J., and Nilsson-Ehle, P., High density lipoprotein concentrations increase after stopping smoking, *Br Med J*, 284, 1511, 1982.
69. Allen, S.S., Hatsukami, D., and Gorsline, J., Cholesterol changes in smoking cessation using the transdermal nicotine system. Transdermal Nicotine Study Group, *Prev Med*, 23, 190, 1994.
70. Quensel, M., et al., High density lipoprotein concentrations after cessation of smoking: the importance of alterations in diet, *Atherosclerosis*, 75, 189, 1989.
71. Thomas, G.A.O., et al., Is transdermal nicotine associated with cardiovascular risk?, *J R Coll Phys*, 29, 392, 1995.
72. Moffatt, R.J., Biggerstaff, K.D., and Stamford, B.A., Effects of the transdermal nicotine patch on normalization of HDL-C and its subfractions, *Prev Med*, 31, 148, 2000.
73. Hatsukami, D.K., et al., Tobacco withdrawal symptoms: an experimental analysis, *Psychopharmacology*, 84, 231, 1984.
74. Hughes, J.R., and Hatsukami, D., Signs and symptoms of tobacco withdrawal, *Arch Gen Psychiatry*, 43, 289, 1986.
75. Gerace, T.A. et al., Smoking cessation and change in diastolic blood pressure, body weight, and plasma lipids. MRFIT Research Group, *Prev Med*, 20, 602, 1991.
76. Oeser, A., et al., Plasma leptin concentrations and lipid profiles during nicotine abstinence, *Am J Med Sci*, 318, 152, 1999.

77. Collins, L.C. et al, Effect of caffeine and/or cigarette smoking on resting energy expenditure, *Int J Obes*, 18, 551, 1994.
78. Collins, L.C., Walker, J, and Stamford, B.A., Smoking multiple high- versus low-nicotine cigarettes: impact on resting energy expenditure, *Metabolism*, 45, 923, 1996.
79. Walker, J et al. Potentiating effects of cigarette smoking and moderate exercise on the thermic effect of a meal, *Int J Obes*, 16, 341, 1991.
80. Walker, J. et al., Body fatness and smoking history predict the thermic effect of smoking in fasted men, *Int J Obes*, 17, 205, 1993.
81. Walker, J.et al., The effect of smoking on energy expenditure and plasma catecholamine and nicotine levels during light physical activity, *Nicotine Tobacco Res*, 1, 365, 1999.
82. Niaura, R., et al., Exercise, smoking cessation, and short-term changes in serum lipids in women: a preliminary investigation, *Med Sci Sports Exerc*, 30, 1414, 1998.
83. Benowitz, N.L., Pharmacologic aspects of cigarette smoking and nicotine addiction, *N Engl J Med*, 319, 1318, 1988.
84. Moskowitz, W.B., et al., Univariate genetic analysis of oxygen transport regulation in children: the Medical College of Virginia Study, *Pediatr Res*, 33, 645, 1993.
85. Garland, C., et al., Effects of passive smoking on ischemic heart disease mortality of nonsmokers, *Am J Epidemiol*, 121, 645, 1985.
86. He, Y., et al. Passive smoking at work as a risk factor for coronary heart disease in Chinese women who have never smoked, *Br Med J*, 308, 380, 1994.
87. Helsing, K.J., Heart disease mortality in nonsmokers living with smokers, *Am J Epidemiol*, 127, 915, 1988.
88. Hole, D.J., et al., Passive smoking and cardiorespiratory health in a general population in the west of Scotland, *Br Med J*, 299, 423, 1989.
89. Humble, C., et al., Passive smoking and 20-year cardiovascular mortality among nonsmoking wives, Evans County Georgia, *Am J Publ Health*, 80, 599, 1990.
90. Svedson, K.H., et al., Effects of passive smoking in the multiple risk factor intervention trial, *Am J Epidemiol*, 126, 783, 1987.
91. Glantz, S.A., and Parmley, W.W., Passive smoking and heart disease: epidemiology, physiology, and biochemistry, *Circulation*, 83, 1, 1991.
92. Moffatt, R.J., Stamford, B.A., and Biggerstaff, K.D., Influence of environmental tobacco smoke on serum lipoprotein profiles of female nonsmokers, *Metabolism*, 44, 1536, 1995.
93. Moffatt, R.J., et al., Acute exposure to environmental tobacco smoke reduces HDL-C and HDL_2-C, *Prev Med*, 38, 637, 2004.
94. Neufeld, E.J., et al., Passive cigarette smoking and reduced HDL cholesterol levels in children with high-risk lipid profiles, *Circulation*, 96, 1403, 1997.
95. Feldman, J., et al., Passive smoking alters lipid profiles in adolescents, *Pediatrics*, 88, 259, 1991.
96. Kawachi, I., Pierce, N., Jackson, R.T., Deaths from lung cancer and ischemic heart disease due to passive smoking in New Zealand, *NZ Med J*, 102, 337, 1989.
97. Kushnick, M.R., and Moffatt, R.J., Acute cigar smoking and exposure to environmental cigar smoke adversely effects blood lipid and lipoprotein profiles, unpublished data, 2002.

15

Lipid and Lipoprotein Concentrations in Americans: Ethnicity and Age

Michael R. Kushnick and Lynn B. Panton

CONTENTS

Introduction 316
An Overview of Ethnicity 316
  Asian Americans 317
  American Indians 318
  Hispanics 318
  Black Americans 319
  Summary of Ethnicity and Lipid and Lipoproteins in Adult Americans 320
Lipid and Lipoproteins in Americans through the Life Span 321
  Developmental Stages 322
  Early Childhood 322
    Total Cholesterol and Low-Density Lipoprotein Cholesterol 322
    Triglycerides and High-Density Lipoprotein Cholesterol 323
    Gender and Ethnic Differences 323
  Mid- to Late Adolescence 324
    Total Cholesterol and Low-Density Lipoprotein Cholesterol 324
    Triglycerides and High-Density Lipoprotein Cholesterol 325
    Gender and Ethnic Differences 326
  Middle Age 326
    Total Cholesterol and Low-Density Lipoprotein Cholesterol 327
    Triglycerides and High-Density Lipoprotein Cholesterol 327
    Gender Differences 329
  Advanced Age 331
    Total Cholesterol and Low-Density Lipoprotein Cholesterol 331

Triglycerides and High-Density Lipoprotein Cholesterol......331
Gender Differences......332
Summary of Lipid and Lipoproteins through the Life Span in Adult Americans......332
Conclusions......332
References......334

Introduction

The relationship between plasma lipoproteins, their constituents, and the risk of coronary heart disease (CHD) in adults is well established.[1] Cholesterol plays a central role in the atherosclerotic process and its association with CHD is reported to be continuous and graded.[2] Across ethnicity, increasing cholesterol levels also are linearly related to CHD.[3] Furthermore, there is little dispute that lipid and lipoprotein profiles change over the lifespan, and there is a clear and positive relationship between blood lipid and lipoprotein concentrations during childhood and later in life.[4]

The purpose of this review is to provide an update on the variations in lipid and lipoprotein concentrations and constituents in human plasma in major American ethnic groups of the United States (U.S.) during adulthood. In addition, this review will examine what is currently known about the changes in lipids and lipoproteins through the lifespan. Those requiring a comprehensive review of lipid and lipoprotein metabolism can be found in chapter 4 and elsewhere (5–18).

An Overview of Ethnicity

There is remarkable variation in inter- and intra-individual lipid and lipoprotein concentrations that no doubt is influenced by a combination of genetic and environmental factors.[19,20] This section will summarize the available information on differences in lipid and lipoprotein concentrations of adults of major ethnic American subpopulations and, where evidenced in the literature, discuss potential reasons for these differences. For the purpose of this investigation the following ethnic divisions will be made: Asians (Chinese Americans, Filipino Americans, Japanese Americans, Asian Indian Americans), American Indians, Hispanic (Mexican Americans), non-Hispanic, African Americans (blacks/Black Americans), and non-Hispanic Caucasians (whites/White Americans). These divisions are made with the intent of marking nationality and regional affiliation.

Asian Americans

Asians are one of the fastest-growing groups of immigrants in the U.S. Approximately 11.9 million or 4.2% of the U.S. population indicate "Asian" origin; defined to include any persons having origins in the Far East, Southeast Asia, or Indian subcontinent. The largest of these groups in the U.S. are Chinese Americans (2.7 million) followed closely by Filipino Americans (2.4 million) and then Asian Indian Americans (1.9 million). These combined groups account for nearly 60% of the total U.S. population reporting Asian ethnicity.[21] However, while there is a great deal of research on lipid and lipoprotein concentrations in Asian Indian Americans and Japanese Americans (1.1 million; ranked 6th in population of Asian Americans), far less information on other Asian American subgroups is available in the current literature.[21]

Chinese and Filipino Americans have been shown to have similar levels of total cholesterol (TC).[22] Choi et al. compared samples of a large group of older Chinese Americans against an all-white sample from the Framingham Cohort Study and found that the mean values of TC, low-density lipoprotein (LDL), LDL cholesterol (LDL-C) and apolipoprotein (apo) B were lower than whites; however, they further indicated that high-density lipoprotein (HDL), HDL cholesterol (HDL-C) and apo A-I were also lower than those of their white counterparts.[19,23] Others have suggested that lipoprotein (a) [Lp(a)] levels of Chinese American women are similar to those of white women (17.5 ± 20 and 23.7 ± 29 mg/dl, respectively).[24]

Japanese Americans have lipoprotein profiles that are characterized by greater HDL-C than whites.[25] Interestingly, Japanese American men appear to exhibit a greater frequency of the LIPC promoter T allele polymorphism than other U.S. ethnic groups, which is associated with lower hepatic lipase (HL) activity.[25,26] This polymorphism may help to explain the greater levels of HDL-C exhibited by this group, since HL activity has been demonstrated to be inversely related to HDL-C.[27] An older report on Japanese American men's blood lipid and lipoprotein profiles comes from the Honolulu Heart Program (HHP) which began in 1965 and reported on CHD risk and risk factors of 8006 Japanese American men residing in Hawaii over more than 30 years. The report from the HHP found concentrations of TC and LDL-C were similar to a cohort of age-matched white men from the Framingham Study.[28] However, in contrast to more recent reports, HDL-C concentration was also similar between the Japanese American men and the white men.[28]

Asian Indian American men have higher TC and LDL-C, as well as lower HDL-C than white men.[29,30] However, these differences were not reported in a group of well-educated male physicians of Asian-Indian descent.[31] Asian Indian American women may have greater HDL-C than white women,[29,32] but this too is not always reported.[30]

In addition, Asian Indian American women may have greater Lp(a) than white women who are not using oral contraceptives,[32,33] and both Asian Indian American men and women appear to have a greater relative distribution of small, dense LDL particles as compared to white men and women.[31,34,35] However, it has been reported that the abundance of small, dense LDL may be explained by a greater concentration of triglycerides (TG)[29,30,33,35,36] and a greater visceral accumulation of adipose at similar body mass indices (BMI) in the Asian Indian Americans compared to whites.[36]

American Indians

American Indians and Alaskan Natives were reported under one heading in the 2000 census. Approximately 4.1 million (1.5%) of adults in the U.S. population reported American Indian or Alaskan Native as their ethnicity.[37] Early reports of American Indians suggested that this group had lower CHD mortality rates than the general population.[38] However, these rates appear to be increasing to levels greater than the average of the general U.S. population.[39] These results are likely related to findings of the Strong Heart Study (SHS), an investigation of health in 13 American Indian communities of three geographically diverse regions of the U.S. A major finding of the SHS was that the prevalence of diabetes in adult American Indians was > 70% in Arizona, and > 40% in Oklahoma and North and South Dakota.[39,40]

American Indians have lower TC and LDL-C than the white adult U.S. average.[39,41–46] An analysis by Robbins et al.[46] suggested that the mean LDL-C concentration of American Indians with diabetes was similar to that of nondiabetics of this population. Comparisons to the NHANES III data[44,45] and other data[47,48] suggest that HDL-C may be lower in American Indians with or without diabetes as compared to whites. Furthermore, American Indians have 3–1.5 times lower concentrations of Lp(a) than those of whites (6.1–6.4 mg/dl),[49] and 10–5 times lower concentrations than those of blacks (21.5–24 mg/dl).[50] In fact, only a small percentage of American Indians from the SHS (1.73%, 7.37% and 4.34% in Arizona, Oklahoma, and the Dakotas) had Lp(a) concentrations > 30 mg/dl (the clinical reference considered to be elevated and at risk for greater CHD events in the current literature).[50] Unlike white and black ethnic groups, however, Lp(a) may be lower in American Indians with diabetes than those without diabetes.[49,51]

Another feature of American Indians' lipoprotein profile is a preponderance of small, dense LDL particles as compared to whites.[52] Interestingly, greater fasting insulin levels, obesity and elevated TG concentrations have also been reported in American Indians.[39,46,52,53] These factors are suggestive of the increase in insulin resistance and its association to chronic changes in LDL distribution in this group of Americans.[52,54]

Hispanics

The 2002 Current Population Survey (CPS) suggests that 37.4 million Hispanic individuals reside in the U.S., representing greater than 13% of the population.[55] Approximately 67% of these Hispanics (or Latinos) are of

Mexican origin (Mexican American). Hispanics in the U.S. have been reported to have similar or lower rates of CHD[56] as compared to whites. However, more recent reports from the San Antonio Heart Study have not supported these figures.[57,58] The primary difference has been termed the "healthy migrant effect" by Wei et al.[58] to suggest that U.S.-born Mexican Americans have a greater BMI, a greater prevalence of diabetes and a higher overall mortality rate than whites or Mexican-born individuals.[59,60]

Mexican Americans tend to exhibit greater obesity and concomitant elevations in TG and reduced HDL-C,[61–67] and these findings are reinforced by similarly lower levels of apo A-I.[68–70] Results from NHANES III suggest that Mexican American men have greater age-adjusted TC concentrations than white men.[71] Among women, however, the Mexican Americans have lower TC than white women.[71] Others have reported similar levels of TC and LDL-C,[64,65,70,72,73] as well as Lp(a) when compared with white men and women.[70,72,74]

Mexican Americans, without diabetes, also have been reported to have lower levels of LDL-C than whites.[56] However, Mexican Americans have a greater prevalence of small, dense LDL particles.[65,75,76] While the small LDL size in Mexican Americans is significantly related to greater adiposity,[67,76] it has also been demonstrated that Mexican Americans may have greater activity of cholesteryl ester transfer protein (CETP), potentially helping to promote these greater levels of small, dense LDL particles.[67]

Black Americans

Black Americans represent approximately 36.4 million or 13% of the U.S. population.[37] A good deal of literature has been compiled, and our knowledge of the lipid and lipoprotein profile of blacks is well documented. These profiles would suggest lower CHD risk than whites. However, this is not the case, as blacks are reported to have the highest overall CHD mortality rate of any group in the U.S. indicative of other factors besides lipids and lipoproteins increasing their relative risk.[77,78]

Black Americans have lower levels of TC and TG and higher levels of HDL-C than whites as well as a lower prevalence of hypercholesterolemia.[44,79–83] The concentrations of apo B and apo A-I are also consistent with these findings (lower in the former; greater in the latter).[68,81]

Another consistent finding in blacks is greater concentrations of Lp(a) than whites.[50,70,74,84] Howard et al. reported on 4125 participants of the Coronary Artery Risk Development in Young Adults (CARDIA) study (> 1/2 black men and women).[50] This investigation suggested that approximately 80% of the blacks had levels of Lp(a) that were higher than the median value for the whites. The median values of Lp(a) in black men and women were 21.5 and 23.9 mg/dl, respectively, compared to 6.1 and 6.4 mg/dl in the white men and women, respectively.[50]

Blacks are also reported to have greater overall adiposity,[85–87] but lower accumulation of visceral adiposity than whites.[81,88] However, lipid and lipoprotein differences are still reported to exist between blacks and whites after adjusting for adiposity indicating a true biologic difference.[89] Interestingly, excess visceral adiposity is often related to reductions in HDL-C through alterations in HL and lipoprotein lipase (LPL) activity.[85] In fact, this may explain why blacks are often observed to have greater LPL activity, lower HL activity,[81,90,91] and greater HDL_2-C concentrations than whites.[80,81,91,92]

More recently, investigations have determined that blacks may have a greater mean LDL particle size,[65,83] and a smaller portion of small, dense LDL particles than whites.[83] However, we were recently unable to confirm this in a group of sedentary black and white men. This result may be due to a smaller number and younger group of subjects, the lack of a statistical difference in TG concentrations between our white and black groups, and/or greater CETP activity in the black men, despite greater HDL-C concentrations.[93]

Summary of Ethnicity and Lipid and Lipoproteins in Adult Americans

Table 15.1 provides an overview of the available data on differences in plasma lipid and lipoprotein concentrations of the major American ethnic groups as compared to White Americans.[94] Coronary heart disease is the

TABLE 15.1

Overview of the Differences in Lipid and Lipoprotein Concentrations of American Ethnic Groups Compared to White Americans

Ethnic Group	TC	LDL-C	TG	HDL-C	Lp (a)	LDL size	Other
Asian Americans							
Chinese Americans	↓	↓	–	↓	↔	–	↓apoB
Filipino Americans	↓	–	–	–	–	–	–
Japanese Americans	↔	↔	–	↔↑	–	–	↓HLa
Asian Indian Americans	↑↔^{A}	↑↔^{A}	↑	↓↔^{A} /↑↔^{B}	↑	↓	–
American Indians	↓	↓		↓	↓	↓	–
Mexican Americans	↑↔^{A}/↓↔^{B}	↓	↑	↓	↔	↓	↓apoA-I; ↑CETPa
Black Americans	↓	↓	↓	↑	↑	↑↔	↑LPLa; ↑HDL_2-C; ↓Hla

↑, higher than White Americans; ↓, lower than White Americans; ↔, equal to White Americans; ^{A} in men; ^{B} in women; LPLa, lipoprotein lipase activity; HLa, hepatic lipase activity; CETPa, cholesteryl ester transfer protein activity; TC, total cholesterol; LDL-C, low-density lipoprotein cholesterol; TG, triglycerides; HDL-C, high-density lipoprotein cholesterol; Lp(a), lipoprotein (a); LDL size, low-density lipoprotein particle size; apo, apolipoprotein.

Source: Adapted from Watson, K.E., *Curr. Cardiol. Rep.*, 5, 483, 2003. With permission.

leading cause of death among all ethnic groups in the U.S.[95] The relationship between plasma lipoproteins, their constituents, and the risk of CHD in adults has been established.[1] In fact, across ethnicity, increasing concentrations of TC are linearly related to the risk of CHD.[3] The current literature provides only a brief synopsis of lipid and lipoprotein concentrations in ethnic groups of the U.S. and the current review provides an overview and reference when considering ethnicity. However, the current literature is limited in that there are only a few studies that include ethnic populations of the U.S., and in most cases, they fail to take into consideration important factors such as social and environmental issues, and age and gender differences that may further impact lipid and lipoprotein levels. Additionally, the mechanisms that drive biological differences among ethnic groups are largely unknown.

Lipid and Lipoproteins in Americans through the Life Span

Plasma lipid and lipoprotein profiles change over the life span, and these changes begin early in development of the growing fetus and continue into older age. In fact, it has been demonstrated that lipid and lipoprotein measurements obtained in childhood and adolescence (ages 8–18 years) are highly predictive of adult levels of TC and LDL-C.[4] Lauer et al. reported that of the children whose TC ranked in the 90th percentile on at least one measurement between ages 8–18 years, 43% were found to have greater than the 90th percentile of TC at ages 20–30 years.[96] This predictive nature is important, in the fact that the atherosclerotic process has been demonstrated to begin early in life[97,98] and understandably, it has also been suggested that lipid and lipoprotein levels at early ages are indicators of long-term risk of CHD and mortality of CHD.[97,99]

The prevalence of CHD is positively associated with the level of plasma cholesterol in both sexes over a wide range of ages.[1,4,97,99] While lipid and lipoprotein concentrations are dynamic throughout the life span, it is typical to observe the greatest concentrations of LDL-C and TC later in adulthood. A number of potential explanations have been proposed for the age-associated changes in lipoprotein concentrations, including dietary patterns,[100–104] total and abdominal obesity,[103,105–109] aerobic fitness,[103,109,110] number and function of the hepatic LDL receptors,[111,112] and altered insulin sensitivity.[109] However, none of these suggested mechanisms that are driving the age-related changes in lipoprotein levels are well studied or understood.

The next section of the chapter will focus on reviewing the changes in lipid and lipoprotein concentrations associated with each unique stage of life. Differences in prospective versus cross-sectional results, the influence of gender and, where available, the affiliations with various ethnic groups (prior to adulthood) will be indicated.

Developmental Stages

During gestation, intrauterine changes in TC, LDL-C and HDL-C have been noted and concentrations are typically greater than those seen at term.[113,114] In fact, changes in lipoprotein constituents are often linked to the development and growth of specific organs. For example, TC typically declines during gestational weeks 12 through 20 at which time the adrenal glands increase in size nearly 10-fold.[113] This period is followed by a rise in TC through 32 weeks and is characterized by a dramatic developmental increase in the fetal liver. From week 32, a second decline in TC appears as the fetus approaches gestation.[113] Triglyceride levels continue to increase as the fetus develops and approaches full term.[114]

Some maternal factors have been shown to influence lipid and lipoprotein concentrations in the developing fetus and neonate. Maternal hypertension may result in fetal hypercholesterolemia as a consequence of reduced adrenal utilization of LDL-C during the late stages of development.[115] Additionally, illness, such as respiratory distress syndrome in neonates or prematurity has been associated with higher TC, TG, and apo A-I.[116,117] Other factors such as maternal stress at delivery, socioeconomic level, low birth weight, or seasonal differences have been investigated and do not appear to alter lipid or lipoprotein levels.[118] In fact, at birth, healthy infants have TC in the range of 50–100 mg/dl and cholesterol is typically more evenly distributed between HDL-C and LDL-C particles than is found at any other time of life.[100,119]

Early Childhood

Total cholesterol increases somewhat prior to the newborn's first oral meal.[120] Additionally, within hours of the first oral feeding, as well as over the first few days postpartum, LDL-C and HDL-C increase regardless of diet.[120,121] When infants are less than 1 year old, TC and LDL-C are typically found to be higher in breast-fed as compared to bottle-fed (formula) infants.[104,120] Other dietary influences may have a profound effect on the infant's lipid and lipoprotein profile. For example, lowering the intake of saturated fat may reduce TC and LDL-C concentrations in infants and children below 5 years of age; however, this does not appear to impact HDL-C.[101]

Total Cholesterol and Low-Density Lipoprotein Cholesterol

With longitudinal designs, some investigators have reported TC to increase through mid-adolescence, with the greatest rise demonstrated within the first two years of life to levels similar to that seen during young adulthood (~ 170–205 mg/dl).[105,122–126] In a study by Rask-Nissilä et al., TC increased progressively from ages 7 to 48 months (140.8 ± 21.8, 152.4 ± 25.4, 155.6 ± 26.9, 162.6 ± 24.3 mg/dl at 7, 13, 24, 48 months, respectively).[125] Other researchers, however, have noted decrements in TC from ages 1 to 2 years[102] and through 8 years of age.[127] Cross-sectional studies of young children are more variable with respect to TC and LDL-C. Total cholesterol and LDL-C have been shown to rise through age 8 years, with the largest difference of increase typically seen between years 1 and 2 (~ 7 mg/dl).[106,124,127] Total cholesterol and LDL-C have also been shown to decrease[103,128] or not change when reported in cross-sectional research.[129]

To our knowledge no investigations have examined the influence of development (age) during early childhood on LDL particle size. However, Steinbeck et al. compared a group of children (~ 8 ± 1.5 years of age) with their parents and were unable to determine differences in LDL particle size (26.7 ± 0.9 versus 26.6 ± 0.8 nm, in children versus parents, respectively).[130] In addition, few investigations have examined Lp(a) in childhood, and it is likely that Lp(a) concentrations are not related to age, at least prior to adulthood.[131,132]

Triglycerides and High-Density Lipoprotein Cholesterol

Triglycerides are less often reported in younger children and this is primarily because of the 9–12 h fasting requirement. However, when reported, TG may be reduced in children after age 2 years and through 8 years of age.[102,127,133] Cross-sectional studies have not reported differences in TG during these younger ages.[123]

HDL-C may increase with early advancing age when reported cross-sectionally,[103,134] but this has not been a consistent finding.[103,106,127–129] Far fewer longitudinal investigations report on HDL-C in children prior to age 8 years, while most have not seen changes,[102,127] others have found HDL-C to increase.[125,133] For example, Kaitosaari et al. reported that HDL-C increased from 7 months through 7 years of age by greater than 40%[133] and this may be explained by a concomitant increase in lecithin cholesterol acyltransferase (LCAT) activity observed by others in children during this period of life.[135]

Gender and Ethnic Differences

In contrast to older ages, TC and apo B are higher in girls than boys (beginning at 7 months of age), while boys have somewhat higher HDL-C.[129,136,137] Triglycerides are typically higher in young girls as compared to boys, often by as much as 20%[102,106,127] and this may be because of different LPL activity; however, this has not been confirmed in the literature. In addition, Boulton et al. reported that girls increased LDL-C through 8 years of age, while LDL-C of boys remained steady from age 2 to 8 years.[102]

Asayama et al. reported on HDL-C and its subfractions from birth in males and females in a cross-sectional cohort.[134] At birth, boys had significantly greater HDL_3-C than girls, while HDL-C was somewhat higher. Interestingly, in boys HDL_3-C remained constant, while HDL-C and HDL_2-C rose ~ 11 mg/dl from birth to ages 6–10 years and then began to decline into adulthood (> 15 years). In girls, HDL-C and HDL_2-C continued to increase beyond birth (35.6 ± 2.3 and 17.7 ± 1.8 mg/dl, respectively) into late adolescence (15 years of age; 51.8 ± 2.3 and 31.7 ± 2.3 mgl/dl), while HDL_3-C rose immediately after birth (16.2 ± 1.1 mg/dl) and continued to rise until 10 years of age (21.4 ± 1.1 mg/dl).[134] Consistently, most others do not report differences in HDL-C between boys and girls of these ages.[106,127,129]

In addition, the mean LDL particle size has been reported to be larger in young girls than boys (2–3 years),[138] whereas no difference in Lp(a) has been observed during these ages.[131,139] Interestingly, it may be expected that boys at this age would have greater LDL particle sizes than girls, since adults with higher TG concentrations typically have smaller LDL particle sizes.[159,160] However, this suggests that other factors, such as very low-density lipoprotein (VLDL) production and enzyme activity, may be unique at different points in the lifespan.

With regard to ethnic differences, Freedman et al. reported that black children 1–4 years of age had higher TC levels as compared to American Indians, Mexican Americans or whites of the same age.[124] Among Mexican Americans and whites, TC is 2–5 mg/dl greater in girls than boys. In black girls TC was 2–3 mg/dl lower as compared to boys during the first 4 years of life.[124] Younger black boys and girls of the Bogalusa study had TG lower than white girls, but not boys,[127] and greater HDL-C than whites,[127,129] but similar to Mexican American children especially at ages closer to 8 years.[129]

Mid- to Late Adolescence

As children mature, lifestyle preferences that may play a role in modeling lipid and lipoprotein profiles are solidified, and these preferences can have a profound impact on adult life.[140] They are indicated by the fact that obesity acquired in childhood is highly predictive of obesity in adult life,[105,141] smoking habits typically begin by high school,[105,142] regular oral contraceptive use in girls frequently begins by age 15 years,[96,143] and dietary preferences, including the intake of processed food, rich in saturated fats and carbohydrates,[4,144] and patterns of physical activity in childhood may remain constant into adulthood.[145] Due to the overwhelming evidence that the atherosclerotic process begins early,[97,98] and in part, the fact that lifestyle can impact risk factors such as lipid and lipoprotein concentrations, the American Heart Association currently makes recommendations on its primary prevention beginning in mid- to late adolescence.[140,146]

Total Cholesterol and Low-Density Lipoprotein Cholesterol

The current literature suggests that TC and LDL-C decrease during adolescence, continuing through puberty until 18–19 years of age. This is followed by a steady increase in LDL-C that appears to be independent of ethnicity.[126,127] Table 15.2 illustrates mean TC values during these periods.[19]

Guo et al. reported that the concentrations of TC and LDL-C decrease somewhat between 9 and 11 years of age through early adulthood

TABLE 15.2

Plasma Total Cholesterol (mg/dl) in the First Two Decades of Life

Age (years)	n	Mean ± S.E.	Percentile	
			5th	95th
0–4				
Male	238	154.6 ± 1.8	114	203
Female	186	156.0 ± 2.0	112	200
5–9				
Male	1253	159.9 ± 0.7	121	203
Female	1118	163.7 ± 0.7	126	205

Source: Adapted from United States Department of Health, Education, and Welfare, National Heart, Lung, and Blood Institutes, National Institutes of Health, Lipid Research Clinics, Vol. I. The Prevalence Study, Bethesda, MD, 79–1527, 1979.

(17–19 years), reaching their minimum values during pubescence in both boys and girls, and then increasing beyond age 19 years.[147] Others have reported similar patterns whether the studies have been longitudinal[102,127,148–151] or cross-sectional.[103,105,106,123,136,152] Reductions observed in apo B during these periods are consistent with reductions in TC and LDL-C.[68,102,148] In addition, VLDL-C has been reported to remain constant during these years.[127,148]

Triglycerides and High-Density Lipoprotein Cholesterol

After a small rise in TG concentration from 8 to 11 years of age, TG levels remain stable through aging[15,102,127] whereas cross-sectional analyses indicate a progressive rise from 10% to 40% from 11 to 15 years.[106,129,136,153] With regards to HDL-C, most prospective investigations also report increasing concentrations prior to age 11 years,[102] followed by stepwise decrements in HDL-C through 18 years of age.[102,147,148] These changes coincide with reductions reported in apo A-I.[68,102,148] Boulton et al. reported apo A-I concentrations substantially lower at age 15 years as compared to 8 years in both boys (123 ± 16 vs. 199 ± 58 mg/dl) and girls (127 ± 18 vs. 192 ± 55 mg/dl).[102] Cross-sectionally, Bachorik et al. reported lower apo A-I in boys,[68] which may coincide with the reduced HDL-C reported in both genders when investigated by this design.[103,126,129,136,152] Consistent with these findings, Ronnemaa et al. reported that LCAT activity was lowest during these years when compared with early adulthood.[154] Contrary to these reports, others have reported no change in HDL-C in boys and girls[106,123] or increases in HDL-C (most notably, HDL_2-C) in girls of 6–10 years as compared to 11–15 years, but not in boys.[134]

Gender and Ethnic Differences

During mid- to late adolescence lipid and lipoprotein constituents may be different in boys and girls. Total cholesterol and LDL-C are often reported to be greater in girls than boys in some prospective[102,148] and cross-sectional[106,129,152] investigations, and this may be due to changing hormone concentrations.[153] However, greater TC and LDL-C in girls have not been reported in all studies.[123,127,136,147,153,154] Most investigations, regardless of design, have not found HDL-C[102,127,136,147,152,154] or TG concentrations to be different between genders during these years.[102,123,127,147,153,154] However, Bachorik et al. demonstrated that apo A-I concentration was approximately 7% lower in males than females at all ages, and the male-female difference in whites was more pronounced than in other ethnic groups (blacks or Mexican Americans).[68] Overall, apo A-I tends to remain constant with age in boys, while being lowest in women < 20 years old.[68] Furthermore, concentrations of Lp(a) appear to be independent of gender at a young age.[102,131]

Some investigations have reported LDL size to be smaller in boys aged 10–17 years than girls of the same age[153–155] and this is consistent with what is observed in younger children. However, others have reported similar LDL sizes[156] and prevalence of small, dense LDL particles between the genders.[157]

With regards to ethnicity during mid- to late adolescence, greater TC and LDL-C in girls may be especially pronounced in blacks more so than whites.[126] In addition, mean levels of TC are lower in black girls by about 10 mg/dl than in white girls,[127] who also tend to have a slower increase in apo B concentrations from early ages to 19 years of age.[68] The current literature also suggests that adolescent blacks have greater Lp(a) concentrations than whites,[126,131,158] while Freedman et al. identified in these ages that blacks have larger LDL particles than whites.[153] In adults, similar differences have been observed and are explained by greater TG.[159,160] However, in this investigation, despite the white children having greater TG than the black children (boys 96 ± 51 vs. 71 ± 30 mg/dl; girls 101 ± 7 vs. 72 ± 27 mg/dl, in whites and blacks, respectively), TG levels were only weakly correlated to LDL particle size for the entire group of children ($r = -0.21$).[153] Furthermore, most reports indicate that blacks have higher HDL-C and apo A-I than whites[126,127,153] during adolescence, despite a significant drop in its concentration observed from age 9 to 19 years.[129] In addition, after about 12 years of age, TG are reported to be lower in black boys and girls[127] than Mexican Americans and whites who display very similar levels.[129]

Middle Age

It is well recognized that the prevalence of CHD increases with age,[10] and clearly, concomitant changes in lipid and lipoprotein profiles play a significant role in this relationship.[10,161] It is generally accepted that plasma TC, LDL-C and TG increase with advancing age in adulthood[162] while HDL-C may decrease[107,163–166] or stay the same.[109,111,160,162,167–76] While part of the age-related changes are due to normal physiologic alterations associated with aging (i.e., menopause, reduced testosterone and estrogen, reduced muscle mass, secondary to loss of testosterone), a large part of these changes is likely attributed to an increase in adiposity[108,109] and a reduction in physical activity.[81,91,109]

Total Cholesterol and Low-Density Lipoprotein Cholesterol

Early cross-sectional literature reported that changes in TC in adulthood are extreme; from approximately 150 mg/dl at age 20 to 200 mg/dl at age 50, thereon remaining constant to nearly 65 years of age at which time it then begins to decline.[19,167] Others, and more recent investigations, also indicate that TC and LDL-C tend to increase with age in young or middle-aged adults studied both cross-sectionally[19,108–111,160–162,167,173,175,177–181] and prospectively.[107,161,163–166,176,180,182,183] Similar age-related increases during adulthood are reported for apo B.[68,111,160,173] In fact, increases in LDL-C may be explained by reports that indicate the plasma residence time of LDL particles and that the hepatic production of VLDL-apo B100 increase with age.[112,173,184]

Some investigations have also identified that the prevalence of small, dense LDL increases[160] and the mean LDL particle size decreases with age.[156] However, these results are not consistent[130,160,185] and potentially may be explained by the reports of McNamara et al. and Lemieux et al., who suggest that LDL particle size is primarily a reflection of TG concentrations, and therefore, not necessarily age dependent.[159,160]

Few investigations have reported on the potential age-related changes in Lp(a) concentrations during adulthood. While it is recognized that Lp(a) levels are highly dependent on genetics,[186,187] there is limited evidence that they increase with age when compared cross-sectionally.[132,188] Others have not found Lp(a) to increase with age, except with menopausal status[189–191] where concentrations increase unless hormonal replacement therapy (HRT) is started.[191] Furthermore, smaller apo(a) levels have also been reported to be greatest in older individuals.[132,189,190]

Triglycerides and High-Density Lipoprotein Cholesterol

Table 15.3 illustrates the mean fasting values of TG concentrations in adults aged 20–59 years from a sample of men and women (not using exogenous hormones).[19] Age-related increases in TG of adults are typical.[108,109,160,162,173,175,176,191,192] Rifkind and Segal suggest that TG increase progressively in men at approximately 18 mg/dl per decade until age 80, but more slowly in women to the age of 70.[191] These changes are likely due to reductions in LPL activity,[192–194] but have also been correlated to increasing visceral fat accumulation with age.[109,160,181] Prospective research has also indicated that TG increases with advancing age.[195]

Anderson et al. reported on fasting samples of 2433 individuals (men: n = 1342; women: n = 1091) from the Framingham Study between the ages of

TABLE 15.3

Plasma Triglycerides (mg/dl) by Age in Adult Males and Females

Age (years)	n	Mean ± S.E.	Percentile 5th	Percentile 95th
20–24				
Male	882	100.3 ± 1.9	44	201
Female	778	72.4 ± 1.3	36	131
25–29				
Male	2042	115.8 ± 2.3	46	249
Female	1329	74.7 ± 1.0	37	145
30–34				
Male	2444	128.3 ± 2.5	50	266
Female	1569	78.5 ± 1.0	39	151
35–39				
Male	2320	144.9 ± 2.5	54	321
Female	1606	86.3 ± 1.2	40	176
40–44				
Male	2428	151.4 ± 3.0	55	320
Female	1583	98.4 ± 2.1	45	191
45–49				
Male	2296	151.7 ± 2.4	58	327
Female	1515	104.5 ± 1.8	46	214
50–54				
Male	2138	151.8 ± 2.5	58	320
Female	1257	114.8 ± 2.0	52	233
55–59				
Male	1621	141.4 ± 2.2	58	286
Female	1112	125.0 ± 2.3	55	262
60–64				
Male	905	142.3 ± 3.1	58	291
Female	723	127.0 ± 3.3	56	239
65–69				
Male	750	136.7 ± 5.2	57	267
Female	748	131.3 ± 4.5	60	243
70+				
Male	850	129.8 ± 2.7	58	258
Female	748	132.4 ± 3.9	60	237

Triglycerides determined on plasma from fasting, white subjects. Females are non-sex hormone users.

Source: Adapted from United States Department of Health, Education, and Welfare, National Heart, Lung, and Blood Institutes, National Institutes of Health, Lipid Research Clinics, Vol. I. The Prevalence Study, Bethesda, MD, 79-1527, 1979.

25 and 54 years who were not using medications known to alter lipid concentrations.[165] Comparisons were made of lipid profiles 8 years after their first measurement and indicated that HDL-C was unchanged in men and reduced in women.[165] However, others have reported that HDL-C decreases with age in both younger and middle-aged men and women[107,163–166]

although, when examined cross-sectionally, HDL-C has not been reported to change.[19,109,111,160,162,167–176] Similarly, apo A-I, apo A-II,[68,175] or LCAT activity do not appear to change with age in cross-sectional studies.[196]

Gender Differences

The changes that occur in lipids and lipoproteins with age in healthy individuals differ between men and women. In women, this is also dependent on HRT. The concentrations of TC and LDL-C are significantly lower in women than men during adulthood, especially before age 55 years[19,68,162,167,196] and this is associated with higher levels of apo B.[68,73,167] Heiss et al. found that the increase in TC and LDL-C in women occurs at a much slower rate than men.[167] However, by age 55–60, the TC in women is typically equal to that in men.[167,178] In contrast, Connor et al. suggested that TC is somewhat higher in women than in men prior to ages 20–35 years,[122] and this is consistent with the findings reported earlier that TC and LDL-C may be greater in women under the age of 20 years in prospective[102,129,148] and cross-sectional studies.[106,129,152]

Bachorik et al. reported that apo B increased from 20 to 50 years in men, but did not increase further during the years 50 to 69.[68] In contrast, apo B did not plateau until 60 years in women. These findings are consistent with others.[73,175] Furthermore, LDL-C may also plateau earlier in men than women.[68] Interestingly, Saito et al. reported that TC and LDL-C did not differ between young (20–39 years) and older men (40–69 years); however, young women (20–39 years) had lower TC and LDL-C than older women (40–69 years).[175]

No gender-related differences are reported to exist for Lp(a);[197] however, the literature suggests that men have smaller mean LDL particle size than women[185,198–201] regardless of menstrual status,[156,201] and this may be related in part to greater visceral adipose tissue accumulation and TG concentrations.[201]

A large part of the discrepancy in blood lipids and lipoproteins between men and women has to do with the use of exogenous hormones or HRT. As reported earlier, regular oral contraceptive use frequently begins by age 15 years.[96,143] Godsland reviewed literature on HRT and blood lipids and lipoproteins from 1974 through 2000 and surmised that, generally, postmenopausal HRT use increases HDL-C and lowers LDL-C, TC, and Lp(a), while its effects on TG depends on route of administration — oral estrogen tends to increase TG, while transdermal estrogen has little effect.[202]

Estrogen has a direct influence on LDL-C by increasing LDL clearance through an up-regulation in LDL receptor activity.[203] Postmenopausal women not receiving HRT are presumably expressing fewer LDL receptors than their younger counterparts, and this is likely contributing to the rise in LDL-C that occurs at menopause.[180] Conversely, Bachorik et al. demonstrated that when women were separated for use and non-use of HRT, users had significantly greater apo B during ages 20–49 years despite having lower LDL-C.[68] This effect of HRT usage would be consistent with reports indicating an increase in small, dense LDL particles;[201,204] however, these results are not consistent.[205,206] Furthermore, spontaneous menopause,[207,208] metabolically characterized by low estrogen levels, elevates TG (> 10%) and reduces HDL-C (as much as 10%) in conjunction with a reduction in LPL activity.[180,209] Conversely, women at all ages taking oral estrogen have approximately 20–80 mg/dl higher TG than those who are not taking oral estrogen at the same age,[18,167,210] and men on exogenous estrogen also report increased TG.[203] In addition, a benefit of HRT may be that it increases HDL-C and apo A-I either through an increase in apo A-I synthesis[211] or decrease in apo A-I breakdown.[212]

Greater synthesis of TG-rich VLDL particles results in individuals with larger visceral fat accumulation[213] and these results are not gender dependent.[108,109,162] In numerous experimental conditions, it has been demonstrated that individuals with high LPL activity have low TG and high HDL-C.[27] Women typically have lower TG than men through their adult lives.[18,108,162,167,175,196] However, it is well known that men tend to accumulate more visceral fat than women[214] and investigators have demonstrated that LPL activity is greater in women than in men,[194] which may be related to fat distribution.[111,215]

In addition, women have greater HDL-C, $HDL_{2\&3}$-C, and apo A-I than men.[68,73,216,217] However, premenopausal women have lower HDL_3-C and higher HDL_2-C than the postmenopausal women who were not on HRT, although their apo A-I and HDL-C levels are typically similar.[73] Interestingly, HRT appears to influence the age-related changes observed in HDL-C and its subfractions. Women on HRT appear to preferentially increase HDL_3-C and decrease HDL_2-C[176] with age, while the opposite appears to be the case for women who are not on HRT. Estrogens also exert their influence by reducing HL activity,[218–220] which would increase the concentration of HDL-C by inhibiting its clearance from the plasma.[27] For more detail on the topic of HRT and lipoproteins please see chapter in this book.

While estrogen is strikingly beneficial in raising HDL-C, testosterone's influence on HDL-C is not well understood. Interestingly, LCAT activity is reported to be higher in men than in women after puberty (suggesting an influence of testosterone), despite men having lower total HDL-C.[154] Cross-sectional observations show positive relationships between HDL-C and normal physiologic levels of testosterone in adult men,[221] but this has not been confirmed by all studies.[222] However, these findings are in direct contrast with the well-documented findings of HDL-C decrease after exogenous androgen administration of supraphysiologic levels[223] or the immediate reduction of HDL-C (by more than 10 mg/dl) in adolescent males going through puberty when an increase in testosterone levels occurs.[224] In addition, testosterone has been demonstrated to reduce apo A-I synthesis,[216] and it follows that apo A-I concentrations are approximately 5–10% lower in males than females at all ages.[68]

Advanced Age

We have suggested that the prevalence of CHD increases with age;[10] however, the association between cholesterol and CHD may weaken in older individuals.[225] The weakened relationship may be due, in part, to the fact that far fewer investigations have examined the effects of older age (≥ 65 years old) on blood lipids and lipoproteins. This section will review what is currently known about blood lipids and lipoproteins in older individuals.

Total Cholesterol and Low-Density Lipoprotein Cholesterol

Total cholesterol and LDL-C decrease with age ≥ 65 years old in cross-sectional[18,168–172,226–229] and prospective studies.[174,227,228,230,231] In fact, during 8 years of follow-up in older individuals (aged 65–79 years when initial samples were taken) in the Framingham Study, TC declined by 0.9 mg/dl per year.[180] Other, longitudinal-design investigations have reported a greater drop in TC of > 1.5 mg/dl per year for subjects of similar age (Honolulu Heart Program;[230] Rancho Bernardo Study;[229] Zutphen Elderly Study[231]). While Ericsson et al. reported that the fractional catabolic rate of LDL apo B of older men was somewhat lower than younger men; this was balanced by a lower production rate.[112] Furthermore, Ferrara et al. suggested that the reduced TC was not the result of survivor bias, weight loss, or use of medications.[229] It is interesting to note that even in older subjects who gained weight, a reduction in TC was noted[229,230] despite a loss of lean body mass[229] and, although no mechanisms have been proposed to explain this phenomena, this may be related to altered nutritional intake or nutrient absorption.[174,231]

The concentration of apo B is also reduced after age 69 years in men but not in women.[68] Knapp et al. reported that in older men the concentration of Lp(a) was lower with increasing age (7th–9th decades of life).[232] However, others have reported no relationship between Lp(a) and older age.[175,233,234] Moreover, to our knowledge no investigations have evaluated the relationship between aging and changes in LDL particle size in this period of older age. However, Mykkanen et al. investigated the relationship between LDL particle size and risk of CHD in the elderly, and determined there was little association.[235]

Triglycerides and High-Density Lipoprotein Cholesterol

Cross-sectional analyses indicate that TG are reduced in older men and women.[101,112,172,227] However, to our knowledge no longitudinal analyses of TG levels have been reported that have taken place over a long enough period of time to determine the effects of aging on TG in older individuals. One study found that 42% of its sample of older adults significantly increased TG while the other 36% significantly decreased their TG over an 18-month period.[227]

In cross-sectional investigations HDL-C does not change[101,169–172] or does apo A-I during older age.[8] However, the prospective literature is equivocal with regards to the concentration of HDL-C during older age, where investigations have reported HDL-C to decrease,[68] increase[230] or not change.[174]

Gender Differences

While few investigations have been reported in older individuals with regards to age-related changes in lipid and lipoprotein profiles, far fewer have reported gender differences. In older age, TC and LDL-C may be greater in women by about 10%, with no differences in TG as compared to men.[172,227] Additionally, HDL-C has been reported to increase in men, but not women in cross-sectional studies, closing the gap between the levels reported in prior age groups.[172,175,227,229]

Summary of Lipid and Lipoproteins through the Life Span in Adult Americans

The prevalence of CHD is positively associated with the level of plasma cholesterol throughout the life span.[1,4,97,99] Plasma lipid and lipoprotein profiles change over the life span, and these changes begin early in development of the growing fetus and continue into older age. It has been demonstrated that lipid and lipoprotein measurements obtained in childhood and adolescence are predictive of adult lipid and lipoprotein profiles.[4,96]

Many factors can influence lipid and lipoprotein profiles and this makes it difficult to truly isolate the effects of aging. Furthermore, while changes in lipid and lipoprotein concentrations over the life span do occur, the mechanisms that drive these changes are not fully understood because social and environmental issues including education, economic status, nutrition, physical activity, obesity, tobacco use, total and abdominal obesity, and biological issues such as activity of hepatic lipoprotein receptors, altered insulin sensitivity, and hormonal changes have a profound influence over lipid and lipoprotein levels and their metabolism. Table 15.4 illustrates some of the major changes in plasma lipid and lipoprotein constituents in stages from (1) gestation to birth; (2) birth to early childhood; (3) early childhood to late adolescence; (4) late adolescence to middle age; and (5) middle age to advanced age.

Conclusions

Lipid and lipoprotein concentrations and their constituents are highly variable within and among individuals.[18,20] The current literature provides

TABLE 15.4

Summary of Major Changes in Plasma Lipid and Lipoprotein Constituents over the Lifespan

Stage I. Gestation to Birth

TC ↓ during weeks 12 through 20 of gestation
TC ↑ during weeks 20 through 32 of gestation
TC at birth between 50–100 mg/dl, however more evenly distributed between HDL-C and LDL-C than at any other time in life

Stage II. Birth to Early Childhood

TC and LDL-C ↑↓↔
TG ↓↔
HDL-C ↑ ↔; may be explained by ↑ LCAT
TC girls > boys and HDL-C girls < boys
LDL size girls > boys

Stage III. Early Childhood to Late Adolescence

TC and LDL-C ↓
HDL-C ↑
TG ↑
TC and LDL-C girls > or = boys
TG and HDL-C = in girls and boys
LDL size girls > boys

Stage IV. Late Adolescence to Middle Age

TC and LDL-C ↑
LDL size ↓
Lp(a) may ↑
TG ↑; likely related to ↓ LPLa
HDL-C ↓↔
TC and LDL-C women < men
Lp(a) men = women
TG women < men; LPLa women > men
HDL-C women >men; HLa women < men

Stage V. Middle Age to Advanced Age

TC and LDL-C ↓
TG ↓
HDL-C ↑ ↓↔
TC and LDL-C women > men

↑, increase during this stage; ↓, decrease during this stage; ↔, does not change during this stage; >, greater; <, lesser; LPLa, lipoprotein lipase activity; HLa, hepatic lipase activity; TC, total cholesterol; LDL-C, low-density lipoprotein cholesterol; TG, triglycerides; HDL-C, high-density lipoprotein cholesterol; Lp(a), lipoprotein(a); LDL size, low-density lipoprotein particle size; apo, apolipoprotein; LCAT, lecithin cholesterol acyltransferase. (Adapted from K. Watson, Plasma Lipoproteins Concentrations in Ethnic Populations, Current Cardiol. Rep. 2003. Published by *Current Medicine*.)

epidemiologic and prospective evidence to suggest that across ethnic groups and throughout the life span, lipid and lipoprotein concentrations are associated with CHD. The information provided in this chapter summarizes lipid and lipoprotein differences and changes across ethnic groups in the United States and throughout the life span. This information may be used by the reader to recognize general trends and key age-related changes in lipid and lipoprotein profiles that may identify individuals at greater risk for developing CHD.

References

1. Kannel, W.B., Lipids, diabetes, coronary heart disease: insights from the Framingham Study, *Am. Heart J.*, 110, 1100, 1985.
2. Stamler, J., Wentworth, D., and Neaton, J.D., Is the relationship between serum cholesterol and risk of premature death from coronary heart disease continuous and graded?, *J.A.M.A.*, 256, 2823, 1986.
3. Verschuren, W.M., Jacobs, D.R., Bloemberg, B.P., et al., Serum total cholesterol and long-term coronary heart disease mortality in cultures. Twenty-five-year follow-up of the Seven Countries Study, *JAMA*, 274, 131, 1995.
4. Knuiman, J.T., Hermus, R.J., and Hautvast, J., Serum total and HDL-cholesterol concentrations in rural and urban boys from 16 countries, *Atherosclerosis*, 36, 529, 1980.
5. Mayes, P.A. Lipid transport and storage and cholesterol synthesis, transport, and excretion, in *Harper's Biochemistry*, 24th ed., Murray, R.K., Granner, D.K., Mayes, P.A., Eds., Appleton and Lange, Stamford, CT, 1996.
6. Dupont, J., Lipids, in *Present Knowledge in Nutrition*, 2nd ed., International Life Sciences, Washington, DC, 1990.
7. Yokayama, S., Release of cellular cholesterol: molecular mechanisms for cholesterol homeostasis in cells and in the body, *Biochim. Biophys. Acta*, 1529, 231, 2000.
8. Jian, B., de la Llera-Moya, M., Ji, Y., et al., Scavenger receptor BI promotes high density lipoprotein-mediated cellular cholesterol efflux, *J. Biol. Chem.*, 272, 20982, 1998.
9. National Cholesterol Education Program (NCEP), Expert Panel on Detection, Evaluation, and Treatment of High Blood Cholesterol in Adults, Executive summary of the third report of the National Cholesterol Education Program (NCEP) Expert Panel on Detection, Evaluation, and Treatment of High Blood Cholesterol in Adults (Adult Treatment Panel III), *J.A.M.A.*, 285, 2486, 2001.
10. Castelli, W.P., Anderson, K., Wilson, P.W., and Levy, D., Lipids and risk of coronary heart disease. The Framingham Study, *Ann. Epidemiol.*, 2, 23, 1992.
11. Durstine, J.L., Crouse, S.F., and Moffatt, R.J., Lipids in exercise and sports, in *Energy Yielding Macronutrients and Energy Metabolism in Sports Nutrition*, Driskell, J.A., Wolinksy, I., Eds., CRC Press, Boca Raton, FL, chap. 6, 2000.
12. Choy, P.C., Sio, Y.L., Myin, D., and Karmin, O. Lipids and atherosclerosis, *Biochem. Cell Biol.*, 82, 212, 2004.

13. Jong, M.C., Hofker, M.H., and Havekes, L.M., Role of ApoCs in lipoprotein metabolism: functional differences between apoC1, apoC2, and apoC3, *Arterioscler. Thromb. Vasc. Biol.*, 19, 472, 1999.
14. Rassart, E., Bedirian, A., Carmo, D.O., et al., Apolipoprotein D, *Biochim. Biophys. Acta*, 1482, 185, 2000.
15. Bocksch, L., Stephens, T., Lucas, A., and Singh, B., Apolipoprotein E: possible therapeutic target for atherosclerosis, *Curr. Drug Targets Cardiovasc. Haematol. Disord.*, 1, 93, 2001.
16. Stan, S., Delvin, E., Lambert, M., et al., Apo A-IV: an update on regulation and physiologic functions, *Biochim. Biophys. Acta*, 1631, 177, 2003.
17. Walldius, G., and Junger, I., Apolipoprotein B and apolipoprotein A-I: risk indicators of coronary heart disease and targets for lipid modifying therapy, *J. Intern. Med.*, 255, 188, 2004.
18. Rader, D.J. Regulation of reverse cholesterol transport and clinical implications, *Am. J. Cardiol.*, 92, 42, 2003.
19. United States Department of Health, Education, and Welfare, National Heart, Lung, and Blood Institutes, National Institutes of Health, Lipid Research Clinics, Vol. I. The Prevalence Study, Bethesda, MD, 79-1527, 1979.
20. Smith, S.J., Cooper, G.R., Myers, G.L., Sampson, E.J., Biological variability in concentrations of serum lipids: sources of variation among results from published studies and composite predicted values, *Clin. Chem.*, 39, 1012, 1993.
21. Barnes, J.S., and Bennett, C.E., The Asian population: census 2000 brief. U.S. Census Bureau, www.census/gov/population/cen2000/briefs, 2002.
22. Klatsky, A.L., and Armstrong, M.A., Cardiovascular risk factors among Asian Americans living in Northern California, *Am. J. Public Health*, 81, 1423, 1991.
23. Choi, E.S.K., McGandy, R.B., Dallal, G.E., et al., The prevalence of cardiovascular risk factors among elderly Chinese Americans, *Arch. Intern. Med.*, 150, 413, 1990.
24. Sowers, M.F., Crawford, S.L., Cauley, J.A., Stein, E. Association of lipoprotein(a), insulin resistance, and reproductive hormones in a multiethnic cohort of pre- and perimenopausal women (the SWAN Study), *Am. J. Cardiol.*, 92, 533, 2003.
25. Carr, M.C., Brunzell, J.D., Deeb, S.S., Ethnic differences in hepatic lipase and HDL in Japanese, black and white Americans: role of central obesity and LIPC polymorphisms, *J. Lipid Res.*, 45, 466, 2004.
26. Zambon, A., Deeb, S.S., Hokanson, J.E., et al., Common variants in the promoter of the hepatic lipase gene are associated with lower levels of hepatic lipase activity, buoyant LDL, and higher HDL2 cholesterol, *Arterioscler. Thromb. Vasc. Biol.*, 18, 1723, 1998.
27. Despres, J.P., Ferland, M., Moorjani, S., et al., Role of hepatic-triglyceride lipase activity in the association between intra-abdominal fat and plasma HDL-C in obese women, *Arteriosclerosis*, 9, 485, 1989.
28. Reed, D., Yano, K., and Kagan, A., Lipids and lipoproteins as predictors of coronary heart disease, stroke, and cancer in the Honolulu Heart Program, *Am. J. Med.*, 80, 871, 1986.
29. Kalhan, R., Puthawala, K., Agarwal, S., et al., Altered lipid profile, leptin, insulin and athropometry in offspring of South Asian Immigrants in the United States, *Metabolism*, 10, 1197, 2001.

30. Lear, S.A., Toma, M., Birmingham, C.L., and Frohlich, J.J., Modification of the relationship between simple anthropometric indices and risk factors by ethnic background, *Metabolism*, 52, 1295, 2003.
31. Abate, N., Garg, A., and Enas E.A. Physico-chemical properties of low density lipoproteins in normolipidemic Asian Indian Men, *Horm. Metab. Res.*, 27, 326, 1995.
32. Palaniappan, L., Anthony, M.N., Mahesh, C., et al., Cardiovascular risk factors in ethnic minority women aged ≤30 years, *Am. J. Cardiol.*, 89, 524, 2002.
33. Kamath, S., Hussain, E.A., Amin, D., et al., Cardiovascular disease risk factors in 2 distinct ethnic groups: Indian and Pakistani compared with American premenopausal women, *Am. J. Clin. Nutr.*, 69, 621, 1999.
34. Kooner, J.S., Balgia, R.R., Wilding, J., et al., Abdominal obesity, impaired non-esterified fatty acid suppression, and insulin-mediated glucose disposal are early metabolic abnormalities in families with premature myocardial infarction, *Arterioscler. Thromb. Vasc. Biol.*, 18, 1021, 1998.
35. Kulkarni, K.R., Markovitz, J.H., Nanda, N.C., Segrest, J.P., Increased prevalence of smaller and denser LDL particles in Asian Indians, *Arterioscler. Thromb. Vasc. Biol.*, 19, 2749, 1999.
36. Raji, A., Seely, E.W., Arky, R.A., and Simonson, D.C., Body fat distribution and insulin resistance in healthy Asian Indians and Caucasians, *J. Clin. Endocr. Metab.*, 86, 5366, 2001.
37. Grieco, E.M., and Cassidy, R.C., Overview of race and Hispanic origin: census 2000 brief, U.S. Census Bureau, www.census.gov/population/www/socdemo/hispanic.html, 2001.
38. Nelson, R.G., Sievers, M.L., Knowler, W.C., et al., Low incidence of fatal coronary heart disease in Pima Indians despite high prevalence of non-insulin dependent diabetes, *Circulation*, 81, 987, 1990.
39. Howard, B.V., Lee, E.T., Cowan, L.D., et al., Rising tide of cardiovascular disease in American Indians. The Strong Heart Study, *Circulation*, 99, 2389, 1999.
40. Knowler, W.C., Pettitt, D.J., Hamman, R.F., and Miller, M., Diabetes incidence and prevalence in Pima Indians: a 19-fold greater incidence than in Rochester, Minnesota, *Am. J. Epidemiol.*, 108, 497, 1978.
41. Page, I.H., Lewis, L.A., and Gilbert, J., Plasma lipids and proteins and their relationship to coronary disease in Navajo Indians, *Circulation*, 13, 675, 1956.
42. Seivers, M.L. Serum cholesterol levels in southwestern American Indians, *J. Chronic Dis.*, 21, 107, 1968.
43. Gillum, R.F, Gillum, B.S., and Smith, N., Cardiovascular risk factors among urban American Indians: blood pressure, serum lipids, smoking habits, health knowledge and behavior, *Am. Heart J.*, 197, 765, 1984.
44. Johnson, C.L., Rifkind, B.M., Sempos, C.T., et al., Declining serum total cholesterol levels among U.S. adults. The National Health and Nutrition Examination Surveys, *J.A.M.A.*, 269, 3002, 1993.
45. Welty, T.K., Lee, E.T., Yeh, J., et al., Cardiovascular disease risk factors among American Indians: the Strong Heart Study, *Am. J. Epidemiol.*, 142, 269, 1995.
46. Robbins, D.C., Welty, T.K., Wang, W.Y., et al., Plasma lipids and lipoprotein concentrations among American Indians: comparisons with the U.S. population, *Curr. Opin. Lipidol.*, 7, 188, 1996.
47. Hu, D., Hannah, J., Gray, R.S., et al., Effects of obesity and body fat distribution on lipids and lipoproteins in nondiabetic American Indians: the Strong Heart Study, *Obes. Res.*, 8, 411, 2000.

48. Welty, T.K., Rhoades, D.A., Yeh, F., et al., Changes in cardiovascular disease risk factors among American Indians. The Strong Heart Study, *Ann. Epidemiol.*, 12, 97, 2002.
49. Wang, W., Hu, D., Lee, E.T., et al., Lipoprotein(a) in American Indians is low and not independently associated with cardiovascular disease: the Strong Heart Study, *Ann. Epidemiol.*, 12, 107, 2002.
50. Howard, B.V., Le, N.E., Belcher, J.D., et al., Concentrations of Lp(a) in black and white young adults: relations to risk factors for cardiovascular disease, *Ann. Epidemiol.*, 4, 341, 1994.
51. Heller, F.R., Jamart, J., Honore, P., et al., Serum lipoprotein(a) in patients with diabetes mellitus, *Diabetes Care*, 16, 819, 1993.
52. Gray, R.S., Robbins, D.C., Wang, W., et al., Relation of LDL size to insulin resistance syndrome and coronary heart disease in American Indians, *Arterioscler. Thromb. Vasc. Biol.*, 17, 2713, 1997.
53. Freedman, D.S., Serdula, M.K., Percy, C.A., et al., Obesity, levels of lipids and glucose, and smoking among Navajo adolescents, *J. Nutr.*, 127, 2120, 1997.
54. Howard, B.V., Cowan, L.D., Go, O., et al., Adverse effects of diabetes on multiple cardiovascular disease risk factors in women and men, *Diabetes Care*, 21, 1258, 1998.
55. Ramirez, R.R., and de la Cruz, G.P., The Hispanic population in the United States: population characteristics. U.S. Census Bureau, www.census.gov/population/www/socdemo/hispanic.html, 2003.
56. Mitchell, B.D., Haffner, S.M., Hazuda, H.P., Patterson, J.K., and Stern, M.P., Diabetes and coronary heart disease risk in Mexican Americans. *Ann. Epidemiol.*, 2, 101, 1992.
57. Wei, M., Mitchell, B.D., Haffner, S.M., and Stern, M.P., Effects of cigarette smoking, diabetes, high cholesterol, and hypertension on all-cause mortality and cardiovascular disease mortality in Mexican Americans. The San Antonio Heart Study, *Am. J. Epidemiol.*, 144, 1058, 1996.
58. Wei, M., Valdez, R.A., Mitchell, B.D., et al., Migration status, socioeconomic status, and mortality rates in Mexican Americans and non-Hispanic whites: the San Antonio Heart Study, *Ann. Epidemiol.*, 6, 307, 1996.
59. Hamman, R.F., Marshall, J.A., Baxter, J., et al., Methods and prevalence of non-insulin dependent diabetes mellitus in a biethnic Colorado population: the San Luis Valley Diabetes Study, *Am. J. Epidemiol.*, 129, 295, 1989.
60. Haffner, S.M., Hazuda, H.J.P., Mitchell, B.D., et al., Increased incidence of type II diabetes mellitus in Mexican Americans, *Diabetes Care*, 14, 102, 1991.
61. Haffner, S.M., Stern, M.P., Hazuda, H.P., et al., The role of behavioral variables and fat pattern in explaining ethnic differences in lipid and lipoproteins, *Am. J. Epidemiol.*, 123, 830, 1986.
62. Burchfiel, C.M., Hamman, R.F., Marshall, J.A., et al., Cardiovascular risk factors and impaired glucose tolerance: the San Luis Valley Diabetes Study, *Am. J. Epidemiol.*, 131, 57, 1990.
63. Hanis, C.L., Hewett-Emmett, D., Douglas, T.C., et al., Effects of the apolipoprotein E polymorphism on levels of lipids, lipoproteins, and apolipoproteins among Mexican-Americans in Starr County, Texas, *Arterioscler. Thromb. Vasc. Biol.*, 11, 362, 1991.

64. Batey, L.S., Goff, D.C., Tortolero, S.R., et al., Summary measures of the insulin resistance syndrome are adverse among Mexican-American versus non-Hispanic white children: the Corpus Christi Child Heart Study, *Circulation*, 96, 4319, 1997.
65. Haffner, S.M., D'Agostino, R., Goff, D., et al., LDL size in African Americans, Hispanics, and non-Hispanic whites: the Insulin Resistance Atherosclerosis Study, *Arterioscler. Thromb. Vasc. Biol.*, 19, 2234, 1999.
66. Ford, E.S., Giles, W.H., and Dietz, W.H., Prevalence of the metabolic syndrome among U.S. adults: findings from the Third National Health and Nutrition Examination Survey, *J.A.M.A.*, 287, 356, 2002.
67. Greaves, K.A., Going, S.B., Fernandez, M.L., et al., Cholesteryl ester transfer protein and lecithin:cholesterol acyltransferase activities in Hispanic and Anglo postmenopausal women: associations with total and regional body fat, *Metabolism*, 52, 282, 2003.
68. Bachorik, P.S., Lovejoy, K.L., Carroll, M.D., and Johnson, C.L., Apolipoprotein B and AI distributions in the United States, 1988–1991: results of the National Health and Nutrition Examination Survey III (NHANES III), *Clin. Chem.*, 43, 2364, 1997.
69. Jeng, J.S., Sacco, R.L., Kargman, D.E., et al., Apolipoproteins and carotid artery atherosclerosis in an elderly multiethnic population: the Northern Manhattan Stroke Study, *Atherosclerosis*, 165, 317, 2002.
70. Paultre, F., Tuck, C.H., Boden-Albala, B., et al., relation of apo(a) size to carotid atherosclerosis in an elderly multiethnic population, *Arterioscler. Thromb. Vasc. Biol.*, 22, 141, 2002.
71. Ford, E.S., Mokdad, A.H., Giles, W.H., and Mensah, J.A., Serum total cholesterol concentrations and awareness, treatment, and control of hypercholesterolemia among U.S. adults: findings from the National Health and Nutrition Examination Survey, 1999 to 2000, *Circulation*, 107, 2185, 2003.
72. Reaven, P., Nader, P.R., Berry, C., and Hoy, J., Cardiovascular Disease Insulin Risk in Mexican-American and Anglo-American Children and Mothers. *Pediatrics*, 101, e12, 1998.
73. Gardner, C.D., Tribble, D.L., Young, D.R., et al., Population frequency distributions of HDL, HDL2, and HDL3 cholesterol and apolipoproteins A-I and B in healthy men and women and associations with age, gender, hormonal status and sex hormone use: the Standford Five City Project, *Prev. Med.*, 31, 335, 2000.
74. Wu, H.D., Berglund, L., Dimayuga, C., et al., High lipoprotein(a) levels and small apolipoprotein(a) sizes are associated with endothelial dysfunction in a multiethnic cohort, *J. Am. Coll. Cardiol.*, 43, 1828, 2004.
75. Haffner, S.M., Mykkanen, L., Valdez, R.A., et al., LDL size and subclass pattern in a biethnic population, *Arterioscler. Thromb.*, 13, 1623, 1993.
76. Rainwater, D.L., Mitchell, B.D., Comuzzie, G., and Haffner, S.M., Relationship of low-density lipoprotein particle size and measures of adiposity, *Int. J. Obes.*, 23, 180, 1999.
77. Barnett, E., and Halverson, J., Disparities in premature coronary heart disease mortality by region and urbanicity among black and white adults ages 35–64, 1985–1995, *Publ. Health Rep.*, 115, 52, 2000.
78. United States Department of Health and Human Services, National Heart, Lung, and Blood Institute, Report of the Working Group on Research in Coronary Heart Disease in Blacks, Bethesda, MD, 94-1, 1994.

79. Jacobs, D.R., Burke, G.L., Liu, K., et al., Relationships of low density lipoprotein cholesterol with age and other factors: a cross-sectional analysis of the Cardia Study, *Ann. Clin. Res.*, 20, 32, 1988.
80. Metcalf, P.A., Sharrett, A.R., Folsom, A.R., et al., African-American-white differences in lipids, lipoproteins, and apolipoproteins, by educational attainment, among middle-aged adults: the Atherosclerosis Risk in Communities Study, *Am. J. Epidemiol.*, 148, 750, 1998.
81. Despres, J.P., Couillard, C., Gagnon, J., et al., Race, visceral adipose tissue, plasma lipids, and lipoprotein lipase activity in men and women: the Health, Risk Factors, Exercise Training, and Genetics (HERITAGE) Family Study, *Arterioscler. Thromb. Vasc. Biol.*, 20, 1932, 2000.
82. Clark, L.T., Ferdinand, K.C., Flack, J.M., et al., Coronary heart disease in African Americans, *Heart Dis.*, 3, 97, 2001.
83. Kral, B.G., Becker, L.C., Yook, R.M., et al., Racial differences in low-density lipoprotein particle size in families at high risk for premature coronary heart disease, *Ethn. Dis.*, 11, 325, 2001.
84. Randall, O.S., Feseha, H.B., Illoh, K., et al., Response of lipoprotein(a) levels to therapeutic life-style changes in obese African-Americans, *Atherosclerosis*, 172, 155, 2004.
85. Despres, J.P., Moorjani, S., Lupien, P.J., et al., Regional distribution of body fat, plasma lipoproteins, and cardiovascular disease, *Arterioscler*, 10, 497, 1990.
86. Folsom, A.R., Burke, G.L., Byers, C.L., et al., Implications of obesity for cardiovascular disease in blacks: the CARDIA and ARIC studies, *Am. J. Clin. Nutr*, 53, 1604, 1991.
87. Maurtaugh K.H., Borde-Perry, W.C., Campbell, K.L., et al., Obesity, smoking, and multiple cardiovascular risk factors in young adult African Americans, *Ethn. Dis.*, 1, 331, 2002.
88. Bowers, J.F., Deshaises, Y., Pfeifer, M., et al., Ethnic differences in postprandial triglyceride response to a fatty meal and lipoprotein lipase in lean and obese African American and Caucasian women, *Metabolism*, 51, 211, 2002.
89. Glueck, C.J., Gartside, P., Laskarzewski, P.M., et al., High-density lipoprotein cholesterol in blacks and whites: potential ramifications for coronary heart disease, *Am. Heart J.*, 108, 815, 1984.
90. Vega, G.L., Clark, L.T., Tang, A., et al., Hepatic lipase activity is lower in African American men than in white American men: effects of 5 flanking polymorphism in the hepatic lipase gene (LIPC). *J. Lipid Res.*, 39, 228, 1998.
91. Bergeron, J., Couillard, C., Despres, J.P., et al., Race differences in the response of postheparin plasma lipoprotein lipase and hepatic lipase activities to endurance exercise training in men: results from the HERITAGE Family Study, *Atherosclerosis*, 159, 399, 2001.
92. Srinivasan, S.R., Segrest, J.P., Elkasabany, A.M., and Berenson, G.S., Distribution and correlates of lipoproteins and their subclasses in black and white young adults. The Bogalusa Heart Study, *Atherosclerosis*, 159, 391, 2001.
93. Kushnick M.R., Bodin, W., Tackett, J., Kingsley, D., et al., LDL particle size and distribution in white and black untrained men following acute treadmill walking [abstract], *Med. Sci. Sport Exerc.*, 36, 143, 2004.
94. Watson, K.E., Plasma lipoprotein concentrations in ethnic populations, *Curr. Cardiol. Rep.*, 5, 483, 2003.
95. Watkins, L.O., Epidemiology and burden of cardiovascular disease, *Clin. Cardiol.*, 27, 2, 2004.

96. Lauer, R.M., Lee, J, and Clarke, W.R., Predicting adult cholesterol levels from measurements in childhood and adolescence: the Muscatine Study, *Bull. N.Y. Acad. Med.*, 65, 1127, 1989.
97. Berenson, G.S., Wattigney, W.A., Tracy, R.E., et al., Atherosclerosis of the aorta and coronary arteries and cardiovascular risk factors in persons aged 6 to 30 years and studied at necropsy (the Bogalusa Heart Study), *Am. J. Cardiol.*, 70, 851, 1992.
98. Berenson, G.S., Srinivasan, S.R., Bao, W., et al., Association between multiple cardiovascular risk factors and atherosclerosis in children and young adults: the Bogalusa Heart Study, *N. Engl. J. Med.*, 338, 1650, 1998.
99. Kannel, W.B., D'Agostino, R.B., and Belanger, A.J., Concept of bridging the gap from youth to adulthood, *Am. J. Med. Sci.*, 310, 15, 1995.
100. Innis, S.M., and Hamilton, J.J., Effects of developmental changes and early nutrition on cholesterol metabolism in infancy: a review, *J. Am. Coll. Nutr.*, 11, 63, 1992.
101. Schaefer, E.J., Lichtenstein, A.H., Lamon-Fava, S., et al., Lipoproteins, nutrition, aging, and atherosclerosis, *Am. J. Clin. Nutr.*, 61, 726, 1995.
102. Boulton, T.J.C., Magarey, A.M., and Cockington, R.A., Serum lipids and apolipoproteins from 1 to 15 years: changes with age and puberty, and relationships with diet, parental cholesterol and family history of ischaemic heart disease, *Acta Paediatr.*, 84, 1113, 1995.
103. Porkka, K.V., Raitakari, O.T., Leino, A,, et al., Trends in serum lipid levels during 1980–1992 in children and young adults. The Cardiovascular Risk in Young Finns Study, *Am. J. Epidemiol.*, 146, 64, 1997.
104. Owen, C.G., Whincup, P.H., Odoki, K., et al., Infant feeding and blood cholesterol: a study in adolescents and a systematic review, *Pediatrics*, 110, 597, 2002.
105. Lauer, R.M., Lee, J., and Clarke, W.R., Factors affecting the relationship between childhood and adult cholesterol levels: the Muscatine Study, *Pediatrics*, 82, 309, 1988.
106. Yamayoto, A., Horibe, S., Sawada, M., et al., Serum lipid levels in elementary and junior high school children and their relationship to relative weight, *Prev. Med.*, 17, 93, 1988.
107. Berns, M.A., DeVries, J.H.M., and Katan, M.B., Increase in body fatness as a major determinant of change in serum total cholesterol and high density lipoprotein cholesterol in young men over a 10 year period, *Am. J. Epidemiol.*, 130, 1109, 1989.
108. Seirvogel, R.M., Wisemandle, W., Maynard, L.M., et al., Serial changes in body composition throughout adulthood and the relationships to changes in lipid and lipoprotein levels. The Fels Longitudinal Study, *Arerioscler. Throm. Vasc. Biol.*, 18, 1759, 1998.
109. DeNino, W.F., Tchernof, A., Dionne, I.J., et al., Contribution of abdominal adiposity to age-related differences in insulin sensitivity and plasma lipids in healthy nonobese women, *Diabetes Care*, 24, 925, 2001.
110. Nicklas, B.J., Ryan, A.S., and Katzel, L.I., Lipoprotein subfractions in women athletes: effects of age, visceral obesity and aerobic fitness, *Int. J. Obes. Relat. Metab. Disord.*, 23, 41, 1999.
111. Lemieux, S., Prud'homme, D., Moorjani, S., et al., Do elevated levels of abdominal visceral adipose tissue contribute to age-related differences in plasma lipoprotein concentrations in men?, *Atherosclerosis*, 118, 155, 1995.

112. Ericsson, S., Berglund, L., Frostegard, J., et al., The influence of age on low density lipoprotein metabolism: effects of cholestyramine treatment in young and old healthy male subjects, *J. Intern. Med.*, 242, 329, 1997.
113. Johnson, H.J., Simpson, E.R., Carr, B.R., et al., The levels of plasma cholesterol in the human fetus throughout gestation, *Pediatr. Res.*, 16, 682, 1982.
114. Lane, D.M., and McConathy, W.J., Factors affecting the lipid and apolipoprotein levels of cord sera, *Pediatr. Res.*, 17, 83, 1983.
115. Parker, C.R., Hankins, G.D.V., Carr, B.R., et al., The effect of hypertension in pregnant women on fetal adrenal function and fetal plasma lipoprotein cholesterol metabolism, *Am. J. Obstet. Gynecol.*, 150, 263, 1984.
116. Lane, D.M., McConathy, W.J., McCaffree, M.A., and Hall, M., Cord serum lipid and apolipoprotein levels in preterm infants with the neonatal respiratory distress syndrome, *J. Matern. Fetal Neonatal Med.*, 11, 118, 2002.
117. Mortaz, M., Fewtrell, M.S., Cole, T.J., and Lucas, A., Cholesterol metabolism in 8 to 12-year-old children born preterm or at term, *Acta Paediatr.*, 92, 525, 2003.
118. Frerichs, R.R., Srinivasan, S.R., Webber, L.S., et al., Serum lipids and lipoproteins at birth in a biracial population: the Bogalusa Heart Study, *Pediatr. Res.*, 12, 858, 1978.
119. Parker, C.R., Carr, B.R., Simpson, E.R. and MacDonald, P.C., Decline in the concentration of low-density lipoprotein cholesterol in human fetal plasma near term, *Metabolism*, 32, 919, 1983.
120. Rafstedt S., Serum lipids and lipoproteins in fullterm newborns during the first few days of life, *Acta Paediatr.*, 44, 26, 1955.
121. Rafstedt S., and Swahn, B. Studies on lipids, proteins and lipoproteins in serum from newborn infants, *Acta Paediatr.*, 43, 221, 1954.
122. Connor, S.L., Connor, W.E., Sexton, G., et al., The effects of age, body weight and family relationships on plasma lipoproteins and lipids in men, women and children of randomly selected families, *Circulation*, 65, 1290, 1982.
123. Porkka, K.V., Viikari, J.S., and Akerblom, H.K., Tracking of serum HDL-C and other lipids in children and adolescents: the Cardiovascular Risk in Young Finns Study, *Prev. Med.*, 20, 713, 1991.
124. Freedman, D.S., Lee, S.L., Byers, T., et al., Serum cholesterol levels in a multiracial sample of 7,439 preschool children from Arizona, *Prev. Med.*, 21, 162, 1992.
125. Rask-Nissilä, L., Jokinen, E., Rönnemaa, T., et al., Prospective, randomized, infancy-onset trial of the effects of a low-saturated-fat, low-cholesterol diet on serum lipids and lipoproteins before school age: the Special Turku Coronary Risk Factor Intervention Project (STRIP), *Circulation*, 102, 1477, 2000.
126. Nicklas, T.A., von Duvillard, S.P., and Berenson, G.S., Tracking of serum lipids and lipoproteins from childhood to dyslipidemia in adults: the Bogalusa Heart Study, *Int. J. Sports Med.*, 23, 39, 2002.
127. Webber, L.S., Srinivasan, S.R., Wattingney, W.A. and Berenson, G.S., Tracking of serum lipids and lipoproteins from childhood to adulthood. The Bogalusa Heart Study, *Am. J. Epidemiol.*, 133, 884, 1991.
128. Brontons, C., Ribera, A., Perich, R.M., et al., Worldwide distribution of blood lipids and lipoproteins in childhood and adolescence: a review study, *Atherosclerosis*, 139, 1, 1998.
129. Hickman, T.B., Briefel, R.R., Carroll, M.D., et al., Distributions and trends of serum lipid levels among United States children and adolescents ages 4–19 years: data from the Third National Health and Nutrition Examination Survey, *Prev. Med.*, 27, 879, 1998.

130. Steinbeck, K.S., Bermingham, M.A., Mahahan, D., and Baur, L.A., Low-density lipoprotein subclasses in children 10 years of age, *J. Paediatr. Child Health*, 37, 550, 2001.
131. Shumacher, M., Kessler, A., Meier, A., et al., Lipoprotein(a) concentrations in cord blood and capillary blood from newborns, and in serum from inpatient children, adolescents and adults. *Eur. J. Clin. Chem. Clin. Biochem.*, 32, 341, 1994.
132. Nago, N., Kayaba, K., Hiraoka, J., et al., Lipoprotein(a) levels in the Japanese population: influence of age and sex, and relation to atherosclerotic risk factors, *Am. J. Epidemiol.*, 141, 815, 1995.
133. Kaitosaari, T., Ronnemaa, T., Raitakari, O., et al., Effect of 7-year infancy-onset dietary intervention on serum lipoproteins and lipoprotein subclasses in healthy children in the prospective, randomized Special Turku Coronary Risk Factor Intervention Project for children (STRIP) Study, *Circulation*, 108, 672, 2003.
134. Asayama, K., Miyao, A., and Kato, K., High-density lipoprotein (HDL), HDL2, and HDL3 cholesterol concentrations determined in serum of newborns, infants, children, adolescents, and adults by use of a micromethod for combined precipitation ultracentrifugation, *Clin. Chem.*, 36, 129, 1990.
135. Dobiasova, M., Stozicky, F., and Kopecka, J., Lecithin-cholesterol acyltransferase activity in children in the early neonatal period, *Biol. Neonate*, 45, 165, 1984.
136. Armstrong, N., Balding, J., Gentle, P., and Kirby, B., Serum lipids and blood pressure in relation to age and sexual maturity, *Ann. Human Biol.*, 19, 477, 1992.
137. Niinikoski, H., Viikari, J., Ronnemaa, T., et al., Prospective randomized trial of a low-saturated-fat, low-cholesterol diet during the first 3 years of life: the STRIP Baby Project, *Circulation*, 94, 1386, 1996.
138. Shea, S., Aymong, E., Zybert, P., et al., Fasting plasma insulin modulates lipid levels and particle sizes in 2- to 3-year-old children, *Obes. Res.*, 11, 709, 2003.
139. DeSimone, M., Verrotti, A., Cappa, M., et al., Lipoprotein(a) in children: correlations with family history of cardiovascular disease, *J. Endocrinol. Invest.*, 26, 414, 2003.
140. Kavey, R.E., Daniels, S.R., Lauer, R.M., et al., American Heart Association guidelines for primary prevention of atherosclerotic cardiovascular disease beginning in childhood, *Circulation*, 107, 1562, 2003.
141. Ogden, C.L., Carroll, M.D., and Flegal, K.M., Epidemiologic trends in overweight and obesity, *Endocrinol. Metab. Clin. North Am.*, 32, 741, 2003.
142. Centers for Disease Control and Prevention, Trend in cigarette smoking among high school students — United States, 1991–2001, *Morbid. Mortal. Wkly. Rep.*, 51, 409, 2002.
143. United States Department of Health and Human Services, Health in the United States, Bethesda, MD, 87-123, 1986.
144. Westenhoefer, J., Establishing dietary habits during childhood for long-term weight control, *Ann. Nutr. Metab.*, 1, 18, 2002.
145. Tammelin, T., Nayha, S., Laitinen, J., et al., Physical activity and social status in adolescence as predictors of physical inactivity in adulthood, *Prev. Med.*, 37, 375, 2003.
146. Williams, C.L., Hayman, L.L., Daniels, S.R., et al., Cardiovascular health in childhood: a statement for health professionals from the Committee on Atherosclerosis, Hypertension, and Obesity in Young (AHOY) of the Council on Cardiovascular Disease in Young, American Heart Association, *Circulation*, 106, 143, 2002.

147. Guo, S., Beckett, L., Chumlea, W.C., et al., Serial analysis of plasma lipids and lipoproteins from individuals 9–21 y of age. *Am. J. Clin. Nutr.*, 58, 61, 1993.
148. Stozicky, F., Slaby, P., and Volenikova, L., Longitudinal study of serum cholesterol, apolipoproteins and sex hormones during puberty, *Acta Paediatr. Scand.*, 80, 1139, 1991.
149. Levy, P.S., Hamill, P.V.V., Heald, F.P., and Roland, M., National Center for Health Statistics. Total serum cholesterol levels of youths, 12–17 years, *Vital Health Stat.*, 156, 1, 1976.
150. Abraham, S., National Center for Health Statistics, Total serum cholesterol levels of children 4–17 years, *Vital Health Stat.*, 207, 1, 1978.
151. Viikari, J., Ronnemaa, T., Seppanen, A., et al., Serum lipid and lipoproteins in children, adolescents and young adults in 1980–1986, *Ann. Med.*, 23, 53, 1991.
152. Twisk, J.W., Kemper, H.C., Mellenbergh, G.J., and van Mechelen, W., Relation between the longitudinal development of lipoprotein levels and biological parameters during adolescence and young adulthood in Amsterdam, the Netherlands, *J. Epidemiol. Commun. Health*, 50, 505, 1996.
153. Freedman, D.S., Bowman, B.A., Otvos, J.D., et al., Levels and correlates of LDL and VLDL particle sizes among children: the Bogalusa Heart Study, *Atherosclerosis*, 152, 441, 2000.
154. Ronnemaa T., Viikari, J., and Marniemi, J. Lecithin: cholesterol acyltransferase activity in children and young adults, *Atherosclerosis*, 77, 7, 1989.
155. Ohta, T., Kakiuti, Y., Kurahara, K., et al., Fractional esterification rate of cholesterol in high density lipoprotein is correlated with low density lipoprotein particle size in children, *J. Lipid Res.*, 38, 139, 1997.
156. Williams, P.T., and Krauss, R.M., Association of age, adiposity, menopause, and alcohol intake with low-density lipoprotein subclasses, *Arterioscler. Thromb. Vasc. Biol.*, 17, 1082, 1997.
157. Arisaka, O., Fujiwara, S., Yabuta, K., et al., Characterization of low-density lipoprotein subclasses in children, *Metabolism*, 46, 146, 1997.
158. Okosun, I.S., Dever, G.E., and Choi, S.T., Low birth weight is associated with elevated serum lipoprotein(a) in white and black American children ages 5–11 y, *Public Health*, 116, 33, 2002.
159. McNamara, J.R., Jenner, J.L., Li, Z., et al., Change in LDL particle size is associated with change in plasma triglyceride concentration, *Arterioscler. Thromb.*, 12, 1284, 1992.
160. Lemieux, I., Pascot, A., Tchernof, A., et al., Visceral adipose tissue and low-density lipoprotein particle size in middle aged versus young men. *Metabolism*, 48, 1322, 1999.
161. Kannel, W.B., and Vokonas, P.S., Demographics of the prevalence, incidence, and management of coronary heart disease in the elderly and in women, *Ann. Epidemiol.*, 2, 5, 1992.
162. Heitmann, B., The effects of gender and age on associations between blood lipid levels and obesity in Danish men and women aged 35–65 years, *J. Clin. Epidemiol.*, 45, 693, 1982.
163. Clark, D., Allen, M.F., and Wilson, F.H., Longitudinal study of serum lipids, *Am. J. Clin. Nutr.*, 20, 743, 1967.
164. Hershcopf, R.J., Elahi, D., Andres, R., et al., Longitudinal changes in serum cholesterol in men: an epidemiological search for an etiology, *J. Chron. Dis.*, 35, 101, 1982.

165. Anderson, K.M., Wilson, P.W.F., Garrison, R.J., and Castelli, W.P., Longitudinal and secular trends in lipoprotein cholesterol measurements in a general population sample: the Framingham Offspring Study, *Atherosclerosis*, 68, 59, 1987.
166. Hubert, H.D., Eaker, E.D., Garrison, R.J., and Castelli, W.P., Life-style correlates of risk factor change in young adults: an eight-year study of coronary heart disease risk factors in the Framingham Offspring, *Am. J. Epidemiol.*, 125, 812, 1987.
167. Heiss, G., Tamir, I., Davis, C.E., et al., Lipoprotein-cholesterol distributions in selected North American populations: the Lipid Research Clinics program prevalence study, *Circulation*, 61, 302, 1980.
168. Abbott, R.D., Garrison, R.J., Wilson, P.W., et al., Joint distribution of lipoprotein cholesterol classes: the Framingham Study, *Arteriosclerosis*, 3, 260, 1983.
169. Laurenzi, M., Mancini, M., Plasma lipids in elderly men and women, *Eur. Heart J.*, 9, 69, 1988.
170. Kromhout, D., Nissinen, A., Menotti, A., et al., Total and HDL cholesterol and their correlates in elderly men in Finland, Italy, and the Netherlands, *Am. J. Epidemiol.*, 131, 855, 1990.
171. Wallance, R.B., and Colsher, P.L., Blood lipids distributions in older persons: prevalence and correlates of hyperlipidemia, *Ann. Epidemiol.*, 2, 15, 1992.
172. Ettinger, W.H., Wahl, P.W., Kuller, L.H., et al., Lipoprotein lipids in older people: results from the Cardiovascular Health Study, *Circulation*, 82, 858, 1992.
173. Millar, J.S., Lichtenstein, A.H,. Cuchel, M., et al., Impact of age on metabolism of VLDL, IDL and LDL apolipoprotein B-100 in men, *J. Lipid Res.*, 36, 1155, 1995.
174. Garry, P.J., Hunt, W.C., Koehler, K.M., et al., Longitudinal study of dietary intakes and plasma lipids in healthy elderly men and women, *Am. J. Clin. Nutr.*, 55, 682, 1992.
175. Saito, K., Sakurabayashi, I., and Manabe, M., Serum lipoprotein lipase in healthy subjects: effects of gender and age, and relationships to lipid parameters, *Ann. Clin. Biochem.*, 35, 733, 1998.
176. Stevenson, J.C., Crook, D., and Godsland, I.F., Influence of age and menopause on serum lipids and lipoproteins in healthy women, *Atherosclerosis*, 98, 83, 1993.
177. Moulopoulos, S.D., Adamopoulos, P.N., Diamantopoulos, E.I., et al., Coronary heart disease risk factors in a random sample of Athenian adults. The Athens Study, *Am. J. Epidemiol.*, 126, 882, 1987.
178. Carroll, M., Sempos, C., Briefel, R., et al., Serum lipids of adults 20–74 years: United States 1976–1980, *Vital Stat.*, 242, 1, 1993.
179. Schaefer, E.J., Lamon-Fava, S., Cohn, S.D., et al., Effects of age, gender and menopausal status on plasma low density lipoprotein cholesterol and apolipoprotein B levels in the Framingham Offspring Study, *J. Lipid Res.*, 35, 779, 1994.
180. Wilson, P.W.F., Anderson, K.M., Harris, T., et al., Determinants of change in total cholesterol and HDL-C with age: the Framingham Study, *J. Gerontol.*, 49, 252, 1994.
181. Denti, L., Pasolini, G., Sanfelici, L., et al., Aging-related decline of gonadal function in healthy men: correlation with body composition and lipoproteins, *J. Am. Geriatr. Soc.*, 48, 51, 2000.
182. Criqui, M.H., Fankville, D.D., Barrett-Connor, E., et al., Change and correlates of change in high and low density lipoprotein cholesterol after six years: a prospective study, *Am. J. Epidemiol.*, 118, 52, 1983.

183. Eberle, E., Doering, A., and Keil, U., Weight change and change in total cholesterol and high-density lipoprotein cholesterol: results of the MONICA Augsburg Cohort Study, *Ann. Epidemiol.*, 1, 487, 1991.
184. Grundy, S.M., Vega, G.L., and Bilheimer, D.W., Kinetic mechanisms determining variability in low density lipoprotein levels and rise with age, *Arteriosclerosis*, 5, 623, 1985.
185. Nikkila, M., Pitkajarvi, T., Koivula, T., et al., Women have a larger and less atherogenic low-density lipoprotein particle size than men, *Atherosclerosis*, 119, 181, 1996.
186. Thillet, J., Doucet, C., Chapman, J., Herbeth, B., et al., Elevated lipoprotein(a) levels and small apo(a) isoforms are compatible with longevity: evidence from a large population of French centenarians, *Atherosclerosis*, 136, 389, 1998.
187. Marcovina, S.M., and Koschinsky, M.L., Lipoprotein(a): structure, measurement and clinical significance, in *Handbook of Lipoprotein Testing*, 2nd ed., Rifai, N., Warnick, G.R., Dominiczak, M.H., Eds., AACC Press, Washington, DC, pp 345–385, 2000.
188. Akita, H., Matsubara, M., Shibuya, H., Fuda, H., and Chiba, H., Effect of ageing on plasma lipoprotein(a) levels, *Ann. Clin. Biochem.*, 39, 237, 2002.
189. Sandkamp M., and Assman, G., Lipoprotein(a) in PROCAM participant and young myocardial infarction survivors, in *Lipoprotein(a)*, Scanu, A.M., Ed., Academic Press, San Diego, pp 205–209, 1990.
190. Nabulsi, A.A., Folsom, A.R., and White, A., Association of hormone-replacement therapy with various cardiovascular risk factors in postmenopausal women, *N. Engl. J. Med.*, 328, 1069, 1993.
191. Berg, G., Mesch, V., Boero, L., Sayegh, F., et al., Lipid and lipoprotein profile in menopausal transition. Effects of hormones, age and fat distribution, *Horm. Metab. Res.*, 36, 215, 2004.
192. Sun, Z., Larson, I.A., Ordovas, J.M., et al., Effects of age, gender, and lifestyle factors on plasma apolipoprotein A-IV concentrations, *Atherosclerosis*, 151, 381, 2000.
193. Jackson, K.G., Knapper-Francis, J.M.E, Morgan, L.M., et al., Exaggerated postprandial lipemia and lower post heparin lipoprotein lipase activity in middle-aged men, *Clin. Sci.*, 105, 457, 2003.
194. Huttunen, J.K., Ehnholm, C., Kekki, M., and Nikkila, E.A., Post-heparin plasma lipoprotein lipase and hepatic lipase in normal subjects and in patients with hypertriglyceridaemia: correlations to sex, age and various parameters of triglyceride metabolism, *Clin. Sci. Mol. Med.*, 50, 249, 1976.
195. Zmuda, J.M., Cauley, J.A., Kriska, A., et al., Longitudinal relation between endogenous testosterone and cardiovascular disease risk factors in middle-aged men. A 13-year follow-up of former Multiple Risk Factor Intervention Trial participants, *Am. J. Epidemiol.*, 146, 609, 1997
196. Albers, J.J., Bergelin, R.O., Adolphson, J.L., and Wahl, P.W., Population-based references values for lecithin:cholesterol acyltransferase (LCAT), *Atherosclerosis*, 43, 369, 1982.
197. Jenner, J.L., Ordovas, J.M., Lamon-Fava, S., et al., Effects of age, sex, and menopausal status on plasma lipoprotein(a) levels. The Framingham Offspring Study, *Circulation*, 87, 1135, 1993.
198. McNamara, J.R., Campos, H., Ordovas, J.M., et al., Effect of gender, age, and lipid status on low density lipoprotein subfraction distribution. Results from the Framingham Offspring Study, *Arteriosclerosis*, 7, 483, 1987.

199. Li, Z., McNamara, J.R., Fruchart, J.C., et al., Effects of gender and menopausal status on plasma lipoprotein subspecies and particle sizes, *J. Lipid Res.*, 37, 1886, 1996.
200. Carr, M.C., Hokanson, J.E., Zambon, A., et al., The contribution of intraabdominal fat to gender differences in hepatic lipase activity and low/high density lipoprotein heterogeneity. *J. Clin. Endocrinol. Metab.*, 86, 2831, 2001.
201. Lemieux, I., Pascot, A., Lamarche, B., et al., Is the gender difference in LDL size explained by the metabolic complications of visceral obesity?, *Eur. J. Clin. Invest.*, 32, 909, 2002.
202. Godsland, I.F., Effects of postmenopausal hormone replacement on lipid, lipoprotein and apolipoprotein (a) concentrations: analysis of studies published from 1974–2000, *Fertil. Steril.*, 75, 898, 2001.
203. Eriksson, M., Berglund, L., Rudling, M., et al., Effects of estrogen on low density lipoprotein metabolism in males. Short-term and long-term studies during hormonal treatment of prostatic carcinoma, *J. Clin. Invest.*, 84, 802, 1989.
204. Wakatsuki, A., Ikenoue, N., and Sagara, Y., Estrogen-induced small low-density lipoprotein particle in postmenopausal women, *Obstet. Gynecol.*, 91, 234, 1998.
205. Griffin, B., Farish, E., Walsh, D., et al., Response of plasma low density lipoprotein subfractions to estrogen replacement therapy following surgical menopause, *Clin. Endocrinol. (Oxf.)*, 39, 463, 1993.
206. Hermenegildo, C., Garcia-Martinez, M.C., Tarin, J.J., et al., The effect of oral hormone replacement therapy on lipoprotein profile, resistance of LDL to oxidation and LDL particle size, *Maturitas*, 38, 287, 2001.
207. Jensen, J., Nilas, L., and Christiansen, C., Influence of menopause on serum lipids and lipoproteins, *Maturitas*, 12, 321, 1990.
208. Bush, T., Cowan, L., Heiss, G., et al., Ovarian function and lipid/lipoprotein metabolism. Results from the Lipid Research Clinics Program, *Am. J. Epidemiol.*, 120, 489, 1984.
209. Mead, J.R., Irvine, S.A., and Ramji, D.P., Lipoprotein lipase: structure, function, regulation, and role in disease, *J. Mol. Med.*, 80, 753, 2002.
210. Kasim, S., Cholesterol changes with aging: their nature and significance, *Geriatrics*, 42, 79, 1987.
211. Schaefer, E.J., Foster, D.M., Zech, L.A., et al., The effects of estrogen administration on plasma lipoprotein metabolism in premenopausal females, *J. Clin. Endocrinol. Metab.*, 57, 262, 1983.
212. Hazzard, W.R., Haffner, S.M., Kushwaha, R.S., et al., Preliminary report: kinetic studies on the modulation of high-density lipoprotein, apolipoprotein, and subfraction metabolism by sex steroids in a post menopausal woman, *Metabolism*, 33, 779, 1984.
213. Couillard, C., Bergeron, N., Prud'homme, D., et al., Gender differences in postprandial lipemia, *Arterioscler. Thromb. Vasc. Biol.*, 19, 2448, 1999.
214. Williams, C.M., Lipid metabolism in women, *Proc. Nutr. Soc.*, 63, 153, 2004.
215. Kobayashi, J., Tashiro, J., Murano, S., et al., Lipoprotein lipase mass and activity in post-heparin plasma from subjects with intra-abdominal visceral fat accumulation, *Clin. Endocrinol.*, 48, 515, 1998.
216. Hargrove, G.M., Junco, A., and Wong, N.C., Hormonal regulation of apolipoprotein AI, *J. Mol. Endocrinol.*, 22, 103, 1999.
217. Godsland, I.F., Biology: risk factor modification by OCs and HRT lipids and lipoproteins, *Maturitas*, 47, 299, 2004.

218. Sorva, R., Kuusi, T., Dunkel, L., and Taskinen, M.R., Effects of endogenous sex steroids on serum lipoproteins and postheparin plasma lipolytic enzymes, *J. Clin. Endocrinol. Metab.*, 66, 408, 1988.
219. Colvin, P.L., Auerbach, B.J., Case, D., et al., A dose-response relationship between sex hormone-induced change in hepatic triglyceride lipase and high-density lipoprotein cholesterol in postmenopausal women, *Metabolism*, 40, 1052, 1991.
220. Tikkanen, M.J., Nikkila, E.A., Kuusi, T., and Sipinen, S.U., High density lipoprotein2- and hepatic lipase: reciprocal changes produced by estrogen and norgestrel, *J. Clin. Endocrinol. Metab.*, 54, 1113, 1982.
221. Lichtenstein, M.J., Yarnell, Y.W., Elwood, P.C., et al., Sex hormones, insulin, lipids and prevalent ischemic heart disease, *Am. J. Epidemiol.*, 126, 647, 1987.
222. Haffner, S.M., Mykkanen, L., Valdez, V.A., et al., Relationship of sex hormones to lipids and lipoproteins in nondiabetic men, *J. Clin. Endocrinol. Metab.*, 77, 1610, 1993.
223. Glueck, C.J., Ford, S., Steiner, P., et al., Triglyceride removal efficiency and lipoprotein lipase: effects of oxandrolone, *Metabolism*, 22, 807, 1973.
224. Kirkland, R.T., Keenan, B.S., Probstfield, J.L., et al., Decrease in plasma high density lipoprotein cholesterol levels at puberty in boys with delayed adolescence, *J.A.M.A.*, 257, 502, 1987.
225. Gordon, D.J., Rifkind, B.M., Treating high blood cholesterol in the older patient, *Am. J. Cardiol.*, 63, 48, 1989.
226. Curb, D.J., Reed, D.M., Yano, K., et al., Plasma lipids and lipoproteins in elderly Japanese-American men, *J. Am. Gerentol. Soc.*, 34, 773, 1986.
227. Frishman, W.H., Ooi, W.L., Derman, M.P., et al., Serum lipids and lipoprotein in advanced age: intraindividual changes, *Am. J. Epidemiol.*, 2, 43, 1992.
228. Newschaffer, C.J., Bush, T.L., and Hale, W., Aging and total cholesterol levels: cohort, period and survivorship effects, *Am. J. Epidemiol.*, 136, 23, 1992.
229. Ferrara, A., Barrett-Connor, E., and Shan, J., Total, LDL and HDL cholesterol decrease with age in older men and women: the Rancho Bernardo Study 1984–1994, *Circulation*, 96, 37, 1997.
230. Abbott, R.D., Sharp, D.S., Burchfiel, C.M., et al., Cross-sectional and longitudinal changes in total and high-density-lipoprotein cholesterol levels over a 20-year period in elderly men: the Honolulu Heart Program, *Ann. Epidemiol.*, 7, 417, 1997.
231. Drewnowski, A., and Shultz, J.M., Impact of aging on eating behaviors, food choices, nutrition, and health status, *J. Nutr. Health Aging*, 5, 75, 2001.
232. Knapp, R.G., Schreiner, P.J., Sutherland, S.E., et al., Serum lipoprotein (a) levels in elderly black and white men in the Charleston Heart Study, *Clin. Genet.*, 33, 225, 1993.
233. Simmons, L., Friedlander, Y., Simmons, J., and McCallum, J., Lipoprotein(a) is not associated with coronary heart disease in the elderly: cross-sectional data from the Dubbo Study, *Atherosclerosis*, 99, 87, 1993.
234. Zulianai, G., Dader, G., Imbastaro, T., et al., Lipoprotein(a) plasma levels and apo(a) isoforms are not associated with longevity or disability in a sample of Italian octo-nonagenarians, *Aging Clin. Exp. Res.*, 7, 385, 1995.
235. Mykkanen, L., Kuusisto, J., Haffner, S.M., et al., LDL size and risk of coronary heart disease in elderly men and women, *Arterioscler. Thromb. Vasc. Biol.*, 19, 2742, 1999.

Index

A

Abbasi studies, 158
ABCA1, *see* Adenosine triphosphate-binding cassette-A1 (ABCA1)
ACEII Receptor 1 blockers, 86
Acetyl coenzyme (CoA), 39
Acetylecholine, 65
ACS, *see* Acute coronary syndrome (ACS)
Acute coronary syndrome (ACS), 104
Acylation-stimulating pathway (ASP), 159–162
Acylation-stimulating protein (ASP), 148
Acylglycerides, 32, *32*
Adams studies, 102
Adenosine diphosphate, 65
Adenosine triphosphate-binding cassette-A1 (ABCA1), 55
Adiponectin, 158–159
Administration, pharmacological treatments
  bile acid-binding resins, 194, 196
  nicotinic acid, 198
  statins, 191
Advanced age, 331–332
Adventitia, 64
African Americans, *see* Black Americans
Alaskan Natives, *see* American Indians
Albers, Warnick and, studies, 127
ALERT trial, 192
Alhassan studies, 117–142
Almonds, 230
Alpha-adrenergic agonists, 65
Alpha-Tocopherol, Beta-Carotene Cancer Prevention Study, 222
American Diabetes Association, 247
American Heart Association, 226, 247, 300, 324
American Indians, 318
Americans, adult, *320*, 320–321
AMPK, *see* AMP-kinase (AMPK)
AMP-kinase (AMPK), 156–158
Anderson studies, 225, 235, 327
Angelopoulos studies, 173–178
Angiotensin II, 97
Animal studies
  acylation-stimulating pathway, 162
  AMPK stimulation, 157
  endothelial function and exercise training, 89–91
Anitschkow, N, 67
Anti-atherogenic roles, HDL, 58
Anti-inflammation, 101
Apolipoproteins
  acute changes induced by exercise, 291–292
  basics, 48
  concentration quantification, 123
  exercise, impact, *268*, 270–271
L-arginine, 86
Arterial ischemia, pre-symptomatic, 23
Artery, anatomical structure, 63–64, *64*
Asayama studies, 323
Asian Americans, 244, 317–318
Asian Indian Americans, *see* Asian Americans
ASP, *see* Acylation-stimulating pathway (ASP); Acylation-stimulating protein (ASP)
Assay linearity, 140–141
Assay procedures, 137–138, 141
Atherogenic lipid phenotype, 148
Atheroma, 76
Atherosclerosis
  artery, anatomical structure, 63–64, *64*
  basics, 6–7, 61–62, *62–63*, 77
  chronic endothelial injury hypothesis, 66–67
  endothelial dysfunction, 64–66
  fatty streak formation, 68–71, *70–71*
  foam cell formation, 72
  immune responsiveness, 74–75, *75*
  intracellular lipid accumulation, 72
  LDL-mediated atherogenesis, 68, *69–70*
  LDL oxidative modification, 68–71, *70–71*
  lipid accumulation, 68, *69–70*
  lipid hypothesis, 67–68
  macrophages, 72
  pathogenesis theories, *66*, 66–68
  plaque formation, *75*, 75–77

reverse cholesterol transport, 54
risk factors, *63*
smoking, 302
smooth muscle cell immigration, *73*, 73–74
soldier autopsies, 61–62
stages, 68–77
Atherosclerotic cardiovascular disease, 14–15, *14–15*
Atkins diet, 235–236
Atorvastatin, 192, 196, 202, 204
ATP III guidelines, 20
ATTICA Study, 232

B

Babies, *see* Early childhood
Bachorik studies, 325–326, 329
Barley, 224, 230
Barter studies, 57–58
Bazzano studies, 223
Beard studies, 267
Belardinelli studies, 95
Ben-Ezra studies, 147–163
Bergholm studies, 96
Berglund studies, 241
Bile acid-binding resins, 194–197
Black Americans, 150–152, 244–245, 319–320
Blood-brain barrier, 308
Blood lipids, *see* Lipids
Blood pressure, high, *see* Hypertension
BMI, *see* Body mass index (BMI)
Body mass index (BMI)
adiponectin, 158
cardiovascular disease predictor, 173–174
metabolic syndrome, 149
obesity, 176
waist circumference, 150–152
Bogalusa Heart Studies, 300, 324
Boulton studies, 323, 325
Brown studies, 68, 72, 224
Butter, 219, 245

C

CACs, *see* Circulating angiogenic cells (CACs)
CAD, *see* Coronary artery disease (CAD)
C3a-des-Arg, *see* Acylation-stimulating pathway (ASP)
Calculations, 138, 141
Callaerta-Vegh studies, 97
Campos studies, 304
Canadian Heart Health Survey, 151
Canola oil, 202
Caramori studies, 104
CARDIA study, Coronary Artery Risk Development in Young Adults (CARDIA)
Cardiovascular disease (CVD), *see also* Heart disease
apolipoproteins, 291
cigarette smoking, 306–307
endothelial function and exercise training, 87, 99, 106
metabolic syndrome, 149
nutrition, 212–213
smoking, 300–301
Cardiovascular disease (CVD), nutrition effects
basics, 212–213, 246, 248, *248*
changing macronutrient profile, 237–240
DASH diet, 233
dietary cholesterol, 222
dietary fiber, 222–225
dietary patterns effect, 228–233, *229*
emerging risk factors, 236–246
fat type dietary intervention, 239–240
fiber type dietary intervention, 239–240
glycemic index/glycemic load, 225–227
HDL particle size, 240–242
heart disease and fiber connection, 222–223
high-fat diets, 237
high-protein diets, 235–237, 239
LDL particle size, 236–237, *238*
Lifestyle Heart Program, 230–231
lipid management, 224–225
lipoprotein (a), 244–246
low-carbohydrate diets, 237, 239
low-fat diets, 234
Mediterranean Diet, 232–233
moderate-fat diets, 234–235, 237
monounsaturated fatty acids, 219–220
multiple dietary strategies, 239–240
NCEP recommendations, 228, 230
n-3 PUFA, 221–222
n-6 PUFA, 220–221
nutrients effect, 213–228, *214–216*
polyunsaturated fatty acids, 220–222
Portfolio diet, 230–231
postprandial TG, 242–244
saturated fatty acids, 217–218
science-based dietary guidelines, 246, *247*
total fat, 213, 215, 217
trans fatty acids, 218–219

weight loss effects, 233–236
Cardiovascular rehabilitation (CVR), 87, 94–95, 98, 103
Cardiovascular risk assessment
atherosclerotic cardiovascular disease, 14–15, *14–15*
basics, 13–14
diabetes, 21, *21*
dyslipidemia, 19–21, *20*
hypertension, 15–18, *16–19*
metabolic syndrome, 21, *21*
multivariable risk assessment, 24–25
novel risk factors, 23–24
obesity, 22, *22*
pre-symptomatic arterial ischemia, 23
preventive implications, 25–26, *26*
risk factors, 15–23
unstable lesions, 23
Carter, R., III, studies, 61–77
Case studies, 102–104
Caucasians
adiponectin, 158
apolipoproteins, 271
lipoprotein (a), 244
post-heparin LPL activity, 273
waist circumference, 150–152
CCR2, *see* Chemokine receptor 2 (CCR2)
CD36, *see* Cluster differentiation 36 surface molecules (CD36) receptors
Cederberg and Enderback studies, 156
Cell permeability, 65
Centers for Disease Control and Prevention, 148
Cerivastatin, 85, 193
Cessation of smoking, 306–308
CETP, *see* Cholesterol/cholesteryl ester transfer protein (CETP)
Chajek-Shaul studies, 302
Change mechanisms, *268*, 272–273, 292–293
Changing macronutrient profile, 237–240
Chang studies, 93
CHD, *see* Coronary heart disease (CHD)
Chelland studies, 299–310
Chemokine receptor 2 (CCR2), 69–70
Chemokines, 69
Cheuvront, S., 77
Children, *see* Early childhood; Mid- to late adolescence
Chinese Americans, *see* Asian Americans
Chlamydia pneumoniae, 65
Chobanian studies, 25
Choi studies, 317
Cholesterol
absorption inhibitors, 200–202
advanced age, 331
atherosclerosis, 6
bile salt conversion, 37
dietary, 37, 222
early childhood, 322–323
ester exchange rate, 139–141
exercise and physical activity, 267
exercise-induced changes, 284, 290–291
middle age, Americans, 327
mid- to late adolescence, 324–325, *325*
nutrition, 213
pharmacological treatments, 183–184
risk factors, 3–4
synthesis regulation, 38–41, *40–41*
Cholesterol/cholesteryl ester transfer protein (CETP)
cigarette smoking, 305
exercise-induced changes, 292
indirect pathway, 57
lipoprotein lipase, 155
post-heparin LPL activity, 273
rate estimation, 139–141
Cholesterol esterase, 120
Cholesterol oxidase, 120
Cholestyramine, 194, 196
Chronic endothelial injury hypothesis, 66–67
Chylomicrons, 50–51, 55, 266
Cianflone studies, 161
Circulating angiogenic cells (CACs), 102
Clarkson studies, 92
Classifications, 32–37, 48–51, *49*
Clinical applications, 274–275
Clinical trials
bile acid-binding resins, 196–197
fibrates, 200
fish oils, 203
nicotinic acid, 198
statins, 194, *195*
Cluster differentiation 36 surface molecules (CD36) receptors, 72
CoA, *see* Acetyl coenzyme (CoA)
Coa studies, 211–248
Colesevelam, 194, 196
Colestipol, 194
Connor studies, 329
Coronary artery disease (CAD)
apolipoproteins, 270
cholesterol relationship, 1–2
endothelial function, 86–87, 91–98, 105–106
exercise and physical activity, 268–269
Japan incidence, 7
lipids and lipoprotein acceptance, 8
metabolic syndrome, 149
pharmacological treatments, 184–187

Coronary artery disease (CAD), exercise training and endothelial function
  animal studies, 88–91
  basics, 85–86, *86*, 104–106, *105*
  case study, 102–104
  dysfunction reversal, 88–91
  human endothelial function, 91–97
  improved endothelial dysfunction, 98–102
  morbidity and mortality, 87
  VLDL particles, 6
  youth endothelial dysfunction, 97–98
Coronary Artery Risk Development in Young Adults (CARDIA), 319
Coronary heart disease (CHD), 148
Coronary Primary Prevention Trial, 3
CP450, *see* Cytochrome P450 (CP450)
Craig studies, 301
C-reactive protein, 24, 149
Crouse studies, 269, 283–295
Curve development, standard, 140–141
CVR, *see* Cardiovascular rehabilitation (CVR)
CY3A4 isoenzyme, 192
CY2C0 isoenzyme, 192
Cycling, postprandial lipemia, 272
Cyclooxygenase, 42
Cyclosporine, 204
CYP3A4 system, 200, 204
Cytochrome P450 (CP450), 192
Cytomegaloviral infections, 65

D

DAG, *see* Diacylglycerol (DAG)
Dark chocolate, 86
DASH Diet, *229*, 233
Dattilo studies, 178
Davey studies, 239
Davis studies, 47–58, 89
Decreased flow-induced vasodilation, 65
DELTA, *see* Dietary Effects on Lipoproteins and Thrombogenic Activity (DELTA)
DeSouza studies, 92
Desroches studies, 239
Developmental stages, Americans, 322
DGAT, *see* Diacylglycerol acyltransferase (DGAT)
Diabetes, *see also* Insulin
  adiponectin, 158
  American Indians, 318
  cardiovascular disease predictor, 174–175
  cardiovascular risk assessment, 21, *21*
  endothelial dysfunction, 65
  endothelial function and exercise training, 92–93
  Hispanic Americans, 319
  obesity, 176
  pharmacological treatments, 187
  VLDL, 5
Diabetic dyslipidemia, 176
Diacylglycerides, 26
Diacylglycerol acyltransferase (DGAT), 159
Diacylglycerol (DAG), 159
Diet and Reinfarction trial, 203
Dietary Approaches to Stop Hypertension (DASH) Diet, *229*, 233
Dietary Effects on Lipoproteins and Thrombogenic Activity (DELTA), 217, 241
Dietary patterns effect, 228–233, *229*
Digestion, lipids, 37–38, *38–39*
Direct pathway, 56–57
Dreon, Krauss and, studies, 237
Dreon studies, 237, 239
Drug interactions, 192, *192*, 196, *see also* Side effects
Drug selection, 204
Dumesnil studies, 237
Dupont studies, 31–44
Durstine and Haskell studies, 178
Durstine studies, 177, 265–275
Dysfunction reversal, 88–91
Dyslipidemias
  acylation-stimulating pathway, 162
  cardiovascular risk assessment, 19–21, *20*
  metabolic syndrome, 148–150
  obesity, 176–178

E

Early childhood, 322–324
Eckel studies, 152
EDD, *see* Endothelium dependent vasodilation (EDD)
Edwards studies, 95
Eicosanoids, 41–42, *42–43*
EID, *see* Endothelial-independent dilation (EID)
Electrophoresis, 48, 128–131
ELISA techniques, 139
Elliason studies, 303
Emerging risk factors, 236–246
Enderback, Cederberg and, studies, 156
Endogenous pathway, 53–54
Endothelial dysfunction, 64–66

Endothelial function
  animal studies, 88–91
  basics, 85–86, *86,* 104–106, *105*
  case study, 102–104
  dysfunction reversal, 88–91
  human endothelial function, 91–97
  improved endothelial dysfunction, 98–102
  morbidity and mortality, 87
  youth endothelial dysfunction, 97–98
Endothelial-independent dilation (EID), 92, 95
Endothelial-leukocyte adhesion molecules, 65
Endothelial nitric oxide synthase (eNOS), 63, 88–89, 101, 105, *see also* Nitric oxide (NO)
Endothelial progenitor cells (EPCs), 91, 101–102, 106
Endothelin-1 (ET-1), 97
Endothelium dependent vasodilation (EDD), 88, 91, 94–95, 98–99, 105
Endurance training, 266–271
eNOS, *see* Endothelial nitric oxide synthase (eNOS)
Environmental tobacco smoke (ETS), 308–309, *see also* Smoking
Enzyme analysis, intravascular, 133–141
EPCs, *see* Endothelial progenitor cells (EPCs)
Erbs studies, 101, 105
Ericsson studies, 331
Essential fatty acids, 41–42, *42–43, see also* Fatty acids; Fish oils; *Trans* fatty acids (TFA)
Estrogen, *see* Hormones
ET-1, *see* Endothelin-1 (ET-1)
Ethnic differences
  atherosclerosis, 62
  early childhood, 323–324
  ethnicity and age, 323–324, 326
  mid- to late adolescence, 326
Ethnicity and age
  advanced age, 331–332
  American Indians, 318
  Americans, adult, *320,* 320–321
  Asian Americans, 317–318
  basics, 316–321, 332, *332,* 334
  Black Americans, 319–320
  developmental stages, Americans, 322
  early childhood, Americans, 322–324
  ethnic differences, 323–324, 326
  gender differences, 323–324, 326, 329–330, 332
  Hispanics, 318–319
  life-span, Americans, 321–332
  middle age, Americans, 326–330
  mid- to late adolescence, Americans, 324–326
ETICA study, 87
ETS, *see* Environmental tobacco smoke (ETS)
Exercise
  apolipoproteins, *268,* 270–271
  basics, 265, 275
  change mechanisms, *268,* 272–273
  clinical application, 274–275
  endurance training, 266–271
  lipids, *266–268,* 266–269
  lipoproteins, 266–269, *268–269*
  physical inactivity, 273–274
  postprandial lipemia, 272
  resistance training, 271
Exercise and obesity
  basics, 173–174, *174,* 178
  dyslipidemias, lifestyle modification, 177–178
  visceral adiposity, 174–177
Exercise-induced changes
  apolipoproteins, 291–292
  basics, 283–284, *286–289,* 294–295
  benefits, 293–294
  blood triglycerides, 285, 290
  change mechanisms, 292–293
  cholesterol, 290–291
  HDL-C and HDL-C subfractions, 284–285
  LDL cholesterol, 290–291
  lipoprotein (a), 291
Exercise training and endothelial function
  animal studies, 88–91
  basics, 85–86, *86,* 104–106, *105*
  case study, 102–104
  dysfunction reversal, 88–91
  human endothelial function, 91–97
  improved endothelial dysfunction, 98–102
  morbidity and mortality, 87
  youth endothelial dysfunction, 97–98
Exogenous pathway, 51–53
Exon 7 polymorphisms, 101, 105
Ezetimibe, 200, 202, 204

F

Familial hypercholesterolemia, 53
Faraj studies, 158, 161
Fat, nutrition effects, 213
Fatty acids, *see also* Essential fatty acids; Fish oils; Free fatty acids (FFA); *Trans* fatty acids (TFA)

basics, 32, *33–35*, 34
cigarette smoking, 303
lipoprotein lipase, 152
Fat-type dietary intervention, 239–240
Fatty streak formation, 68–71, *70–71*
Fenofibrate, 200
Ferrara studies, 331
Ferre studies, 157
FFA, *see* Free fatty acids (FFA)
Fiber, 222–225, 230, 239–240
Fibrates, 199–200, 204
Fibrinogen, 23
Filipino Americans, *see* Asian Americans
Fish oils, 202–203, 221–222, 239, 244–245, *see also* Essential fatty acids; Fatty acids
Flaxseed, 202
Flow-mediated dilation (FMD), 92–93, 95, 98, 100
5-Fluorouracil (5-FU), 91
Fluvastatin, 191–192, 204
FMD, *see* Flow-mediated dilation (FMD)
Foam cell formation, 72
Fogarty studies, 90
Foger studies, 292
Folic acid, 86
Foster studies, 236
Framingham Heart Study
advanced age, 331
Asian Americans, 317
cardiovascular disease, 14, *14–15*, 300
cholesterol relationship, 3
diabetes, *21*, 22
dyslipidemia, 20, *20*
exercise and physical activity, 274
hypertension, 15–17, *16–19*
metabolic syndrome, 149
multivariable risk assessment, 25
obesity, 22
pre-symptomatic arterial ischemia, 23
preventative implications, 26
risk factor, 24
Freedman studies, 324, 326
Free fatty acids (FFA), *see also* Fatty acids
acylation-stimulating pathway, 160–162
cigarette smoking, 303
lipoprotein lipase, 152, 154
Freeman studies, 301, 303
5-FU, *see* 5-Fluorouracil (5-FU)
Fuchsjager-Mayerl, 93
Fukai studies, 99
Future trends, 7

G

Garg studies, 220, 225
Gebauer studies, 211–248
Gel electrophoresis, 48, 128–131
Gemfibrozil, 200
Gender differences
advanced age, 332
early childhood, 323–324
ethnicity and age, 323–324, 326, 329–330, 332
middle age, Americans, 329–330
mid- to late adolescence, 326
Gerhard studies, 235
Gestation, *see* Developmental stages, Americans
GI, *see* Glycemic index/glycemic load
Gidez studies, 127
Gielen studies, 94, 99
GISSI Prevention Study, 221
Glide and Van Bilsen studies, 157
Glomser, Ross and, studies, 6
Glomset, Ross and, studies, 66
Glucose transporters, 160
Glycemic index/glycemic load, 92, 225–227
Glycerol kinase, 120
Glycerol phosphate oxidase, 120
Godsland studies, 329
Gokce studies, 95
Goodarzi studies, 153
Goto studies, 95–96, 106
Graham and Rush studies, 89
Grandjean studies, 117–142
Grape juice, 86
Green studies, 99
Griel studies, 211–248
Griffin studies, 304
Grundy, Mattson and, studies, 220
Grundy and Mattson studies, 220
Guan-Da studies, 93
Guar gum, 224
Guo studies, 324

H

Hagberg studies, 270
Halle studies, 177
Hambrecht studies, 93–94, 98, 100, 103, 105
Hamilton studies, 274
Hammalainen studies, 87
Hammond and Horn studies, 301
Hardman studies, 294
Harris studies, 221

Haskell, Durstine and, studies, 178
Haskell studies, 91
Havel studies, 124
Hayward studies, 91
HDL, *see* High-density lipoprotein (HDL)
HDL-C, *see* High-density lipoprotein (HDL-C) cholesterol and subfractions
Health impact, 8, *see also* Exercise; Nutrition
Health Professionals Follow-Up Study, 221
Heart disease, *see also* Cardiovascular disease (CVD)
  atherosclerosis, 302
  basics, 299–300, 309–310
  carbon monoxide, 308
  cardiovascular disease, 300–301
  cessation of smoking, 306–308
  environmental tobacco smoke, 308–309
  fiber, 222–223
  HDL, 304–306
  LDL, 304
  lipid metabolism, 302–306
  metabolic changes, smoking cessation, 307–308
  nicotine, 308
  triglycerides, 302–304
  VLDL, 302–304
Heart Protection Study, 26
Hedin, Thyberg and, studies, 76
Hegsted studies, 217
Heilbronn studies, 227
Heiss studies, 329
Helicobacter pylori, 65
Hellerstein studies, 303
Henderson studies, 89
Heparin/manganese-chloride ($MnCl_2$) method, 127
Hepatic (triglyceride) lipase (HL/HTGL)
  activities, laboratory methods, 133–138
  endogenous pathway, 53
  exercise-induced changes, 292
Hepatotoxicity, 193
Herpes virus infections, 65
He studies, 153
Higashi studies, 93
High-carbohydrate diet, 234
High-density lipoprotein (HDL)
  basics, 48, 50
  cardiovascular disease, 300
  cholesterol ester transfer protein, 139
  cigarette smoking, 301, 304–308
  exercise-induced changes, 292
  exogenous pathway, 52
  foam cell formation, 72
  formation, 54–56
  indirect pathway, 57
  intravascular formation, 133
  lipid hypothesis, 67
  lipoprotein isolation, 127
  lipoprotein lipase, 155
  metabolic syndrome, 148–149
  nutrition, 212
  obesity, 173–178
  particle size, 240–242
  pharmacological treatments, 184–185
  reverse cholesterol transport, 55–56
  statin effects, 191
High-density lipoprotein (HDL-C) cholesterol and subfractions
  advanced age, 331–332
  basics, 51
  cigarette smoking, 303
  dyslipidemia, 19–20
  early childhood, 323
  exercise and physical activity, 268–269
  exercise-induced changes, 284–285, 292
  foam cell formation, 72
  intravascular formation, 133
  lipoprotein isolation, 127
  metabolic syndrome, 149
  middle age, Americans, 327–329, *328*
  mid- to late adolescence, 325
  nutrition, 213
  pharmacological treatments, 184–185
  post-heparin LPL activity, 273
  resistance training, 271
High-fat, moderate-fat diet effects, 237
Highly sensitive C-reactive protein (hsCRP), 102
High molecular weight (HMW) standards, 129, 131
High-protein diets, 235–237, 239
Hilpert studies, 211–248
Hingorani studies, 101
Hispanic Americans
  ethnicity and age, 318–319
  lipoprotein lipase, 153
  waist circumference, 150–152
Historical developments, 7
Homeostasis Model Assessment (HOMA) of IR, 175
Homocysteine, 24, 62, 102
Honolulu Heart Study, 222, 300, 331
Hormones, 327, 329–330
Horn, Hammond and, studies, 301
Hosakawa studies, 96
Houmard studies, 153
Howard studies, 319
hsCRP, *see* Highly sensitive C-reactive protein (hsCRP)

Human endothelial function, 91–97, *see also* Endothelial function
Hu studies, 218
7α-hydroxylase, 40
Hypercholesterolemia, 65
Hyperlipidemia, 187
Hypertension
  cardiovascular risk assessment, 15–18, *16–19*
  endothelial dysfunction, 65
  endothelial function and exercise training, 92–93
Hypothyroidism, 187

I

IDL, *see* Intermediate-density lipoprotein (IDL)
IL-8, *see* Interleukin-8 (IL-8)
Immune responsiveness, atherosclerosis, 74–75, *75*
Improved endothelial dysfunction, 98–102
Indications
  cholesterol absorption inhibitors, 202
  fibrates, 200
  fish oils, 203
Indirect pathway, 57
Indo-Mediterranean Diet Heart Study, 232
Infants, *see* Early childhood
Inflammation, 65
Insulin, *see also* Diabetes
  adiponectin, 158–159
  cardiovascular disease predictor, 174
  cigarette smoking, 303
  endothelial function and exercise training, 92
  lipoprotein lipase, 154–155
  metabolic syndrome, 148
  obesity, 175–176
  VLDL, 5
Interleukin-8 (IL-8), 70
Intermediate-density lipoprotein (IDL), 5, 50–51
Intracellular lipid accumulation, 72
Intrauterine development, *see* Developmental stages, Americans
Intravascular enzyme analysis, 133–141
Ion chelation, 86
IP-10, 70
Isolating lipoproteins, 123–133, *132*
Israeli population, 220

J

Janssen studies, 152
Japanese Americans, *see* Asian Americans
Jogging, 272
Jones studies, 61–77
Judd studies, 218

K

Kahn and Valdez studies, 151
Kaitosaari studies, 323
Kannel studies, 13–26
Kantor studies, 285
Kaushik, S., 77
Kemi studies, 100
Keys studies, 217
Kildsgaard studies, 161
Kingwell studies, 92
Knapp studies, 331
Kobayashi studies, 95
Kokkinos studies, 177
Kostner studies, 300
Kratz studies, 239
Krauss and Dreon studies, 237
Kris-Etherton studies, 211–248
Kushnick studies, 315–334

L

Laboratory methods, lipid and lipoprotein analysis
  analysis of lipoprotein, 132–133, *133–134*
  apolipoprotein concentration quantification, 123
  assay linearity, 140–141
  basics, 118, 142
  blood lipid concentration quantification, 120–122
  cholesterol ester exchange rate, 139–141
  gel electrophoresis, 128–130
  hepatic lipase activities, 133–138
  intravascular enzyme analysis, 133–141
  isolating lipoproteins, 123–133, *132*
  lipoprotein lipase, 133–138
  lipoprotein precipitation, 126
  NaBr calculation, 126
  neutral lipids, fluorescent intensity, 140–141
  plasma density calculations, 125–126
  plasma preparation, 119–120

pre-electrophoresis procedures, 130–131
separating lipoprotein, 128
sequential ultracentrifugation, 124–126
serum preparation, 119–120
transfer protein activity analysis, 133–141
LaFontaine studies, 85–106
Lamarche studies, 239
Lamon-Fava studies, 291
L-arginine, 86
Latinos, *see* Hispanic Americans
Lauer studies, 321
Laughlin studies, 88–90
Lavrencic studies, 93
Layman studies, 235
LCAT, *see* Lecithin:cholesterol acyltransferase (LCAT)
LDL, *see* Low-density lipoprotein (LDL)
LDL-C, *see* Low-density lipoprotein (LDL-C) cholesterol
Lecithin:cholesterol acyltransferase (LCAT)
cigarette smoking, 305
exercise-induced changes, 292
foam cell formation, 72
indirect pathway, 57
post-heparin LPL activity, 273
reverse cholesterol transport, 56, 293
Left internal mammary artery (LIMA), 100
Lemieux studies, 150–151, 327
Leon studies, 270
Leptin, 156–158, 307–308
Lesions, unstable, 23
Leukocytes
adhesion molecules, 65
atherosclerosis, 74
count, unstable lesion indictor, 23
Levine studies, 301
Lichtenstein studies, 219
Life-span, Americans, 321–332
Lifestyle changes and modifications, 177–178, 186–187
Lifestyle Heart Program
DASH diet, 233
endothelial function and exercise training, 98
nutrition effects, 230–231
summary, *229*
LIMA, *see* Left internal mammary artery (LIMA)
Linke studies, 94, 105
Linoleate, 41
Linoleic acid, 41, 220, 246
-linolenic acid, 41, 243
Lipid and lipoprotein analysis, laboratory methods
analysis of lipoprotein, 132–133, *133–134*
apolipoprotein concentration quantification, 123
assay linearity, 140–141
basics, 118, 142
blood lipid concentration quantification, 120–122
cholesterol ester exchange rate, 139–141
gel electrophoresis, 128–130
hepatic lipase activities, 133–138
intravascular enzyme analysis, 133–141
isolating lipoproteins, 123–133, *132*
lipoprotein lipase, 133–138
lipoprotein precipitation, 126
NaBr calculation, 126
neutral lipids, fluorescent intensity, 140–141
plasma density calculations, 125–126
plasma preparation, 119–120
pre-electrophoresis procedures, 130–131
separating lipoprotein, 128
sequential ultracentrifugation, 124–126
serum preparation, 119–120
transfer protein activity analysis, 133–141
Lipid and lipoprotein metabolism
anti-atherogenic roles, HDL, 58
basics, *47–48*, 49–50
classification, lipoproteins, *49*, 50–51
direct pathway, 56–57
endogenous pathway, 53–54
exogenous pathway, 51–53
HDL formation, 54–56
indirect pathway, 57
reverse cholesterol transport, 54–58, *58*
transport, lipids, 51–54, *52*
Lipid hypothesis, 67–68
Lipid-lowering effects
bile acid-binding resins, 196
cholesterol absorption inhibitors, 202
fibrates, 199
fish oils, 203
nicotinic acid, 197
statins, 190–191, *191*
Lipidology
acylglycerides, 32, *32*
basics, 31
cholesterol synthesis regulation, 38–41, *40–41*
classes, lipids, 32–37
digestion, lipids, 37–38, *38–39*
eicosanoids, 41–42, *42–43*
essential fatty acids, 41–42, *42–43*
fatty acids, 32, *33–35*, 34
peroxidation, lipids, 43–44, *44–45*
phospholipids, 34, 36, *36*
sphingolipids, 34, 36, *36*

steroids and sterols, 36–37, *37*
Lipid Research Clinics, 300
Lipids
accumulation, 68, *69–70*
atherosclerosis, 6–7
basics, 1–2
cholesterol risk factor, 3–4
concentration quantification, 120–122
digestion, 37–38, *38–39*
exercise, impact, *266–268*, 266–269
fluorescent intensity, 140–141
future trends, 7
health impact, 8
historical development, 7
lipoproteins, 4–6
management, nutrition effects, 224–225
smoking, 302–306
Lipoprotein, *see also* High-density lipoprotein (HDL); Low-density lipoprotein (LDL)
basics, 4–6
density, 48
exercise, impact, 266–269, *268–269*
isolating, 123–133
precipitation, 126
separating, 128
Lipoprotein, metabolism, *see also* Metabolic syndrome
atherosclerosis, 302
basics, 299–300, 309–310
carbon monoxide, 308
cardiovascular disease, 300–301
cessation of smoking, 306–308
endothelial dysfunction, 65
environmental tobacco smoke, 308–309
HDL, 304–306
LDL, 304
lipid metabolism, 302–306
metabolic changes, smoking cessation, 307–308
nicotine, 308
triglycerides, 302–304
VLDL, 302–304
Lipoprotein (a)
endogenous pathway, 54
exercise and physical activity, 267
exercise-induced changes, 291
nutrition effects, 244–246
Lipoprotein lipase (LPL)
cigarette smoking, 303–304
exercise-induced changes, 292
exogenous pathway, 52
laboratory methods, lipid and lipoprotein analysis, 133–138
lipid concentrations quantification, 120
metabolic syndrome, 152–155, *154–155*
postprandial lipemia, 272
Lipotoxicity, 156–158
Lithell studies, 152
Liu studies, 223
L-NMMA, 96
Lovastatin, 190–192, 231
Low-density lipoprotein (LDL)
apolipoproteins, 291
atherosclerosis, 62, 68, *69–70*, 70
basics, 50–51
cardiovascular disease, 300
cholesterol ester transfer protein, 139
cigarette smoking, 301–302, 304, 307
dyslipidemia, 19
exercise-induced changes, 290–292
indirect pathway, 57
lipid hypothesis, 67–68
metabolic syndrome, 148–149
nitric oxide, 7
obesity, 173–178
oxidative modification, 68–71, *70–71*
particle size, 236–237, *238*
statin effects, 190–191, *191*
Low-density lipoprotein (LDL-C) cholesterol
advanced age, 331
apolipoproteins, 270
dyslipidemia, 19
early childhood, 322–323
exercise and physical activity, 267–268
exercise-induced changes, 290–291
metabolic syndrome, 149
middle age, Americans, 327
mid- to late adolescence, 324–325, *325*
nutrition, 212–213
pharmacological treatments, 185–186
physical inactivity, 273
resistance training, 271
Low-density lipoprotein (LDL) receptor-related protein (LRP), 53
Low-density lipoprotein (LDL) receptors, 53
Low-fat, high-carbohydrate diets, 213, 215
Low-fat diets, 228, 234
LRP, *see* Low-density lipoprotein (LDL) receptor-related protein (LRP)
Ludmer studies, 65, 104
Luscombe studies, 227
Lymphocytes, 74
Lyon Diet Heart Study, 232–233

M

MACAD, *see* UCLA/Cedar Sinai Mexican American Coronary Artery Disease (MACAD) project
Macronutrient profile, changing, 237–240
Macrophage chemotactic protein 1 (MCP-1), 69–70
Macrophages, 70–72
Maeda studies, 97
Maiorana studies, 92, 99
Margarine, 219
Marine-derived fatty acids, *see* Fish oils
Materials, laboratory methods
  apolipoprotein concentrations, 123
  blood lipid concentrations, 121
  cholesterol ester exchange rate, 139
  gel electrophoresis, 129
  isolation, lipoproteins, 124
  lipase activities, 134–135
  lipoproteins, 124, 127
  precipitation, 127
Maternal factors, *see* Developmental stages, Americans
Matrix metalloproteinases (MMPs), 77
Matrix proteins, 76–77
Matsumoto studies, 96
Mattson, Grundy and, studies, 220
Mattson and Grundy studies, 220
McCall studies, 305
McNamara studies, 327
MCP-1, *see* Macrophage chemotactic protein 1 (MCP-1)
Mechanisms of action
  bile acid-binding resins, 194
  cholesterol absorption inhibitors, 202
  fibrates, 199
  fish oils, 203
  nicotinic acid, 197
  statins, 190
Mediterranean Diet, 219, 228, *229*, 232–233
Menopause, *see* Hormones
Mensink studies, 218
Messenger RNA (mRNA), 273
Metabolic changes, smoking cessation, 307–308
Metabolic syndrome, *see also* Lipoprotein, metabolism
  acylation-stimulating pathway, 159–162
  adiponectin, 158–159
  basics, 147–148, *148–149*, 162–163, *163*
  cardiovascular risk assessment, 21, *21*
  diagnostic criteria, 4
  dyslipidemia, 149–150
  leptin, 156–158
  lipotoxicity, 156–158
  LPL activity, 152–155, *154–155*
  obesity, 22
  PPARs, 156–158
  waist circumference, 150–152, *151*
Metabolism, lipid and lipoprotein
  anti-atherogenic roles, HDL, 58
  basics, *47–48*, 49–50
  classifications, *49*, 50–51
  direct pathway, 56–57
  endogenous pathway, 53–54
  exogenous pathway, 51–53
  HDL formation, 54–56
  indirect pathway, 57
  reverse cholesterol transport, 54–58, *58*
  transport, lipids, 51–54, *52*
Mevalonate, 39
Mexican Americans, *see* Hispanic Americans
Middle age, Americans, 326–330
Mid- to late adolescence, 324–326, *see also* Youth
Miller studies, 226
Minokoshi studies, 156
MMPs, *see* Matrix metalloproteinases (MMPs)
$MnCl_2$ method, *see* Heparin/manganese-chloride ($MnCl_2$) method
Moderate-fat diets, 234–235, 237
Moffatt studies, 1–8, 299–310
Monitoring, 204–205
Monnink studies, 104
Monoacylglycerides, 26
Monocyte recruitment, 69
Monounsaturated fatty acids (MUFA), 212, 217, 219–220
Morbidity and mortality, 87
MRFIT, *see* Multiple Risk Factor Intervention Trials (MRFIT)
mRNA, *see* Messenger RNA (mRNA)
MUFA, *see* Monounsaturated fatty acids (MUFA)
Muller studies, 88
Multiple dietary strategies, 239–240
Multiple Risk Factor Intervention Trials (MRFIT)
  cardiovascular disease, 300
  dyslipidemia, 19
  hypertension, 16
Multivariable risk assessment, 24–25
Mustard and Packham studies, 302
Mykkanen studies, 331

N

NaBr calculation, 126
National Academies, 247
National Academy of Science, 223
National Center for Health Statistics, 148
National Cholesterol Education Program (NCEP)
 cholesterol relationship, 3
 exercise and physical activity, 274
 lipid concentrations quantification, 122
 nutrition, 213, 228
 particle size, 240
 pharmacological treatments, 184
 recommendations, nutrition, 228, 230
National Heart, Lung, and Blood (NHLB) Institute, 3, 247
National Heart Institute, 300
National Institutes of Health (NIH), 3, 247
Navare studies, 183–205
NECP, *see* National Cholesterol Education Program (NCEP)
NEFA, *see* Non-esterified fatty acids (NEFA)
Neibauer studies, 89
Nephrotic syndrome, 187
Nestel studies, 245
Neutral lipids, fluorescent intensity, 140–141
Newborns, *see* Early childhood
NHANES I and III studies
 Hispanic Americans, 319
 metabolic syndrome, 147–148
 nutrition, 222
 waist circumference, 150–152
NHLB, *see* National Heart, Lung, and Blood (NHLB) Institute
Niacin, 163, 205
Niaspan, 196
Niaura studies, 308
Nicklas studies, 178
Nicotinic acid, 197–198, 204
NIH, *see* National Institutes of Health (NIH)
Nitric oxide (NO), *see also* Endothelial nitric oxide synthase (eNOS)
 atherosclerosis, 7, 63
 cigarette smoking, 302
 endothelial dysfunction, 65
 endothelial function, 96, 99
L-NMMA, 96
NO, *see* Nitric oxide (NO)
Non-denaturing polyacrylamide gradient gel electrophoresis, 48
Non-esterified fatty acids (NEFA), 160
Novel risk factors, 23–24
N-3 PUFA, 221–222
N-6 PUFA, 220–221
Nuclear magnetic resonance (NMR), 48, 50–51, 123
Nuclear transcription factors, 157
Nurses' Health Study, 218, 222, 226
Nutrition
 basics, 212–213, 246, 248, *248*
 changing macronutrient profile, 237–240
 DASH diet, 233
 dietary cholesterol, 222
 dietary fiber, 222–225
 dietary patterns effect, 228–233, *229*
 emerging risk factors, 236–246
 fat type dietary intervention, 239–240
 fiber type dietary intervention, 239–240
 glycemic index/glycemic load, 225–227
 HDL particle size, 240–242
 heart disease and fiber connection, 222–223
 high-fat diets, 237
 high-protein diets, 235–237, 239
 LDL particle size, 236–237, *238*
 Lifestyle Heart Program, 230–231
 lipid management, 224–225
 lipoprotein (a), 244–246
 low-carbohydrate diets, 237, 239
 low-fat diets, 234
 Mediterranean Diet, 232–233
 moderate-fat diets, 234–235, 237
 monounsaturated fatty acids, 219–220
 multiple dietary strategies, 239–240
 NCEP recommendations, 228, 230
 n-3 PUFA, 221–222
 n-6 PUFA, 220–221
 nutrients effect, 213–228, *214–216*
 patterns, dietary effect, 228–233
 polyunsaturated fatty acids, 220–222
 Portfolio diet, 230–231
 postprandial TG, 242–244
 saturated fatty acids, 217–218
 science-based dietary guidelines, 246, *247*
 total fat, 213, 215, 217
 trans fatty acids, 218–219
 weight loss effects, 233–236
Nuts, 202

O

Oats, 224–225, 230, 239
Obesity, *see also* Exercise training and endothelial function
 adiponectin, 158
 basics, 173–174, *174*, 178
 cardiovascular risk assessment, 22, *22*

dyslipidemias, 177–178
insulin, 156
leptin, 156
lifestyle modifications, 177–178
metabolic syndrome, 22
visceral adiposity, 174–177
Oeser studies, 307
Okosun studies, 150, 152
Olefsky studies, 157
Olive oil, 219
Omega-3 fatty acids, 202
Oram studies, 56
Owens studies, 158
Oxidation, lipoprotein, 65
Oxidized low-density lipoprotein (oxLDL), 67

P

Packham, Mustard and, studies, 302
PAGE, *see* Polyacrylamide gradient gel electrophoresis (PAGE)
Panton studies, 315–334
Paradoxical vasoconstriction, 93
Particle size
basics, 5–6
HDL, 240–242
LDL, 236–237, *238*
Pathogenesis theories, *66*, 66–68
Patterns, dietary effects, 228–233
PCI, *see* Percutaneous intervention (PCI)
PDE3/4, *see* Phosphodiesterase 3/4 (PDE3/PDE4)-mediated mechanisms
PDGF, *see* Platelet-derived growth factor (PDGF)
Pectin, 224
Pelkman studies, 234
Percutaneous coronary angioplasty (PTCA), 96
Percutaneous intervention (PCI), 104
Permeability, 65
Peroxidase, 120
Peroxidation, lipids, 43–44, *44–45*, 302
Peroxisome proliferator-activated receptors (PPARs), 156–158, 196
Peters and VanSlyke studies, 2
Pharmacological treatments
basics, 183–184, 205
bile acid-binding resins, 194–197
cholesterol absorption inhibitors, 200–202
drug selection, 204
fibrates, 199–200
fish oils, 202–203
lifestyle changes, 186–187
monitoring, 204–205
nicotinic acid, 197–198
pharmacotherapy, 187–189, *188–189*
selection of drug, 204
statins, 189–194
therapy goals, 185, *185–187*
treatment targets, 184–185
Pharmacology
bile acid-binding resins, 194
cholesterol absorption inhibitors, 202
fibrates, 199
nicotinic acid, 197
statins, 189–190, *190*
Pharmacotherapy, 187–189, *188–189*
PHLPL, *see* Post-heparin LPL (PHLPL) activity
Phosphatidic acid, 34
Phosphatidylinositol 3-kinase, 159
Phosphodiesterase 3/4 (PDE3/PDE4)-mediated mechanisms, 159
Phospholipids, 34, 36, *36*
Physical activity
apolipoproteins, *268*, 270–271
basics, 265, 275
change mechanisms, *268*, 272–273
clinical application, 274–275
endurance training, 266–271
lipids, *266–268*, 266–269
lipoproteins, 266–269, *268–269*
physical inactivity, 273–274
postprandial lipemia, 272
resistance training, 271
Physical inactivity, 273–274
Physicians' Health Study, 24, 240
Pietinen studies, 222
Pima Indians, 158
Plant sterols and stanols, 230, 239
Plaque formation, *75*, 75–77
Plasma density calculations, 125–126
Plasma preparation, 119–120
Platelet activation, 65
Platelet-derived growth factor (PDGF), 73
Polyacrylamide gradient gel electrophoresis (PAGE), 129–130
Polyunsaturated fatty acids (PUFA), 217, 220–222
Portfolio diet, *229*, 230–231
Post-heparin LPL (PHLPL) activity, 272–273
Postprandial lipemia, 272
Postprandial TG, 242–244
PPARs, *see* Peroxisome proliferator-activated receptors (PPARs)
Pravastatin, 191–192, 204
Pre-$beta_1$ HDL particle, 55–56

Pre-electrophoresis procedures, 130–131
Preiss-Landl studies, 152
Pre-symptomatic arterial ischemia, 23
Preventive implications, 25–26, *26*
Pritikin Program, 234
Procedures
  apolipoprotein concentrations, 123
  blood lipid concentrations, 121–122, *122*
  cholesterol ester exchange rate, 139–141
  gel electrophoresis, 129
  lipase activities, 135–138
  lipoprotein isolation, 124, *125*
  lipoprotein precipitation, 127–128
  pre-electrophoresis, 130–131
Psota studies, 211–248
Psyllium, 224, 230
PTCA, *see* Percutaneous coronary angioplasty (PTCA)
PUFA, *see* Polyunsaturated fatty acids (PUFA)
Puppione, Schumaker and, studies, 124

R

Rancho Bernardo Study, 331
RANTES, 70
Rask-Nissilä studies, 322
Rauscher studies, 101
Reaven studies, 175–176
Rehman studies, 102
Resistance training, 271–272
Reverse cholesterol transport
  basics, 48
  foam cell formation, 72
  lipid and lipoprotein metabolism, 54–58, *58*
Rhabdomyolysis, 193
Rifkind and Segal studies, 327
Risk assessment, cardiovascular
  atherosclerotic cardiovascular disease, 14–15, *14–15*
  basics, 13–14
  diabetes, 21, *21*
  dyslipidemia, 19–21, *20*
  hypertension, 15–18, *16–19*
  metabolic syndrome, 21, *21*
  multivariable risk assessment, 24–25
  novel risk factors, 23–24
  obesity, 22, *22*
  pre-symptomatic arterial ischemia, 23
  preventive implications, 25–26, *26*
  risk factors, 15–23
  unstable lesions, 23
Risk factors, 3–4, 15–24, 236–246
Rivellese studies, 239
Robbins studies, 318
Robinson, S., 77
Roeters van Lennep studies, 150
Roitmann studies, 85–106
Ronnemaa studies, 325
Ross and Glomser studies, 6
Ross and Glomset studies, 66
Ross studies, 6, 302
Rosuvastatin, 191–192, 204
Rush, Graham and, studies, 89

S

Saito studies, 329
San Antonio Heart Study, 319
Saturated fatty acids (SFA), 212, 217–218
Scavenger receptor A (SR-A), 72
Scavenger receptor class B type I (SR-BI), 56–57
Schaefer studies, 174, 176
Schopenhauer, A., 1
Schumaker and Puppione studies, 124
Science-based dietary guidelines, 246, *247*
Segal, Rifkind and, studies, 327
Seip and Semenkovich studies, 273
Selection, drugs, 204
Selective uptake, 56
Semenkovich, Seip and, studies, 273
Separating lipoprotein, 128
Sequential ultracentrifugation, 124–126
Serotonin, 65
Seven Countries Study, 217, 219–220, 222, 232
SFA, *see* Saturated fatty acids (SFA)
Sharman studies, 239
SHEP trial, 15
Side effects, *see also* Drug interactions
  bile acid-binding resins, 196
  fibrates, 200
  fish oils, 203
  nicotinic acid, 198
  statins, *192*, 193–194
Simvastatin, 190, 192, 204
Sjogren studies, 239
SMCs, *see* Smooth muscle cells (SMCs)
Smoking
  atherosclerosis, 302
  basics, 299–300, 309–310
  carbon monoxide, 308
  cardiovascular disease, 300–301
  cessation of smoking, 306–308
  endothelial dysfunction, 65

environmental tobacco smoke, 308–309
HDL, 304–306
LDL, 304
lipid metabolism, 302–306
metabolic changes, smoking cessation, 307–308
nicotine, 308
triglycerides, 302–304
VLDL, 302–304
Smooth muscle cells (SMCs), *see also* Vascular smooth muscle cells (VSMCs)
basics, 63
immigration, *73*, 73–74
lipid hypothesis, 67–68
Sniderman studies, 149, 161
SOD-1, *see* Superoxide dismutase (SOD-1)
Solutions
gel electrophoresis, 129–130
lipase activities, 135–136
lipoprotein precipitation, 127–128
Soybean oil, 202, 219
Soy protein, 230, 239, 245
Sphingolipids, 34, 36, *36*
Squalene, 40
SR-BI, *see* Scavenger receptor class B type I (SR-BI)
SREBP transcription factors, 72
St-Amand studies, 270
Stamford studies, 1–8, 299–310
Standard curve development, 140–141
Statins
endothelial dysfunction, 65–66
metabolic syndrome, 163
monitoring, 205
pharmacological treatments, 189–194
Portfolio diet, 231
Steffen-Batey studies, 87
Steinbeck studies, 323
Step I and Step II diets, 224, 228, *229*, 230, 237, 241
Steroids and sterols, 36–37, *37*
Stewart studies, 93
Stiebeling studies, 31–44
Substance P, 65
Summer studies, 265–275
Superoxide dismutase (SOD-1), 89, 99
Suvorava studies, 90

T

Taddei studies, 92
Taimela studies, 270
Tanabe studies, 90, 270
Tanaka studies, 92
Tangier Disease, 56
TBARS concentrations, 304
T-786c promoter, 101
Tea, 86
Testosterone, *see* Hormones
Tetrahydrobiopterin, 86
TFA, *see Trans* fatty acids (TFA)
TG, *see* Triglycerides (TG)
Therapeutic Lifestyle Changes, 228, *229*
Therapy goals, 185, *185–187*
Thomas studies, 242
Thompson studies, 183–205, 270, 293
Thrombus formation, 65
Th1 *vs.* Th2 cytokine responses, 74
Thyberg and Hedin studies, 76
TIA, *see* Transient ischemic attack (TIA)
Tissue-type plasminogen activator (t-PA), 99
TNF-α, *see* Tumor necrosis factor alpha (TNF-α)
Tocopherols, 44
Total cholesterol, *see* Cholesterol
Total fat, nutrition effects, 213, 215, 217
t-PA, *see* Tissue-type plasminogen activator (t-PA)
Trans fatty acids (TFA), 34, 218–219, *see also* Essential fatty acids; Fatty acids
Transfer protein activity analysis, 133–141
Transient ischemic attack (TIA), 102
Transplant patients, 192
Transport, lipids, 51–54, *52*
Treatment targets, 184–185
Triacylglycerides, 26
Triglycerides (TG)
advanced age, 331–332
cigarette smoking, 303, 307
early childhood, 323
exercise-induced changes, 284–285, 290, 293
levels defined, 300
middle age, Americans, 327–329, *328*
mid- to late adolescence, 325
nutrition, 212–213
pharmacological treatments, 184–185, 187
smoking, 302–304
statin effects, 191
Troglitazone, 157
Tromso Heart Study, 300
Tumor necrosis factor alpha (TNF-α), 149
Tunica media, 63

U

UCLA/Cedar Sinai Mexican American Coronary Artery Disease (MACAD) project, 153
Ultracentrifugation, sequential, 124–126
Unstable lesions, 23
U.S. Departments of Agriculture/Health and Human Services, 247

V

Vague studies, 173
VA-HIT trial, 26
Valdez, Kahn and, studies, 151
Van Bilsen, Glide and, studies, 157
Van Gaal studies, 178
VanSlyke, Peters and, studies, 2
Vascular cell adhesion molecule-1 (VCAM-1), 71, 74
Vascular endothelial growth factor (VEGF-165), 90
Vascular smooth muscle cells (VSMCs), 76, *see also* Smooth muscle cells (SMCs)
Vasodilation, 65
VCAM-1, *see* Vascular cell adhesion molecule-1 (VCAM-1)
Vegetarian diets, 228
VEGF-165, *see* Vascular endothelial growth factor (VEGF-165)
Very late antigen-4 (VLA-4), 71
Very low-density lipoprotein cholesterol (VLDL-C), 53
Very low-density lipoprotein (VLDL)
  basics, 5, 50–51
  cardiovascular disease, 300
  cholesterol ester transfer protein, 139
  cigarette smoking, 303–304
  exercise and physical activity, 266
  exercise-induced changes, 292
  indirect pathway, 57
  lipid hypothesis, 67
  lipoprotein lipase, 152, 155
  pharmacological treatments, 184
  reverse cholesterol transport, 55
  smoking, 302–304
Visceral adiposity, 174–177
Vitamin C, 85
Vitamin E, 85–86, 221, 304
VLA-4, *see* Very late antigen-4 (VLA-4)
VLDL, *see* Very low-density lipoprotein (VLDL)
VLDL-C, *see* Very low-density lipoprotein cholesterol (VLDL-C)
Vona studies, 96
VSMCs, *see* Vascular smooth muscle cells (VSMCs)

W

Wagganer studies, 47–58
Waist circumference (WC)
  cardiovascular disease predictor, 173
  metabolic syndrome, 148, 150–152, *151*
Walnuts, 86
Walsh studies, 95
Walther studies, 100
Wang studies, 88
Wannamethee studies, 87
Warnick and Albers studies, 127
Waters studies, 302
Watts studies, 98
WC, *see* Waist circumference (WC)
Weight loss effects, 233–236
Wei studies, 319
Western diet, 219, 245
Western Electric Study, 222
Weyer studies, 158, 160
Wheat, 225, 239
Whites, *see* Caucasians
Williams studies, 177, 267, 269
Witt studies, 87
Wolk studies, 222
Women's Health Study, 223
Woodman studies, 88
Woods studies, 269
Wood studies, 270
Woolf-May studies, 177
Woo studies, 98
World Health Organization, 306

X

Xanthomatosis, 1

Y

Yamashita studies, 89
Yeast, 224
Ye studies, 157

Youth, 97–98, *see also* Mid- to late adolescence
Yu-Poth studies, 228

Z

Zeiher studies, 58
Zhang studies, 161
Zhu studies, 151–152
Zutphen Elderly Study, 331